616·891

Working with Serious Mental Illness

DATE DUE

19/11/08			
20/8/10			
22/5/13			

Especially for John

Commissioning Editor: Susan Young
Development Editor: Catherine Jackson
Project Manager: Joannah Duncan
Designer: Judith Wright
Illustrations Manager: Bruce Hogarth

Working with Serious Mental Illness

A manual for clinical practice

SECOND EDITION

EDITED BY

Catherine Gamble BA(Hons) RGN RMN RNT
Consultant Nurse, South West London and St George's Mental Health Care Trust, London, UK

Geoff Brennan BSc(Hons) RNMH RMN
Research Fellow, City University, London, UK

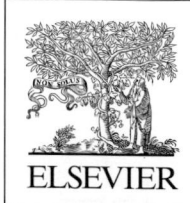

ELSEVIER

EDINBURGH LONDON NEW YORK OXFORD PHILADELPHIA ST LOUIS SYDNEY TORONTO 2006

ELSEVIER

Butterworth-Heinemann
An imprint of Elsevier Limited

First edition published 2000
Reprinted 2000, 2001, 2002, 2003, 2004
Second edition published 2006
Reprinted 2007

ISBN-13: 978–0–7020–2716–1
ISBN-10: 0–7020–2716–2

British Library Cataloguing in Publication Data
A catalogue record for this book is available from the British Library

Library of Congress Cataloging in Publication Data
A catalog record for this book is available from the Library of Congress

Note
Knowledge and best practice in this field are constantly changing. As new research and experience broaden our knowledge, changes in practice, treatment and drug therapy may become necessary or appropriate. Readers are advised to check the most current information provided (i) on procedures featured or (ii) by the manufacturer of each product to be administered, to verify the recommended dose or formula, the method and duration of administration, and contraindications. It is the responsibility of the practitioner, relying on their own experience and knowledge of the patient, to make diagnoses, to determine dosages and the best treatment for each individual patient, and to take all appropriate safety precautions. To the fullest extent of the law, neither the Publisher nor the Editor assumes any liability for any injury and/or damage to persons or property arising out of or related to any use of the material contained in this book.
The Publisher

Printed in China

Contents

Contributors

Dinesh Bhugra MA MSc MBBS FRCPsych MPhil PhD LMSSA
Professor of Mental Health and Cultural Diversity, Institute of Psychiatry
and Honorary Consultant, South London and Maudsley NHS Trust, London

Geoff Brennan BSc(Hons) RNMH RMN
Research Fellow, City University, London

Rahul Bhintade MD
Research Co-ordinator, Nair Hospital, Mumbai, India

Tom KJ Craig MBBS PhD FRC(Psych)
Professor, Social Psychiatry, Institute of Psychiatry, King's College, London

Eric Davis BSc MSc(Dist) PhD Dip Psych AdvDipPsych CertManagement
Consultant Clinical Psychologist, Gloucestershire and South West Regional
Leader for Early Intervention in Psychosis Services

Sharon Dennis BSc(Hons) RMN Dip Family Therapy PG Dip Advanced Practice (Nursing)
CMS RNT
South East Regional Director, Royal College of Nursing; National Patient
Safety Agency

Joanna Denney MSc DipCOT
Clinical Specialist, Psychosocial Interventions for Psychosis, Gloucestershire
Partnership Trust

Jayne Fox BSc(Hons) RMN ENB650
Programme Manager Education, Northern Ireland Clinical and Social Care
Govenance Support Team, DHSS, N. Ireland

Catherine Gamble BA(Hons) RGN RMN RNT
Consultant Nurse, South West London and St George's Mental Health Care
Trust, London

Jood Gibbins RMN
Consultant Nurse (Dual Diagnosis), Dorset Health Care NHS Trust
Addiction Services

Sally Goldspink BSc(Hons) SROT
Lecturer, Homerton School of Health Studies, Cambridge

Helen Healy PhD CPsychol AFBPsS
Trainee Clinical Psychologist, University of Wales

Susan E Kerr BA(Hons) PG Dip RMN Dip (He)
Lecturer, Mental Health, Homerton School of Health Studies, Cambridge

Cheryl Kipping PhD RMN RGN
Consultant Nurse (Dual Diagnosis), South London and Maudsley NHS Trust

Avie Luthra MBChB BSc(Hons) MRCP MRCPsych
South London and Maudsley NHS Trust, London

Kenny Midence CPsychol AFBPsS
Principal Clinical Psychologist, Department of Clinical Psychology,
University of Wales

Jem Mills MscPgDipCT ENB650 ENB870 RMN
Cognitive Behavioural Psychotherapist with an Assertive Outreach team,
East Sussex, and Senior Lecturer, University of Brighton

Paula Morrison BSc(Hons) RMN
Associate Director Public Health, Bromley Primary Care Trust

Rachel Perkins BA MPhil PhD
Director of Quality Assurance and the User/Carer Experience, South West
London and St George's Mental Health NHS Trust

David Reader BSc(Hons) BA(Hons) Diploma in Nursing (Thorn) RMN
Clinical Nurse Specialist, Psychosocial Interventions for Psychosis, North
West Wales NHS Trust

Cliff Roberts MSc BSc(IIons) PGDE RN
Senior Lecturer Psychopharmacology, London South Bank University,
London

Paul Rogers PhD MSc RMN Cert ENB650 Dip Behav Psych
Professor of Forensic Nursing, School of Care Sciences, University of
Glamorgan, Pontypridd, and Caswell Clinic Bro Morgannwg NHS Trust,
Bridgend

Liz Sayce MSc
Director, Policy and Communications, Disability Rights Commission,
London

Lyn Shore BEd(Hons) MSc
Carer Researcher/Trainer

Jacqueline Sin MSc(Nursing) BSc(Hons) Mental Health Nursing (THORN) BNursing BGS
RMN RN(Psy)
Education and Practice Lead in Psychosocial Interventions, Berkshire
Healthcare NHS Trust and Thames Valley University

Andrew M Vidgen MA(Hons) MSc DClinPsy
Clinical Psychologist, Psychology and Counselling Services Directorate and
Clinical Tutor, South Wales Doctoral Course in Clinical Psychology,
Whitchurch Hospital, Cardiff

Nigel Wellman MSc BA(Hons) RMN
Professor of Mental Health Nursing, Thames Valley University; Honorary
Consultant Nurse, Berkshire Healthcare NHS Trust

Preface

Four years have passed since the first edition of this book was published. Much has changed at national, regional and local level during this time. Nationally, the government has set up new institutions and developed numerous policies and guidelines to enhance the delivery of National Health Service mental health provision, for users, carers and the workforce. At regional level, now there are development centres, strategic health authorities and workforce initiatives, while locally there are forums and implementation groups that are strategically placed to disseminate, share and evaluate best practice. Meanwhile, the traditional medical model is being augmented and modified by the influence of new disciplines and humanistic models of care. The basis of all this change is to improve the quality of life of the service user. Consequently, there is a need for all practitioners to continue to place greater emphasis on working with users, using skills that have a sound theoretical, pragmatic basis. As highlighted in the first edition, the underlying aim of this book is to guide practitioners through this process.

Indeed, irrespective of the clinical setting or client group that practitioners are working with, there remains a need for the entire workforce to deconstruct personal and organisational patriarchal attitudes that alienate individual clients. Although it is acknowledged that this alienation has occurred through ignorance rather than malice, there is no longer any justification for it. Clients have long been aware that their needs were, and are still, not being met. Fortunately their voice is now gaining in strength, and their involvement has become a central part of policy and social delivery. Nevertheless, if a moment is taken to consider some positive, personal life events that you personally may have experienced over the last four years, such as succeeding on a course of study; moving house; meeting a new partner; getting married; having children; getting or changing jobs; achieving promotion and/or experiencing exotic holidays, it is possible to realise that users of mental health services continue to struggle to achieve the things that many of us take for granted in today's society. So, although practitioners are attempting to correct past errors, on reflection much has still to be done! Indeed, rather than trusting to intuitive ideas or blindly following charismatic leaders and their individual philosophies, there continues to be a need to challenge and scientifically analyse treatment methodologies. Nevertheless, in this scientific quest (so-called 'evidence based analysis') it should not be forgotten that the best evidence is the personal experience of the user. Collaboration and inclusion should therefore be the cornerstone of current and future practice.

This second edition reflects the changing nature and evolvement of mental health care. While some reflections, interventions and strategies remain, there are some notable updates and new chapters, which include the carer's perspective, social inclusion, relapse prevention and getting support. However, overall, the adaptation of evidence-based treatment methods to suit the individual remains the book's primary concern. Likewise, it seeks to guide, plan and suggest down-to-earth ideas for individuals working with clients on a day-to-day basis.

In summary, to assist the reader the book has been divided up into four sections.

Section 1: Promoting understanding of the manifestations of serious mental illness

As user and carer involvement is now recognised as a central part of policy and service delivery, this opening section is designed to promote reflection on how serious mental illness is perceived and treated. The first chapter focuses on a user experience and asks readers to walk in the footsteps of someone who has a lot to teach us. Chapter 2 introduces the practitioner to the carer's experience of living with and coping with serious mental illness. The third chapter reflects upon the importance of promoting social inclusion and recovery both within individual clinical practice and mental health services generally. The remaining two examine stress vulnerability and introduce the subject of how interventions advocated within this book have developed and been evaluated.

Section 2: Engaging, assessing and formulating care

This section introduces how to build relationships and assess and formulate a client's care. Through lessons learnt from first-hand observation and accounts, Chapter 6 guides practitioners as to how to develop relationships and help clients build on their strengths, abilities and wishes, using Rogerian principles. Chapter 7 examines signs, symptoms and diagnosis. Chapters 8–10 recognise the importance of undertaking collaborative formalised assessment processes and examine how to choose and use some of the tools available. In doing so they identify specific skills in focusing this information towards client's goals and identifying risk factors.

Section 3: Interventions

This forms the main body of the book. To get the best use from this section it is advised that practitioners examine their communication skills, attitudes and beliefs. Chapters 1 and 6 will aid reflection on these issues. Subsequent chapters concern direct interventions and practitioners should match the chapters with the individuals they are working with. For example, if your client is hearing voices and/or experiencing strange thoughts then Chapter 11 will be of most relevance. Many individuals will have complex needs, so it is worth reading the other chapters that pertain to their presentation, dealing with blankness and deadness, family issues, dual diagnosis, anger, offending behaviour, relapse prevention, and medication and cultural issues.

Section 4: Considerations for effective practice

The chapters in this section deal with issues that, although they appear to stand alone, often frame the potential success or failure of interventions. They aim to guide practitioners to reflect on issues such as ethical considerations, professional relationships and getting support.

Acknowledgements

We would like to thank:

- All the contributors for their hard work and patience
- The users, carers and practitioners whose reported experiences have helped shape this 2nd edition
- Neil Brimblecombe for his editorial contributions
- On a personal note, Diana, Sarah, Edward, David, Lynda, Hannah, Fred, Ella and Beth, for their unique family skills!

Section 1

Promoting understanding of the manifestations of serious mental illness

1

Serious mental illness: a view from within

EDITORS' NOTE

This individualised account of an experience of serious mental illness remains unchanged from the first edition. It has purposely been left, as it provides the reader with an opportunity to 'walk in the footsteps' of a person who has encountered mental health services and come out the other side! It does not seek to prescribe or direct practitioners to interventions, attitudes or knowledge but serves as an introduction to this book and its content. It does require the reader to consider the following:

♦ What does this account tell me about the experience of living and coping with a mental health problem?
♦ If I met this person, how would I embrace their knowledge and expertise so they felt listened to and appreciated?
♦ In doing so, how would this promote collaboration and understanding, and endorse therapeutic hope, trustworthiness and respect?

There were several things that influenced my illness:

I was a clumsy child who suffered from dyspraxia.
I was the eldest of four girls and was jealous of my sister who was 18 months younger than me.
I found a few things physically difficult, e.g. riding a bike and knitting.
I had nightmares and sleepwalked.
I had a fixation about death.
I always wanted to please and was very sensitive.
I was a diligent reader and from the age of three I had a vivid imagination.
I had a difficult birth, was paralysed down one side for a few weeks and was shortsighted – I have often asked myself 'Could this have led to brain changes?'
I was picked on at school at the age of 14 and not invited to peers' parties.
I wanted to be a nurse from the age of 12 to help others.
I failed my English A level and was bitterly disappointed.

I did achieve my ambition and started nurse training – unfortunately there were problems straight away. I experienced two people dying while I was giving them bed baths. I remember being 'sent for a coffee break', shocked and upset, as a means of coping. Another time I spent several hours talking to a young girl who was 18 years old like me. She had leukaemia and died. The next day I had a panic attack.

During my psychiatric placement there were two incidents that particularly upset me. First, a lesbian woman made a pass at me, which shocked me as I was only 19. I didn't know how to deal with this. Secondly, I was looking after this gay young man who I became involved with. It all became too much and I completely flipped. I was hysterical, but no one did anything about it. I feel I should have been counselled or offered supervision. Basically the work had stimulated past experiences in my life and this, with other experiences in my nurse training, should have made me give up the training as it was affecting me badly. I continued for another 8 years.

Another factor was I worked on a cancer ward and witnessed lots of deaths including those of young people. As this went on I became scared of death, which led me to become phobic.

At the age of 24, I started local philosophy classes after I had seen the course advertised on the bus. It was run by an organisation called the School of Economic Science. I did not know this was an undercover cult. I attended 17 sessions. I can't really remember them clearly, as we were encouraged to clear our minds of everything and not to tell people, especially our family, what was going on and what we heard. As a consequence I became cut off from my family. My family, however, knew something was wrong.

Eventually a housemate alerted me to the fact that the classes were run by a cult. Luckily I got out, but I became paranoid and frightened that someone from the cult was following me. At this point I became psychotic and suspicious of everyone. I moved in with friends who were into Buddhism and the occult. They lived in a flat decorated in black. At the time I thought nothing of it, but my family were growing more concerned as they didn't know where I was.

I began meditating. I stayed up all night and all day. I starved myself. Around this time, my boyfriend left for Mexico. I began isolating myself and staying in my room. Friends and family rang, but I didn't come out. I started reading books about black magic and the occult. I listened to tapes and heard messages and I experienced double meanings in the books I was reading. Things came to a head when I saw myself on the television conducting an orchestra. I ran to the TV and turned it off. My flatmate didn't know what was happening. He asked 'What do you think you're doing?' I couldn't tell him.

I was left at home on my own. When someone came round I thought they were from the cult and I wouldn't let them in. That was it – I was totally paranoid. I thought I had to get away. In desperation I telephoned my gran and said I was in trouble. This prompted my family to start searching for me. They knew something was very wrong. I wandered around the city with the words 'Come out of the dark, walk into the light' ringing in my head. I thought the cult were following me and I was going to be sacrificed. Throughout the day I tried to call home but I couldn't get through. I thought the city had been shut down by occult means, and my home town no longer existed. I felt I couldn't use any money as I thought the money had been changed.

I then decided I would find my boyfriend. I got on a train to the airport. Once there I went up to one of the ticket desks and asked for a ticket to Mexico. The attendant told me that there were no flights to Mexico from this particular airport and I didn't have my passport on me. I decided to go to a sea port as, coincidentally, I had enough money. On the train I threw all my possessions away. During the journey I was hallucinating. I thought I was on a train to heaven. I remember looking at all the people on the train and deciding if they were going to heaven or hell based on their possessions. For example, I saw people using mobile phones, Filofaxes or Walkmans and these had separate meanings. Eventually I arrived at the sea port, which I had previously visited with a friend, on our way abroad. I queued up at passport control but of course I had no passport or ticket so I was not allowed on the boat.

I also thought I was there to be a martyr and I was to be sacrificed. I began wandering around. I was having visual and auditory hallucinations. I came to a bridge. There were seagulls on either side of me and I thought I was walking into heaven. Suddenly I heard voices and turned to find the police. It was about two in the morning. The police picked me up and took me back to the station. It was terrifying as I thought all men were witch doctors. I kept trying to run out of the room as I thought I was going to be sacrificed. Somehow I remembered my parents' telephone number and the police phoned them. By now it was 4 am. Eventually my parents arrived. I was very anxious and scared of my dad as I felt he was also a witch doctor. It took them quite a while to persuade me to get in the car. I was disorientated and frightened. When we got home I had to have a shower. I think my Mum thought I had been sexually assaulted. I was shown to my parents' bed, as they thought this would help me get some sleep but, as I lay down, I felt an electric shock and refused to get back in. I was crying and screaming hysterically as I still thought my father was a witch doctor and was going to sacrifice me.

I had other psychotic thoughts. I thought all men were in the cult and that my family were part of an undercover species who came to life at night and went into hibernation during the winter. I would not drink tap water because I thought it was poisoned. I felt people with various eye colours were good or bad: blue was good, brown was bad.

Later that morning the general practitioner (GP) came round; I was totally disorientated. I thought I had died and gone to heaven. The doctor said I had to be admitted to the local psychiatric hospital as soon as possible. I didn't want to go but my gran came. Gran was the only one who could persuade me. An ambulance was eventually called and mum came with me. During the journey my mind was racing and I was reliving my childhood life and memories. I thought I had become a child again. We arrived at the hospital, where I was shown into a small room with a clock on the wall and a female doctor was sitting in front of me. I thought it was a concentration camp and my parents were interned with me. The doctor stupidly asked my parents if they wanted to take me home for the weekend. They refused. It had taken all their strength to get me there and they were exhausted.

I remained disorientated and confused. A nurse was assigned to me for 24-hour observations. I was shown to the first bed in a dormitory. I was examined and a blood test was taken. I screamed and shouted, thinking I was being attacked. My parents left to get me some toiletries and clothes. I was alone and I was scared.

I remember sitting in bed on the first night with a nurse by my side, thinking I was going to die. I was very frightened and needed lots of reassurance. I told her I was a Catholic and she said she was one too. I remember drifting off to sleep as the medicine made me drowsy. I woke up next morning and there was tea at the hatch on the main ward. I still had a nurse with me; it was 6 am in the morning. The women in the beds adjacent to me started talking and reassuring me that I would get well and not to be frightened. I became like a small child: vulnerable and quiet.

In the early days, I can remember sitting in the lounge with a nurse by my side. I was experiencing hallucinations. I thought I was in a plane and I was flying to heaven. I suppose I must have started taking Largactil to help with my symptoms. The days began to drift into each other as I had many hallucinations and delusions and remained disorientated. I remember thinking I was a princess and was going to get married. When my family came to see me I thought the hospital was my palace and I was receiving my family. I then used to go to the kitchen and make them a pot of tea.

I became muddled up with past friends. A young man who was a friend became my fiancé in my mind. He came to see me a few times. I thought my dad was my bodyguard and was there to protect me. He would come and see me every day and take me out for drives. My mum used to find it hard to see me suffering and would often burst into tears. My sisters used to come and visit and tried to get some normality into my existence.

I continued to see and hear messages so the medication was increased and increased. Eventually my body began to be affected. I was stiff. I had pains in my legs. My mouth was dry. I shook and could not keep still, so I spent hours pacing the ward. I paced so much that the nurses used to say I would wear the carpet out.

In spite of this, the suspicious thinking continued. I still felt I was being watched and that some patients were in the occult. I also saw myself on TV again. I continued to believe I was in heaven and the hospital was heaven.

I also thought that the hospital was the home of the cult and I had been imprisoned by a relative who was a high teacher within the occult.

My days were comprised of getting up at 6 am and having tea, then a wash, breakfast, watching TV and walking around the hospital. There was a library, shop, coffee, drop-in and lots of grounds. I used to put on my Walkman and go walking. I found this helped to lift my mood. It also helped when I thought the hospital was my palace. I continued to experience side-effects of medication. I could smell rotting flesh, I had severe headaches and was affected by anything electrical. I also saw strange things like the water flowing in the opposite direction when I ran the tap. Of course all this was very frightening. Because of all these symptoms I began to think I was dying. I became even more restless and anxious. I was then prescribed drugs for my side-effects. I began to be so anxious I could not sleep. I would wander around the ward all night or would lie on my bed and writhe. I could not keep still. I did not sleep for 2 weeks. I just wanted to be given an injection to knock me out. It was terrible, truly awful.

After this my medication was changed completely. I started on Stelazine. Then I collapsed as my blood pressure dropped too fast. I hit my head and was allowed to spend the morning in bed. They also tried me on antidepressants as they thought I was depressed, but these made me more depressed and I eventually refused to take them. Interspersed with all this I attended OT (occupational therapy) daily. This was truly an escape from the hell of the ward. In OT I used to do things like word games, typing, cooking, puzzles, relaxation and brass rubbing. I used to enjoy this time and the OTs really encouraged me.

After about 6 weeks I was discharged. Unfortunately things did not work out and I ended up back in hospital three times in 3 months. Lots of my nursing friends came to see me. They were not impressed with the hospital; they thought it was old and run down and did not have a nice atmosphere.

One day I decided I had had enough, so I walked off the ward in my nightie and bare feet. I walked through reception. I walked down the steep slope to the main road and tried to run into the traffic. Luckily a distraught woman rescued me and took me back to the ward. There was a man with me. I think he was a policeman. I remember he was furious and told the nurses to 'lock me up'. The staff and my parents were very surprised at what I had done. My clothes were taken off me for 24 hours.

On another occasion, when I was at home and I felt I could not bear the pains in my head any more, it was so bad I took an overdose. My younger sister found me and couldn't understand why I had done it. 'We love you so much' she said. My stomach was pumped; I was admitted to another hospital and then sent back to the original one.

After all these incidents my family decided I should be transferred to a more renowned psychiatric hospital. A top nurse had been in touch with the consultant there and he agreed to take me on. My room was cleared and I moved the next day. I arrived on the ward with my dad. I was shown into the quiet room. I remember feeling upset and disillusioned as I thought I was never going to get better. I now had the diagnosis of 'paranoid schizophrenic'.

I was shown into my room. It was quite nice. I remember my dad gave me a hug and said 'I like this place. I think this place will help you.' I met my primary nurse and we had a chat. I told him I thought my brain was dead and that there was no hope for me. I didn't know what he must have thought. Things were very different at this hospital. I met the consultant and had to go into the ward round to tell them all about me. As I came out I was told I had done very well. I was started on clozapine 200 mg. With this I needed weekly blood tests. This drug was to help me a lot in the future. I still had delusions. I had nightmares. One night I thought I was being executed. I saw myself flying on the ceiling. I felt my soul left me.

Every day I spent 15 minutes with my morning nurse and time later with my afternoon nurse. Because I was convinced my brain was dead a scan was arranged for me. It was normal. I began OT again and this really helped. I did such things as typing, creative art, pottery, stress management, cookery, gym, swimming, writing and craft. Each ward had its own OT and mine used to spend an hour counselling me, which really helped.

I began going home at weekends. I found it hard to sleep and I often felt anxious. My parents took me out at weekends for drives in the country.

I began to relive my childhood again and had nightmares and fears. These lessened when I returned to the ward.

I was on the ward 9 months. My room became a haven. I put up artwork, psalms, books by my bed and so on. Many other patients would come into my room and be mesmerised. Then they would calm down as they sat on my bed.

Eventually the delusions drifted away and I became more positive. I would go for my daily walk around the grounds. Many friends visited me and my family remained very supportive. I was now ready to leave. But I had nowhere to live so I moved to a hostel. After 3 months a flat was found for me – it was a few minutes away from my parents. I was seen as an outpatient for 6 months.

One side-effect was I had put on a lot of weight, which knocked my confidence. I still have regular blood tests, which means I will always have a tie to the hospital. I developed a feeling of blackness and deadness, which has stayed with me; to this day I have felt I have died inside. I have lost all my inner energy and because of this I have thought I am going to die, which is very frightening.

When I first got discharged I got a job at Dillons book shop, which I found difficult because my medication made me so drowsy. I did this for 18 months. I then got involved in the voluntary services and started a job at a playgroup for children with special needs. I worked there for $4\frac{1}{2}$ years and really enjoyed it. I also became involved in a Clubhouse rehabilitation scheme. I worked in the office, kitchen, took part in meetings and did a 3-week training in America. I spent $4\frac{1}{2}$ years at the Clubhouse.

I am now an education project officer for our local user group on a part-time basis. I run seminars, give presentations and talks to schoolchildren and train nurses about mental health issues. My job carries responsibility and I find it challenging and empowering. I am also involved in a women's Clubhouse. I am on the management committee. In this I do a lot of outreach work, going into the community and meeting women in psychiatric wards or in day centres. I also take part in a 'schizophrenia roadshow' where I travel around the country talking about and sharing my experiences.

I still need medication, and see a psychiatrist. But I feel some good has come out of my illness. I am working and functioning. I am part of the community.

There *is* life after schizophrenia.

2

Inside caring in mental health

Lyn Shore

KEY ISSUES

◆ Carer's journey and experience
◆ The impact of caring
◆ Lessons to be learnt and recommendations

This chapter focuses on the experience of carers and families who support someone with serious mental illness. It draws on my experiences as a carer and as a carers' worker over a period of 9 years.

My family is just one of several hundred thousand families in the UK that support someone made vulnerable by infirmity or disability. It has been estimated that 1.6 million people in the UK are 'carers' and perhaps as many as 11% of this carer population may be supporting people with mental health difficulties (Office for National Statistics 2000). My family's experience cannot, of course, represent the collective experience of carer families any more than any other single family's experience can. It is used here simply to illustrate some of the issues and dilemmas that commonly arise for families living with the impact of serious mental illness in one or more of its members.

INTRODUCTION TO MENTAL HEALTH CARE: A FAMILY PERSPECTIVE

My 'carer's journey' began in 1994 with a series of dramatic and traumatic events that signalled the start of my middle son's first nightmare journey into psychosis. During the summer vacation between his first and second years at university it became apparent to the family and others that he was 'not himself'. As so many families in similar situations do, we found ways of discounting our fears, trying to find rational explanations for his increasingly irrational thoughts and behaviour.

Within a few weeks his mental health had deteriorated to such an extent that it was clear we needed to seek professional help. Unable to recognise that he might have a problem, he refused to visit our GP and eventually I approached the GP myself to seek advice and help. I was astounded and dismayed to be told that he could not do anything unless my son went to see him. I was later to learn from other carers that what I faced then was to be the first in a long series of 'carer's dilemmas'. That my help-seeking on behalf of my son was frustrated in this way was by no means unusual. Other families have faced this problem and many still do (Pinfold & Corry 2003). Certainly I didn't know at that stage that professionals were unable to act until a crisis arose of such magnitude that it was sufficient to trigger a Mental Health Act assessment. Nor did I know that each time my son would relapse in future I would be faced with the same dilemma.

Unable to get any help from our GP, and without a clue where else to seek help, I looked on helplessly as my son deteriorated yet further. We found ourselves living a bizarre and increasingly alarming 24-hour life for several weeks as his descent into psychosis accelerated.

Although I was deeply worried about his state of mind, I was unable to prevent him returning to his university town at the beginning of term. Two weeks later I received the telephone call I had been dreading but half-expecting. He had been apprehended by police and admitted to a psychiatric hospital under section. I received the news in a state of deep shock. I didn't know what 'sectioning' meant and had difficulty grasping the significance of what had happened. At first, I couldn't think of anything to say, then was overwhelmed by a flood of emotions and questions – What had happened to him? How was he? When could I come and see him? What did he need? When could I speak to his doctor? – all the basic questions any family members might ask when someone they love is involved in a medical emergency that requires specialist care in hospital. I imagined that my feelings and questions about my son would be understood and responded to with understanding and support. I was totally unprepared for the response I received.

It was at this stage that I was confronted with a second 'carers' dilemma'. We approached the hospital both to seek information and advice and also to offer ourselves as a resource to help my son. Inexplicably we were turned away and asked not to visit for several days. No explanation was given for this and we were left deeply dismayed that my son would be left in acute distress in a strange place without access to people he knew and trusted. We didn't understand why the little information we received from ward staff seemed to be delivered with reluctance and in a guarded way. Why was it not possible to talk freely to us? We were given to understand that my son's consultant would not wish to speak to us. Nobody told us why. Our phone calls to the ward were actively discouraged. No past medical history or information about events leading up to the crisis was sought from us. Indeed, there seemed to be little acknowledgement of the legitimacy of our family's interest in what was happening to our son and brother. This, I later learned, was also a common experience for families.

When, on our visits to see him, our belongings were searched and our requests for information were turned down 'for confidentiality reasons', we began to wonder whether my son's professional carers had suspicions about the role we played in his life. It increasingly seemed to us that, although we regarded ourselves as a potentially valuable resource for my son, perhaps the professionals involved did not see us as such. For reasons we could not understand, some members of the care team, who did not know us and knew nothing of our relationship with him, seemed to regard us as part of the problem rather than as part of the solution. This apparent distrust of us and our intentions at this time of trauma was deeply unsettling for us all. I have heard many carer families speak of finding themselves in a similar situation.

In the absence of guidance, what were we to make of what was happening to him, and to us, in this fraught and uncertain new environment? We met no other family members at the hospital and knew of nobody then who had faced such problems. We felt uniquely alone, literally overwhelmed by the enormity of what was happening. We were desperate for any snippet of information that would help us make sense of what was going on. Our minds were flooded with questions – Why did this happen? What is happening now? What's going to happen next? Soon these gave way to Why him? Why us? Have we done anything wrong? Later, when we had found ways of coping better with the confusion and the swell of emotions, the distress and self-blame that swamped us, we wanted to know 'What can we do to help him?' Later still, as depression descended in the face of my son's first relapse, a further question formed: 'Why can't you do anything that helps him?'

We found our answers to all these questions eventually but, without access to guidance at this crucial first stage, we found it almost impossible at the time to know how to think about and articulate a response to his distress and our own emotional turmoil. We greeted his discharge from hospital that first time with deep anxiety and a feeling of utter helplessness.

More 'carers' dilemmas' presented themselves in the years that followed, as my son succumbed to four relapses and further admissions to hospital on his way to recovery. Most of the dilemmas were linked in some way with that tricky trinity of issues – consent, confidentiality and capacity.

When I later became a carers' worker, I came across, for the first time, the many published and unpublished narratives of carers, from different parts of the UK and in many countries beyond, that described events, service responses and feelings just like ours. As a worker and a researcher I had the opportunity to be in regular contact with other families like ours. I took part in groups that provided opportunities to hear from other carers that our experiences were by no means unique. What I learned from other carers proved invaluable. It helped make the difference between coping and not coping, between 'hanging on in there' and seeking to disengage from my son because we couldn't face the challenges any more. I feel sure that, had we been put in contact at that early stage with both a skilled professional, who understood and could work with family issues, and an experienced carer, we would have coped much better than we did right from the beginning.

As it was, no guidance was offered and we were left feeling isolated, impotent, powerless, helpless and anxious. We became 'carers', knowing we were ill-equipped to respond effectively to my son's needs and completely unprepared for the challenges that lay ahead.

THE IMPACT OF CARING

We were to find, as many families do, that our new roles as 'carers' involved much trial-and-error learning about how to manage a variety of puzzling mental health events and their consequences. It required a radical and ongoing review of the way family resources (personal, social and material) were used, so as to respond flexibly to whatever occurred in this very uncertain situation. We tried to incorporate complex new tasks and ways of doing things into our everyday patterns of family life to meet each new contingency. All this led to significant change in family roles and had a profound impact on family relationships and dynamics.

Underneath all of our 'doing' we felt a great, great sense of loss – the young man we each loved deeply in our own way as a son or a brother was, for long periods, unrecognisable, unreachable and seemingly condemned to a life of desolation and despair. This uniquely painful life event has been described by some as a form of bereavement. It has certainly felt just like that at times for him and for us. He lost his sense of who he was. He lost his place in the world. His plans, hopes and dreams for the future had to be relinquished one by one. So, too, did ours. This single major life event began to radically reshape the life trajectories of us all.

Each of us, to a greater or lesser extent, felt the impact at a personal, family and community level. We were all, I think, influenced by the way society stigmatises mental illness and people who experience it. And all of us felt the effects of the change that were required in everyday family life. Individually, though, we coped in different ways. Some of us were more defensive and emotion-focused, others were more active and problem-solving in our approach. A full range of different sibling coping strategies – collaborative, crisis oriented and detached approaches (Lefley 1996) was evident in the responses of my other adult children.

Importantly, our individual ways of coping changed over time in ways that I now know reflect the stages of adjustment that have been identified in other similar family situations (Nolan et al 1996, Terkelson 1987) This has significantly influenced our readiness to take on new information and learn ways of doing things over the years.

WHERE WE ARE NOW

Nine years on, our family picture is rosier than we could have expected in those dark, early days. Despite four relapses, my son's underlying trend line is upwards. He is working creatively on optimising his recovery and we all have reason to be optimistic about his future.

Like us, mental health services seem to have moved on. Psychological therapies are now more widely available, and access to atypical medications has made pharmacological intervention seemingly more acceptable to service users. Much very good work is also now being done with and for families. Useful explanations and responses to issues arising in family care now abound in the clinical, social care and social policy literatures. A wealth of robust evidence on the usefulness and effectiveness of family interventions in psychosis is available. This provides a clear rationale for working supportively with families to optimise therapeutic outcomes for service users. The thorny problems of information-sharing and confidentiality are at last being tackled by research and through development of new tools and approaches, including information-sharing contracts (NHS Executive 2001) and advance directives.

Positive change for family carers is well under way and families coming in contact with mental health services for the first time today report far fewer negative experiences than was the case 9 years ago. Increasing commitment to carers at policy level (e.g. Department of Health 1999a, b), at practice level (e.g. NICE guidelines) and a continuing programme of research on specific areas of concern in work with carers should ensure further positive developments.

WORKING WITH CARERS – A CARERS' WORKER PERSPECTIVE

Working with carers: what do we know?

As a carers' worker I have become familiar with the now extensive evidence base on carers and caregiving. The map of research on informal care includes contributions from several literatures. Figure 2.1 illustrates some of the major contributions from each:

Clinical/health literatures

Family risk factors for serious mental illness
Influence of families/carers on onset, course and outcome in mental illness, inc. EE
Family/carer assumptions, attributions, beliefs about MI
Impact of MI on families, inc. stigma and discrimination
Health impacts of caring, inc. stress and 'burden'
Carer coping - appraisal, responses, strategies, skills, styles
Resources and needs of families/carers
Caregiving and caring styles
Carers in different family roles
Culture and ethnicity issues for families/carers
Interventions and services for families/carers
Issues in working with families/carers
Nature and characteristics of informal care
Carers - who they are, what they do and why
Impact of caring - identities, roles, life transitions
Social impacts of caring over time

Social care and social policy literatures

Figure 2.1 The evidence base on families and carers in mental health.

Caring and stress

It has been said that 'to care is to experience stress' (Opie 1994). Certainly much of what carers say about their experience of supporting someone with a serious mental illness focuses on issues of coping and stress. The literature includes many studies which explore carers' coping (including resources, strategies and skills), coping overwhelm (including subjective and objective 'burden') and the association of these with caregiver stress. The social impact of caring on carers has also been written about extensively.

Individuals manage stresses in different ways, and some carers cope with caregiving more successfully than others. But it has been suggested many carers experience some of the characteristic consequences of caregiving stress described by Heron (1998):

◆ Emotional disturbance (including grief, guilt, frustration, anger)
◆ Personal stress
◆ Relationship stress
◆ Overburden and burnout (including 'stress addiction')
◆ Mental and physical health problems

- Life limitations (including job loss, social isolation, stigma)
- Exploitation or abuse (by the carer or by the cared-for)
- Positive outcomes (including enhanced closeness of carer and cared-for).

The American psychiatrist, Harriet Lefley (1996) has constructed a map of caregiver stress that includes three categories of stress that are particularly significant for carers of people with serious mental illness. She assigns the types of stresses that carers live with on a daily basis to three 'domains':

- Situational (i.e. related to the mental health condition, its events and consequences)
- Societal (i.e. to do with the responses and attitudes of institutions and communities to the expression of mental illness, including stigma and discrimination)
- Iatrogenic (i.e. arising from contacts with mental health services).

She doesn't herself rank the domains in terms of their relative stress-inducing capacity, but a visitor to a mental health carer support group would be likely to come away with the impression that carers' concerns about their relationships with mental health services rank at least as highly as the stresses arising in the other two domains.

Lefley also includes in her map a list of the known outcomes for carers of accumulations of such stresses. She describes the consequences of unrelieved carer stress as: confusion, frustration, grief, anger, self-blaming, guilt and defensive coping.

It can be very difficult at times for carers to manage the very powerful emotions triggered by the events and consequences of serious mental illness. Perhaps it is not surprising that in contacts with professionals, whom carers see as the primary source of help, it can sometimes become difficult for carers to contain their feelings. Carers are hugely appreciative of those practitioners who understand the reasons behind any emotion-focused coping and work constructively with it. But occasionally, they may find the pressures unbearable and this can cause misunderstandings and conflicts to arise. Lefley explores some of the ways in which carers may sometimes wittingly or unwittingly impede the delivery of professional care and the reasons that such problems occur. What is clear now is that access to skilled family workers and carers' support workers who have expertise in responding to issues arising can do much to reduce the risks associated with such difficulties.

Carers' needs

That carers sometimes need a break from caring has been widely recognised, particularly in the introduction of carers' assessments and the funding of respite breaks through the carers' special grant. However, when asked about their needs, carers often rank provision of quality services for the person they care for as their highest priority (Hogman & Pearson 1995, Muijen et al 1994). Regular contact with professionals, information and training in how to care are also highly ranked, along with recognition of the carer's role in the partnership of care and meaningful involvement in care-planning around the service user.

It has long been national policy to include carers in this way wherever possible, but a recent study (Pinfold & Corry 2003) suggests that this is still not happening routinely. The survey of 1400 carers found that:

◆ One in four carers (27%) had been denied access to help in the past 4 years
◆ 92% of carers want contact with professionals but just 49% have that contact.

What carers value in professionals

Carers value professionals who:

◆ Understand the carer's situation
◆ Are aware of the history and complexity of the caring relationship
◆ Can be relied on to listen to the carer's point of view
◆ Have respect for other people's way of life (beliefs, fears and aspirations as well as language, culture and religion)
◆ Construct with them an 'ethic of care' unique to their situation.

What information, guidance and support is most valuable to carers?

◆ Recognition of their caring role
◆ Information (about the mental health condition, treatments, services, sources of support)
◆ Regular and meaningful contact with the care coordinator
◆ Involvement in decision-making and care-planning
◆ Education and skills training (e.g. problem-solving, communicating effectively)
◆ Opportunities to share experiences with other carers
◆ Respite breaks.

[From Rethink reports *The Silent Partner* (Rethink 1995) and *Who Cares?* (Rethink 2003).]

Why involve carers at all?

A considerable body of literature now illustrates that, with time and experience, families acquire considerable expertise in their varied roles as care manager, planner, direct care provider, advocate, problem solver and gatekeeper. Investigations of the coping strategies families use to deal with different demands and circumstances show that coping is best when families can draw from a repertoire of coping strategies and match strategies to particular demands. Being able to exploit problem solving and cognitive reframing to the full, instead of using reactive stress reduction tactics is generally more helpful. A capacity to make sense of what can often be non-normative circumstances appears to be a consistent factor in successful coping. Finally, drawing from different trusted sources of support to help at appropriate times can make the difference between sinking, surviving and swimming.

Grant 2002, p. 105

To conclude, I would like to offer two approaches to answering this question, one that makes reference to national research and the other that makes use of my family experience.

In 2002, Carers UK, the leading national voluntary agency for carers, published the findings of research that estimated the monetary value of the support provided by informal family carers (Carers UK 2002). It was able to show that carers save the country a staggering £57.4 billion every year. If we take the government's estimates for the numbers of carers who support people with mental health difficulties as approximately 11% of the total number of carers, this suggests that the support provided by the national population of mental health carers each year is worth £6 billion. Carers are a valuable resource indeed!

The grid in Table 2.1 describes the support that is provided within my carer family. It is a numerical representation of our family's experience of mental health care over time. The information included was compiled by my son and me from family-held records – diaries, appointment letters, care plans and other documents. The grid was completed 3023 days after my son's first admission to hospital for the first time. One of our records is incomplete, but as far as we can tell this is an accurate account of his (and our) experience thus far.

The table identifies the amount of time spent in each care delivery 'domain'. The number of hours shown under Community Mental Health Team refers to actual contact hours, i.e. the amount of time spent in contact with members of the care team.

Our experience, as expressed in the table, is not dissimilar to that of many other carers I've known and worked with. I hope the figures it contains will largely speak for themselves.

My son and I were 'knocked sideways' by what we discovered when it was completed. Neither he nor I had fully understood how much of the

Table 2.1 Formal and informal care: one family's experience

Phase	Total care (days)	Acute inpatient level	CMHT aftercare (h)/CPA level (h)	Day centre (h)	Supported accommodation (days)	Primary care (GP appointments) (days)	Self-care (client chose to live independently) family (days)	Family care (client chose to live with family) (days)
First (acute episode 1994)	614	147 (formal)	14 Psychiatrist outpatient appointments				253	214
Second (acute episode 1996)	718	119	10 Psychiatrist outpatient appointments				354	245
Third (acute episode 1998)	1368	136	9 Complex CPA ↓ as recovery sustained		98	5	341	793
Fourth (acute episode 2002)	142	28 (informal)	10 Enhanced CPA†				93	21
Fifth (acute episode 2002)	181	38 (formal)	28 Enhanced CPA†	69			22	121
Total	3023 days	468 days	71 h	69 h	98 days	5 visits	1063‡ days	1394 days

Late in 1998, client chose to leave supported accommodation to return to family home. In 1999, with family support, found part-time then full-time job for 3+ years; positive appraisals led to promotion. Moved into own flat 2001. Relapse and job loss followed 6 months after s. 117 discharge into primary care when GP advised withdrawal from medication (risperidone)

Discharged from s. 117 'care complete'

Client wary of psychiatric services following deeply traumatic first admission to hospital. Assertive outreach/crisis resolution teams not operational locally until late 2002.

† No relapse/contingency/crisis planning done (interventions in relapse not achieved until 7–9 weeks after family identified early-warning signs and notified services in phases 1, 3, 5.
‡ With enhanced contact with family.
CMHT, Community Mental Health Team; CPA, Care Programme Approach.

responsibility for managing his situation was 'down to us'. It raised many questions for both of us about why people like us were not routinely offered information, education or training and support to help us manage such a complex and puzzling condition on a day-to-day basis.

My son's comment on completion of the grid was rueful – 'Is it any wonder I kept relapsing? How on earth were we supposed to know what to do...?' For this reason, and for all of the above, it seems important to fully acknowledge carers as the vital resource they are in the provision of mental health care ... and ensure they have all the means available to continue providing support effectively and safely.

References

Carers UK 2002 Without us ... Calculating the cost of carers' support, London

Department of Health 1999a Caring about carers: a national strategy. Department of Health, London

Department of Health 1999b A national service framework for mental health. The Stationery Office, London

Office for National Statistics 2000 General Household Survey. The Stationery Office, London

Grant G 2002 Caring families: their support or empowerment? In: Stalker K (ed) Reconceptualising work with carers: new directions for policy and practice, research highlights in social work. Jessica Kingsley, London

Heron C 1998 Working with carers. Jessica Kingsley, London, pp 43–60

Hogman G, Pearson G 1995 The silent partners: the needs and experiences of people who care for people with severe mental illness. National Schizophrenia Fellowship, Kingston-upon-Thames

Lefley H 1996 Family caregiving in mental illness. Sage, Thousand Oaks, CA, p 66

Muijen M et al 1994 Relative values. the differing views of users, family carers and professionals on services for people with schizophrenia in the community. Sainsbury Centre for Mental Health, London

NHS Executive/Social Services Inspectorate, Carers Advisory Group 2001 Working with carers: a handbook for professionals working with those who provide help and support to people with mental health problems

Nolan M, Grant G, Keady J 1996 Understanding family care. Open University, Buckingham

Opie 1994 as cited by Nolan M, Grant G, Keady J (eds) 1996 Understanding family care. Open University, Buckingham

Pinfold V, Corry P 2003 Who cares? The experiences of mental health carers accessing services and information. Rethink, Kingston upon Thames, London 2003

Terkelson K G 1987 The evolution of family responses to mental illness through time. In: Hatfield A B, Lefley H P (eds) Families of the mentally ill: coping and adaptation. Guilford, New York, pp 151–166

Further reading

Carers UK 2002 Paying the price: carers, poverty and social exclusion. Child Poverty Action Group, London

National Institute for Clinical Excellence 2002 Schizophrenia guideline: core interventions in the treatment and management of schizophrenia in primary care and secondary care. National Institute for Clinical Excellence, London

3

Social inclusion

Rachel Perkins and Liz Sayce

KEY ISSUES

- ◆ Social inclusion
- ◆ Challenging negative assumptions and attitudes
- ◆ Employment and improving self esteem
- ◆ Support and assistance
- ◆ Case study

'Schizophrenics go home' read the slogan daubed on a van outside a new residential facility for people with mental health problems (Repper et al 1997). But where is 'home'? The experience of people who experience serious mental health problems is often one of having no 'home': belonging nowhere, being rejected, despised, ridiculed, feared by those around them.

When boxer Frank Bruno was admitted to hospital in 2003 the headline in the *Sun* read 'Bonkers Bruno locked up'. Following complaints, anxious executives changed the headline in the second edition to 'Hero Bruno in mental home'; and members of the public left flowers at the hospital gate. Empathetic responses are still, however, not the automatic response to people experiencing mental health problems. On this occasion the affection in which Frank Bruno is held may have prompted goodwill; but goodwill can still never be assumed in relation to users of mental health services in general. Not every black man escorted to hospital by the police could expect such a positive public response.

Mental health problems carry with them not only distressing symptoms but all the prejudice, discrimination and exclusion that accompany diagnoses such as schizophrenia and manic depression. An ordinary life seems impossible. Dreams of a nice home, a decent job, family, friends are shattered by the images of 'the mentally ill' that are so often portrayed in the media and popular culture (Dunn 1999, Sayce 2000, Repper & Perkins 2003). On the one hand you are seen as incompetent, unable and unfit to participate fully in society, in need of others to look after you, make decisions for you. On the other hand you are seen as unpredictable, dangerous, responsible for the 'rising tide of killings', one of the 'nuts' who should be 'caged for life' to protect others. Despite the fact that the proportion of homicides committed by people with mental health problems fell from 35% in 1967 to 11.5% in 1996 (Taylor & Gunn 1999), the 'psycho-killer' image continues to reign supreme.

> *The media make people afraid of us. One person is violent and it's all over the press and then people think it applies to everyone who has been in hospital. If you're a big man like me it's worse. People cross the street to avoid me.*

(Cited in Rose 1966)

People with mental health problems have the same range of needs and ambitions as any other citizens – somewhere decent to live, someone to love, something worthwhile to do, to be a part of the communities in which they live. The prejudice and discrimination that flow from popular images of mental health problems are at least as important in preventing people pursuing these goals as the symptoms of mental health problems themselves.

> *Mental health problems are not a full time job – we have lives to lead. Any services, or treatments, or supports must be judged in these terms – how much they allow us to lead the lives we wish to lead.*

(Perkins 2000)

The task of mental health practitioners is to help people who experience serious mental health problems to rebuild their lives, and this requires that we move beyond our traditional focus on symptoms and medication and explore how we can reduce the discrimination and social exclusion that prevent people from doing the things they want to do. Even if symptoms can be completely eliminated, people are often denied access to economic and social opportunities because they have a history of mental health problems. This means that it is never enough simply to treat the symptoms of mental health problems: we must pay equal attention to promoting participation and inclusion.

Social inclusion is about having the opportunity to participate fully as equal citizens (Disability Rights Commission 2001). It is about value, opportunity and rights: having the opportunity to do the things you want to do, being valued and respected as a citizen alongside other citizens and having the same rights as other citizens. But, while the idea of social inclusion may be relatively straightforward, ensuring that it is a reality for people with mental health problems is altogether more complex.

In order to understand how practitioners might promote participation and inclusion, it is important to first understand the experience of exclusion and the mechanisms by which it is maintained. (For a more detailed description of ways in which practitioners might promote social inclusion and enable people to do the things they want to do see Repper & Perkins 2003.)

DISCRIMINATION AND EXCLUSION SPAN ALL AREAS OF LIFE

In the ordinary round of everyday life, prejudice and exclusion are commonplace. Sometimes this is quite subtle: people treating you differently or avoiding you.

> *Friends, family, people you meet every day – people treat you differently. Like they are treading on eggshells ... they think that if they say something wrong you're going to flare up or whatever.*

> (Cited in Repper et al 1998)

Sometimes rejection is more explicit.

> *Friends avoided me and would not let their children play with my children any more.*

> (Cited in Read & Baker 1996)

> *When I went into psychiatric hospital the minister didn't come and visit me. He always visits people when they are in hospital. But he didn't visit me.*

> *My in-laws wouldn't have me in the house for 10 years after my mental illness. My wife and daughter visited them, but I was not permitted.*

> (Cited in Sayce 2000)

And sometimes it takes on a more frightening and sinister form. Read & Baker (1996) cite numerous examples of people who have been attacked in the street, had eggs thrown at them and had dog faeces put through their letter box simply because they were known to have mental health problems. As one 71-year-old man recounted: 'Various gangs in the district call me "nutter" and spit on me. The gangs on the estate know I was a psychiatric patient and so I'm teased and harassed' (Read & Baker 1996).

The social isolation that results from loss of friends and social contacts is often exacerbated by unemployment and poverty. Being able to work – contribute to the communities in which we live – is central to inclusion: it links us with the communities in which we live, gives us a purpose and meaning in life, and is protective against a range of physical and mental health problems (Rowland & Perkins 1988, Shepherd 1989, Repper & Perkins 2003, Royal College of Psychiatrists 2003). 'It boosts self-esteem and provides a sense of purpose and accomplishment. Work enables people to enter, or re-enter, the mainstream after hospitalisation' (Rogers 1995).

The majority of surveys repeatedly show that the majority of people with mental health problems would like to work, yet they are the most disadvantaged group in relation to employment. Only 21% of people with long-term mental health problems are in employment compared with 49% of disabled people more generally (Office for National Statistics 2003). The literature is replete with accounts of people who have been denied employment because of their mental health problems (Dunn 1999, Sayce 2000, Repper & Perkins 2003).

I had a cleaning job for three years, but when I mentioned an appointment with a psychiatrist I received a letter the next week to say that my services were no longer required.

Last year I was offered a position as a graduate programmer and I was pleased with the prospect of working in industry using the skills and knowledge I had gathered from my time at university. I was devastated to be told a week later that the offer had been withdrawn because my security clearance was not accepted due to me suffering a mental illness.

(Cited in Read & Baker 1996)

And these people are not being 'paranoid'. Research conducted by the Department of Work and Pensions (2001) shows that, in the face of labour shortages, while 62% of employers were prepared to consider employing people with physical impairments only 37% said they would consider those with mental health difficulties. Neither are these high unemployment rates a result of the symptoms themselves. There is now a wealth of research evidence that as many as 60% of people with serious mental health problems can work if they are provided with the right ongoing support and opportunities (Bond et al 1997, 2001, Crowther et al 2001).

Unemployment is also associated with poverty and this exacerbates social exclusion: people simply do not have the money to avail themselves of the opportunities that are available.

Out of the blue your job has gone, and with it any financial security you may have had. At a stroke, you have no purpose in life, and no contact with other people. You find yourself isolated from the rest of the world. No-one telephones you. Much less writes. No-one seems to care if you are alive or dead.

(Bird 2001)

The literature is also replete with examples of people being excluded from all manner of goods and services like leisure activities and facilities, clubs and community organisations, access to justice and physical health services.

I've changed my church because at the last one they were terrible about mentally ill people.

The man was sexually harassing me and I went to the police station for help. I said I wanted to take out an injunction. They said I couldn't because I was a mental patient.

(Cited in Rose 1996)

When I fill in an insurance form I have to put down about my depression. I got refusals from three companies I tried.

(Cited in Dunn 1999)

It took longer to diagnose my chest pains as heart disease because my symptoms were thought to be 'all in the mind'.

(Cited in Disability Rights Commission 2003)

Such exclusion from appropriate physical health care is particularly serious, and potentially fatal. Harris & Barraclough (1998) have shown that mental disorder is as strongly associated with premature death as smoking.

THE ROOTS OF EXCLUSION

Link & Phelan (2001) have described how exclusion begins with the *distinguishing and labelling of human differences*. Some differences – like food preferences, height or hair colour are relevant in relatively few situations, but others – like sexuality, IQ, skin colour and mental health status – are highly salient. With differences such as these, labelling is followed by *stereotyping: the linking of labelled people to undesirable characteristics*. So the label of 'mental illness' has been associated with a number of undesirable characteristics: dangerousness, unpredictability, incompetence. This stereotyping then forms the basis of the *separation of 'them' from 'us'*. Those to whom negatively loaded labels are applied are separated from the rest of society: come to be seen as a separate class of person. There are 'them' (who have mental health problems) and 'us' (who do not). People *have* cancer or heart disease, but remain one of 'us' who is ill. But people *are* 'schizophrenics', 'manic depressives' and are very definitely not one of 'us'. During this process the negative attributes associated with 'them' are elaborated and extended and this forms the basis of a rationale for *loss of status, discrimination* and *exclusion.* It makes sense to exclude a group of people who are dangerous, unpredictable and unable to participate in ordinary community life.

Most importantly, discrimination and exclusion are dependent on social, economic and political power (Link & Phelan 2001): the power to determine which differences are salient in a society, the power to separate 'them' from 'us', and the power to deny 'them' jobs, decent housing, an adequate income, etc. People with mental health problems do not have such power.

Sometimes this process has been described as a process of stigmatisation (Link & Phelan 2001); however, there may be problems with the concept of 'stigma'. Different terms lead to different understandings of where the 'problem' lies and therefore to different prescriptions for changing the situation (Sayce 1998). The term 'stigma' focuses attention on the person who is the recipient of the rejection and exclusion rather than on those who perpetuate the unjust treatment. This leads to a focus on the impact of stigma on the individual (they cannot get a job, are socially isolated, etc.) rather than the mechanisms that result in these disadvantages (Oliver 1990, Sayce 2000, Chamberlin 2001). Chamberlin (2001) argues that the term 'stigma' is in itself stigmatising because it implies that there is something wrong with the person and places the onus on them to change, while the terms 'prejudice' and 'discrimination' put the onus where it belongs, on the individuals, groups and social structures that practise it.

In the mental health arena, the shortcomings of using the concept of stigma can be seen in a number of arenas. For example, within mental health services there has been a focus on changing the individual – reducing their symptoms, helping them to change their behaviour or develop skills – so that they can 'fit in' and participate, be included. In addition, therapeutic approaches have been proposed to reduce the psychological impact of stigma on the individual rather than reducing the barriers that prevent their participation and maintain their exclusion (Hayward & Bright 1997).

The importance of reducing discrimination and exclusion is recognised in Standard 1 of the mental health National Service Framework (Department of Health 1999), which places an obligation on mental health services to decrease the discrimination experienced by people with mental health problems and promote their social inclusion. The remainder of this chapter will be directed towards a consideration of what mental health practitioners might be able to do to contribute to this agenda.

CHALLENGING DISCRIMINATION AND PROMOTING INCLUSION: WHAT CAN MENTAL HEALTH PRACTITIONERS DO?

Link & Phelan (2001) have identified three levels at which discrimination operates to ensure that people are excluded from the ordinary social and economic opportunities that non-disabled citizens expect: individual discrimination, structural discrimination and discrimination that results from the person's own beliefs and behaviour. These provide a useful framework for exploring ways in which practitioners might promote social inclusion. (For a more detailed description of ways in which practitioners might promote social inclusion and enable people to do the things they want to do see Repper & Perkins 2003.)

Throughout, it is important to remember that attempts to promote inclusion and participation must be tailored to the needs and wishes of the person. Different things are meaningful and valuable to different people and people have preferences about the type of help they would like to receive.

Individual discrimination and exclusion

This occurs when people are, for example, turned down for a college course, rejected by friends, taunted in the street because they are known to use mental health services or not taken seriously by their doctor when they report physical complaints. Traditionally, mental health practitioners have attempted to decrease the exclusion resulting from such individual rejection by 'changing' the individual so that they can 'fit in' better. This might include a number of approaches, for example:

◆ Medication and psychological treatments to reduce symptoms
◆ A range of approaches to modify unusual behaviour
◆ Helping people to develop the skills they need
◆ Reducing anxiety and lack of confidence that might prevent people from engaging in activities they value.

While these may all be important, approaches based on changing the individual have significant limitations. First, pervasive prejudice ensures that, even if a person's symptoms can be reduced and their skills and confidence increased, they often remain excluded because of their history of mental health problems – 'What happens if they go mad again?' Second, it remains the case that there are many problems that people experience that cannot be eliminated by treatment, therapy and training. If opportunity is contingent on a person ceasing to have difficulties, those who have ongoing or recurrent problems will remain excluded.

We would never dream of saying that a person with a broken spine could only have access to the things they want to do if they are enabled to walk again. Instead we think about the supports and adaptations that might enable them to do the things they want in the presence of their continuing mobility impairments. Ensuring this for people who have the cognitive and emotional impairments commonly associated with serious mental health problems requires a similar approach – a shift away from helping the person to 'fit in' to changing the environment in which they operate so that it can accommodate them: the psychiatric equivalents of wheelchairs, personal assistants, ramps and hearing loops.

Support and assistance – the psychiatric equivalent of the wheelchair and the personal assistant

There are a number of ways in which mental health practitioners can provide people with the assistance they need in order to do things they want to do. These might include:

◆ *Practical assistance* such as help to get up in the morning, transport, money to register for the college course.
◆ *Having someone to do things with you*, to help you to do what you want to do. Such assistance may be provided by the mental health worker, but it may also be provided by a friend, family member or a peer with mental health difficulties – it is important to remember the enormous amount of support and help that people with mental health problems can give each other. Alternatively, it might be provided by someone else who is also engaged in the activity: a fellow student, workplace mentor, a member of the local church or football team.
◆ *Relieving the person of responsibility for some things that they do not greatly value in order to enable them to do things they want to do.* Sometimes an implicit hierarchy operates in which it is assumed that a person must wash their socks and do their domestic chores before they can go out to the pub or go to work. This is unhelpful. Often a person's impairments make it difficult for them to do all that is expected of them. If this is the case then it may be desirable to relieve them of responsibility for activities that they do not value greatly (perhaps domestic chores) in order to enable them to devote their energies and resources to things that give their life meaning (perhaps going to college, to work or out with friends).

Adjustments in what is expected of the person so that they are able to meet those expectations – the psychiatric equivalent of ramps and lifts

Often, when we think about adjustments, we think about ways of changing the physical environment so that it is accessible for people who have mobility or sensory impairments: Braille lift buttons, ramps, etc. However, similar adjustments are possible to facilitate access for people with mental health difficulties. Sometimes this may involve adjustments in the physical environment (such as reducing distractions that may interrupt a person) but more often the necessary adjustments are in role expectations. It is important to remember that the roles that people occupy in any social, family, leisure, work or education setting are not fixed – there is no set of skills or behaviours that defines the role of worker or son or student. This means that they can be renegotiated to accommodate the person's limitations and enable them to participate. This may involve negotiations with families, friends, employers, tutors.

For example, one young man was unable to continue living in his own flat because of his mental health problems and returned to his parents' home. This forced a renegotiation of roles. From leaving home and living independently he returned to dependence on his parents. Initially, his role became one of a young child: his parents did everything for him and made decisions on his behalf. This did not allow him to use the abilities he had, so the family were assisted to renegotiate their expectations of each other once again. The young man took on a range of tasks to help his ageing parents (shopping, decorating, doing the heavy garden jobs). Similarly, it may be possible to negotiate with a college for someone to have extra time to complete their course or assignments or to do some work at home rather than always having to go into college.

Esso Leete (1989), who has a diagnosis of schizophrenia, has enumerated a range of adjustments that enable her to work despite the continuing presence of symptoms. These include:

◆ having a highly structured daily schedule and writing lists of what she must do
◆ asking others to communicate in a clear way and break down tasks into steps
◆ sitting with her back to the wall and facing the door because she sometimes believes that the police will surprise her
◆ having the possibility of withdrawing to another room if she feels overwhelmed when there are a large number of people around
◆ working in a quiet area where distractions are minimised.

Other people may require slight adjustments in hours, or flexi-time, or time off for appointments. Adjustments are highly individual things and must be tailored to the needs of the individual and the specific work, social, education or leisure situation.

Sometimes it is assumed that any assistance or adjustments that a person requires will be time-limited – helping them to engage in an activity until they are able to do so unaided. This is a mistake. 'Independence' from support is less important than what a person is able to achieve with that support. If a person can only continue to participate with ongoing assistance then it would be a grave mistake to withdraw support. Just as someone with a physical impairment may need a wheelchair or a personal assistant on an ongoing basis, so someone with cognitive and emotional impairments may need support indefinitely.

In helping people to do the things they want to do it is important to consider whether the help or adjustments draw negative attention to the person – whether they make them feel stupid or look odd or incompetent in the eyes of others. Arriving at college in an ambulance is likely to single a person out in a negative fashion, while arriving in a taxi is not. If a young man goes to the pub or pool hall with an older female mental health worker it can look rather as if he is being taken there by his mother – which is likely to do little for the way he is seen in the eyes of others. Perhaps it would be better if he went with his brother, or another client or volunteer of the same age? The way in which help is offered can also be important: holding someone's hand when crossing the street or giving instructions in a loud voice makes clear the distinction between 'them' and 'us'.

Structural discrimination and exclusion

Much of the work of mental health practitioners to reduce social isolation is likely to occur at an individual level but it is important to recognise some of the structural barriers that exist. There may be problems with the benefits system that make it difficult for a person to work without risking their income. There is a tendency for employers to require references from current employers and look suspiciously on gaps in employment history. Also, the tendency for poverty to accompany mental health problems means that a person may lack the resources to engage in social and leisure activities or be forced to live in a high-crime area where 'hard to let' public housing is available.

While it may be difficult for mental health practitioners to address such structural discrimination in their day-to-day work, three things may be possible:

◆ *Supporting employers, colleges and the providers of goods and services.* If a worker gets to know what is available in their local community, and the people who provide various services, then this can serve to break down barriers and dispel myths. If employers or colleges or leisure facilities are provided with the support they need – or think they need – to accommodate someone who has mental health problems then they may be more willing to allow them to participate. This can be as simple as giving them a number to ring if they have difficulties.

◆ *Individual advocacy and support.* It may be possible for a worker to advocate for a person with an employer, course or leisure activity, extolling their virtues, negotiating any adjustments they may need and dispelling any fears that the people running the agency may have.

◆ *Helping people to understand and secure their rights.* The 1995 Disability Discrimination Act (DDA) makes it illegal to discriminate against people on the basis of their mental health problems and places an obligation on employers, educators and the providers of goods and services to make 'reasonable adjustments' to enable them to participate. People with mental health problems have a right to adjustments at work, at college and in using other services and facilities. Mental health professionals can assist in informing people of their rights, helping them to identify and negotiate such adjustments, reminding employers, colleges and the providers of goods/services of their obligations, and helping people to seek assistance if they experience discrimination. The Disability Rights Commission provide information, advice and a casework service to help people who have experienced discrimination to obtain redress (see www.drc-gb.org or contact the Disability Rights Commission helpline, 08457 622633).

Mental health workers also have an important role in ensuring that people can access other entitlements, such as housing and the all-important state benefits that are, for many, the major source of income. The benefits system is complex and difficult to negotiate and many fail to get their entitlements, either because they are unaware of them or because they find the process of securing them insurmountably difficult.

Exclusion resulting from the person's own beliefs and behaviours

Widespread individual and structural discrimination, combined with negative stereotypes of people with mental health problems, sap the confidence of many who have serious mental health problems and cause many to give up trying to participate. If you are turned down repeatedly it is easy to believe you are incapable of working and give up trying to get a job; stop trying to make friends because you have been rejected so many times in the past; give up going to the GP because you know that they will write off everything you report as a symptom of your mental health problems. In the face of repeated failure and humiliation it is easy to give up believing in the possibility of a decent future.

The accounts of people who have experienced mental health problems consistently emphasise the importance of hope in enabling them to rebuild their lives (Deegan 1988, 1993, 1996, Spaniol & Koehler 1994, Young & Ensing 1999) – a perspective that is shared by an increasing body of professional research. It has long been recognised that hope is central to successful psychotherapy (Menninger 1959, Frank 1968) and a number of studies have shown that hope is central if people with schizophrenia are to rebuild their lives (Anthony et al 1990, Woodside et al 1994, Kirkpatrick et al 1995, Kanwal 1997, Russinova 1999, Landeen et al 2000). Aguilar et al (1997) have shown that higher levels of 'hopelessness' during a person's first episode of serious mental health problems are predictive of poor outcome.

Hope – a belief in the possibility of a valued and valuable life – is critical if people are to participate in their communities. Yet many people have described ways in which mental health services have contributed to their feelings of hopelessness and despair. Mental health workers have a central role in fostering (or diminishing) hope (Kirkpatrick et al 1995, 2001, Russinova 1999, Repper & Perkins 2003). If we always focus on people's deficits and dysfunctions – the things that people cannot do – then we foster despair. If those who are helping a person can see no possibility for a valuable life, what hope is there? Practitioners must be able to hold on to hope when a person is unable to believe in their own possibilities and help them to retain a vision of possibilities through the setbacks and relapses that many with mental health problems experience.

'Giving up', apathy and indifference can be a way of protecting oneself from further disappointment – protecting 'the last vestiges of the wounded self' (Deegan 1990). Restoring hope – shedding the protection afforded by apathy and withdrawal – is a risky journey. The person must risk further disappointment and failure and dare to trust people again. People with serious mental health problems have identified four things as important in 'igniting and nurturing their hope' (Kirkpatrick et al 2001):

◆ *Experiencing success.* This may be via recognising personal achievements, achieving personally valuable goals or seeing the things that other people with similar difficulties have experienced. People may have contact with others who have experienced similar challenges either directly or through their writing (Leete 1988, 1989, Deegan 1989, Spaniol & Koehler 1994, Reeves 1998, Read & Reynolds 2001 and journals such as *Schizophrenia Bulletin*). 'My suggestion is to get as many success stories as possible from those who have schizophrenia to give a sense of hope to those just beginning their journey' (Kirkpatrick et al 2001).
◆ *Taking control.* Gaining understanding and control over problems and symptoms that at first seem uncontrollable. There is a wealth of evidence that people can monitor and gain control over the symptoms they experience (Repper & Perkins 2003). 'I have more control over my illness

than I ever realised .... Knowing that gives me more hope because I know the next time when I start to get ill I can turn it around. You don't have to let your illness run your life' (Kirkpatrick et al 2001).
◆ *Finding meaning.* People need ways of finding meaning and value in their lives with mental health problems; 'feeling like there is some purpose in life. I'm not just a person here on earth meant to take, take, take, but I have something to give' (Kirkpatrick et al 2001).
◆ *Maintaining relationships.* Hope cannot exist in a vacuum: it is difficult to maintain a belief in yourself and your own possibilities when all around can see no value in your life. Relationships with mental health practitioners can be critical in enabling people to hold on to hope but such relationships will always have their limitations because their very context is devaluing: the worker is only there because they are paid to be there – it is their job. The success of a relationship between practitioner and client might best be judged in terms of the extent to which it enables people to maintain and regain other hope-inspiring and valued relationships with friends, relatives, neighbours, colleagues and peers with mental health problems. 'He listens to me and understands I am not well and that there are things I can and cannot do, but he always has the utmost faith in me' (a participant speaking of his relationship with his brother, cited in Kirkpatrick et al 2001).

(For a more detailed description of ways in which mental health workers can foster hope see Repper & Perkins 2003.)

SOCIAL INCLUSION, ILLNESS AND DISABILITY

Promoting social inclusion is about enabling people with mental health problems to do the things they want to do – things that give their life meaning and value; to be a valued part of their communities and to contribute to their communities. Frequently there is an emphasis on treatment and care, but this is only a part of what people with mental health problems need. Always being the 'poor unfortunate' who is on the receiving end of the ministrations of others is demeaning and dispiriting. If people with serious mental health problems are to rebuild their lives, the opportunity to contribute is at least as important. In this chapter we have outlined some of the ways in which this might be achieved. However, the ways in which we conceptualise people's difficulties and possibilities is equally critical.

A number of anti-stigma campaigns organised by the World Psychiatric Association, the Royal College of Psychiatrists and the Department of Health have focused on educating the public that 'mental illness is an illness like any other'. The assumption is that, if people can come to see that mental illness is a disease of the brain, then people with mental health problems will be viewed in the same way as someone with heart disease, diabetes or asthma, negative stereotypes will be eroded and people will not be blamed for their difficulties. But does the belief that mental illness is an illness like any other reduce discrimination and exclusion? There is an increasing body of evidence that it does not, and may even have the reverse effect (Sayce 2000, Read & Harré 2001). On the basis of research conducted in Switzerland, Nordt et al (2001) concluded that 'Anti-stigma campaigns that focus on the recognition of illness and its particular symptoms run the risk of increasing discrimination'.

It is popularly assumed that if someone is ill – whether their ailment is physical or psychiatric – they should be relieved of responsibilities at work or college and suspend social and leisure activities – tucked up in bed – until they are well again. This is all very well for time-limited physical and mental health problems, but what about those whose 'illnesses' are ongoing? If they are deemed to be ill, they risk being permanently excluded from social and economic life.

And does the public really view 'diseases of the brain' as being like any other illnesses of the body? In the popular conception, diseases of the brain render a person unable to think properly, unable to take responsibility for their actions and likely to be unpredictable and perhaps dangerous – precisely the negative stereotypes that underlie the discrimination that people with mental health problems experience. At best, such an approach is likely only to replace blame and fear with pity. And being 'the poor unfortunate' is no basis for inclusion on equal terms with other citizens.

Sayce (2000) has suggested that the concept of 'illness' for people with enduring mental health problems should be replaced with one of 'disability'. Illness calls for the often illusive 'cure' whereas 'disability' moves beyond symptom removal to a focus on the adjustments and accommodations that people need to participate in their communities. Within the social model of disability developed by the broader disability movement, people are not disabled by their specific mobility, sensory, cognitive or emotional impairments, but by the way in which society views and treats people with such impairments. If people are disabled, then the challenge is to ensure that they have access to the things they want to do and the Disability Discrimination Act (1995) affords them rights to participate and to adjustments that will enable them to participate.

Social inclusion is about enabling people to participate in, contribute to, and become valued members of the communities in which they live. If this is to become a reality then two ingredients are key: hope and opportunity. Without hope there is no point in trying to rebuild a meaningful and valued life. But hope cannot be sustained without opportunity: the chance to do the things you want to do, the things that give your life meaning and purpose. The following case study summarises what can be learnt from this chapter:

Case study – Fred

In his second year at college Fred started having great difficulty studying. He could not go out because he believed that his fellow students were plotting against him … so he stayed in his room all day, venturing out only at night when there was no-one else around. His fellow students were worried about him. They tried to help but he would not speak to them. Eventually the doctor was called and Fred was compulsorily admitted to hospital, where he was treated for schizophrenia.

An all too common scenario
The college did not really know what was happening. No-one contacted them. Debts mounted for Fred's fees and rent in the hall of residence. He failed to show up for lectures and examinations and was expelled. His friends drifted away – they did not know what was happening. Only his worried parents kept in touch – they did not know what to do for the best and could not understand what had happened to their son, who had been so successful at school. When Fred left hospital he went back to live with his parents and did little but sit in his room playing records and smoking.

Another way
With Fred's permission, his care coordinator contacted the college and said that he was ill, arranging for him to take some time out and to give up the tenancy of his room to avoid running up further debts.

To start off with, Fred did not want to see anyone or talk to his college tutor. He was convinced that there was no hope of him ever finishing his course or obtaining a degree. He believed that all was hopeless and that his life was over.

His care coordinator arranged for him to speak to another client who had a similar diagnosis and had been successful in returning to college. Fred was initially sceptical but agreed reluctantly to see him. After a number of meetings Fred became a little less pessimistic – he agreed that there might be an outside chance of his going back to college but was worried that his friends would never want to speak to him again.

His named nurse suggested that he might write to his friends and explain what had happened. He helped him to write a letter and send it … and within a week he received a card from his closest friend.

Throughout his time in hospital Fred's worried parents kept in regular contact. His care coordinator spent time with them explaining the problems that Fred was experiencing. Initially, they were very hopeless about their son's prospects but the care coordinator was able to help them with information and support – he told them about Fred's rights under the Disability Discrimination Act – and gradually they became more optimistic. The care coordinator also suggested various websites where they might get more information.

Case study – Fred (cont'd)

When he was feeling a bit better, his named nurse encouraged Fred to call one of his close friends and invite him to come and visit. With the help of his named nurse he explained what was wrong with him. Initially his friend was a bit uneasy but as Fred got better the pair went out to the pictures together and arranged for Fred to get together with some of his other mates.

When Fred was discharged from hospital he returned to live with his parents and his care coordinator continued to help him to pursue his aim of getting back to college and finishing his degree.

He arranged a meeting with Fred, his parents and his college tutor. Initially his tutor was convinced that Fred would never be able to resume his studies but, after discussing the position with Fred, his nurse and his psychiatrist, he was eventually convinced that a return to college might be possible. The named nurse gave Fred's tutor some information about the impact of mental health problems on studying and some of the types of 'adjustment' Fred might need – and pointed out the college's obligations under the Disability Discrimination Act. His tutor contacted the Student Support Service, who met with Fred and his care coordinator, and together they made a plan.

Fred would take the rest of the year off college and return in the following October. In the meantime his tutor would arrange to send him some books and assignments that he could work on at home to keep his hand in and agreed to meet with him every couple of months to see how he was doing. In order to help him get back to mixing with other people, Fred registered for a photography course at the local college – he was a keen photographer – and arranged to meet his friends from college socially.

Fred did go back to college. It was hard to start off with and he needed help from the Student Support Service, his care coordinator, his psychiatrist and his parents. The Student Support Service arranged for additional help with studying and some flexibility around assignments. Fred's care coordinator provided encouragement and assisted him in monitoring and managing some of his remaining symptoms. His psychiatrist adjusted his medication to ensure that he was not too sedated at college. His parents provided a great deal of support and encouragement and help with day-to-day tasks. Fred decided to continue to live at home while he was at college and his parents assisted him with his assignments. He did go through some pretty rough patches and on one occasion was briefly re-admitted to hospital … but he did manage to finish his degree.

References

Aguilar E J, Haas G, Manzanera F J et al 1997 Hopelessness and first episode psychosis: a longitudinal study. Acta Psychiatrica Scandinavica 96:25–30

Anthony W A, Cohen M, Farkas M 1990 Psychiatric rehabilitation. Center for Psychiatric Rehabilitation, Boston, MA

Bird L 2001 Poverty, social exclusion and mental health: a survey of people's personal experiences. A Life in the Day 5:3

Bond G R, Drake R E, Meuser K T, Becker D R 1997 An update on supported employment for people with severe mental illness. Psychiatric Services 48:335–346

Bond G R, Becker D R, Drake R E, Rapp C A, Meisler N, Lehman A F, Bell M D & Blyler C R 2001 Implementing supported employment as an evidence based practice. Psychiatric Services 52:313–322

Chamberlin J 2001 Equal rights not public relations. World Psychiatric Association Conference 'Together Against Stigma', Leipzig, September 2001

Crowther R E, Marshall M, Bond G R, Huxley P 2001 Helping people with severe mental illness to obtain work: systematic review. British Medical Journal 322:204–208

Deegan P 1988 Recovery: the lived experience of rehabilitation. Psychosocial Rehabilitation Journal 11:11–19

Deegan P 1989 Consumer empowerment and recovery: the new horizon. Paper presented at the conference 'From the New Frontier to the Next Horizon: Mental Health Directions in the Decade Ahead', Stamford, CT

Deegan P 1990 How recovery begins. Paper presented at the eighth Annual Education Conference Alliance for the Mentally Ill of New York State, Binghamton, NY

Deegan P 1993 Recovering our sense of value after being labeled. Journal of Psychosocial Nursing 31:7–11

Deegan P 1996 Recovery as a journey of the heart. Psychosocial Rehabilitation Journal 19:91–97

Department of Health 1999 A national service framework for mental health. The Stationery Office, London

Department for Work and Pensions 2001 Recruiting benefits claimants: quantitative research with employers in ONE pilot areas. Research series paper 150. Department for Work and Pensions, London

Disability Rights Commission 2001 Who we are and what we do. Disability Rights Commission, London

Disability Rights Commission 2003 Coming together. Mental health service users and disability rights. Disability Rights Commission, London

Dunn S 1999 Creating accepting communities: report of the Mind inquiry into social exclusion and mental health problems. Mind Publications, London

Frank J 1968 The role of hope in psychotherapy. International Journal of Psychiatry 5:383–395

Harris E C, Barraclough B 1998 Excess mortality of mental disorder. British Journal of Psychiatry 173:11–53

Hayward P, Bright J A 1997 Stigma and mental illness: a review and critique. Journal of Mental Health 6:345–354

Kanwal G S 1997 Hope, respect and flexibility in the psychotherapy of schizophrenia. Contemporary Psychoanalysis 33:133–150

Kirkpatrick H, Landeen J, Byrne C et al 1995 Hope and schizophrenia: clinicians identify hope-instilling strategies. Journal of Psychosocial Nursing and Mental Health Services 33:15–19

References (cont'd)

Kirkpatrick H, Landeen J, Woodside H, Byrne C 2001 How people with schizophrenia build their hope. Journal of Psychosocial Nursing 39:146–153

Landeen J, Pawlick J, Woodside H et al 2000 Hope, quality of life and symptom severity in individuals with schizophrenia. Psychiatric Rehabilitation Journal 23:3464–3469

Leete E 1988 The treatment of schizophrenia: a patient's perspective. Hospital and Community Psychiatry 385:486–491

Leete E 1989 How I perceive and manage my illness. Schizophrenia Bulletin 15:197–200

Link B G, Phelan J C 2001 Conceptualising stigma. Annual Review of Sociology 27:363–385

Menninger K 1959 Hope. American Journal of Psychiatry 116:481–491

Nordt C, Falcato L, Lauber C, Rossler W 2001 Recognition increases social distance: a dilemma for anti-stigma strategies. World Psychiatric Association Conference 'Together Against Stigma', Leipzig, September 2001

Office for National Statistics 2003 Labour force survey August 2003. The Stationery Office, London

Oliver M 1990 The politics of disablement. Macmillan, Basingstoke

Perkins R 2000 I have a vision …. Paper presented at BRIJ Conference 'Meeting the Challenge of the 21st Century', Nottingham, 15 March

Read J, Baker S 1996 Not just sticks and stones: a survey of the stigma, taboos and discrimination experienced by people with mental health problems. Mind Publications, London

Read J, Harré N 2001 The role of biological and genetic causal beliefs in the stigmatisation of 'mental patients'. Journal of Mental Health 10:223–235

Read J, Reynolds J 1996 Speaking our minds. Macmillan, Basingstoke

Reeves A 1998 Recovery: a holistic approach. Handsell Publishing, Runcorn, Cheshire

Repper J, Perkins R 2003 Social inclusion and recovery: a model for mental health practice. Baillière Tindall, London

Repper J, Sayce L, Strong S, Willmot J, Haines M 1997 Tall stories from the backyard: a survey of 'nimby' opposition to community mental health facilities experienced by key service providers in England and Wales. Mind Publications, London

Repper J, Perkins R, Owen S 1998 'I wanted to be a nurse … but I didn't get that far': women with serious ongoing mental health problems speak about their lives. Journal of Psychiatric and Mental Health Nursing 5:505–513

Rogers J 1995 Work is key to recovery. Psychosocial Rehabilitation Journal 18:5–10

Rose D 1996 Living in the community. Sainsbury Centre for Mental Health, London

Rowland L A, Perkins R E 1988 You can't eat drink and make love eight hours a day: the value of work in psychiatry. Health Trends 20:75–79

Royal College of Psychiatrists 2003 Employment opportunities for people with psychiatric disabilities. Council report. Royal College of Psychiatrists, London

Russinova Z 1999 Providers' hope-inspiring competence as a factor optimizing psychiatric rehabilitation outcomes. Journal of Rehabilitation 16:50–57

Sayce L 1998 Stigma, discrimination and social exclusion: what's in a word? Journal of Mental Health 7:331–343

References (cont'd)

Sayce L 2000 From psychiatric patient to citizen: overcoming discrimination and social exclusion. Macmillan, London

Shepherd G 1989 The value of work in the 1980s. Psychiatric Bulletin 13:231–233

Spaniol L, Koehler M 1994 (eds) The experience of recovery. Center for Psychiatric Rehabilitation, Boston, MA

Taylor P, Gunn J 1999 Homicides by people with mental health problems: myth and reality. British Journal of Psychiatry 174:9–14

Woodside H, Landeen J, Kirkpatrick H et al 1994 Hope and schizophrenia: exploring attitudes of clinicians. Psychosocial Rehabilitation Journal 8:140–144

Young S L, Ensing D S 1999 Exploring recovery from the perspective of people with psychiatric disabilities. Psychiatric Rehabilitation Journal 22:219–231

Useful websites

Boston University Centre for Psychiatric Rehabilitation: www.bu.educ/cpr
Provides information for educators, employers and students about the impact of mental health problems at work/college and the sorts of adjustment people might need,

Disability Rights Commission: www.drc-gb.org
Provides information to disabled people, including people with mental health problems, and educators, employers and the providers of goods and services,

Skill: The National Bureau for Disabled Students: www.skill.org
Provides information and advice to disabled students, including those with mental health problems,

Annotated further reading

Disability Rights Commission 2003 Disability equality: making it happen. First review of the Disability Discrimination Act 1995. Disability Rights Commission, London

Link B G, Phelan J C 2001 On the nature and consequences of stigma. Annual Review of Sociology 27:363–385

This paper provides an excellent analysis of the development and impact of stigma, discrimination and exclusion in relation to people with mental health problems.

Repper J, Perkins R 2003 Social inclusion and recovery: a model for mental health practice. Baillière Tindall, London

This book provides a description of the impact of discrimination and exclusion and the recovery process. It offers a detailed exploration of the practical ways in which direct care professionals can support the recovery journey of individuals with mental health problems, promote their social inclusion and help them to rebuild meaningful and satisfying lives.

Sayce L 2000 From psychiatric patient to citizen. Overcoming discrimination and social exclusion. Macmillan, London

Drawing on a comprehensive review of the research literature, this book provides an analysis of the discrimination and social exclusion of people with mental health problems and ways in which these might best be reduced through legal rights, communications campaigns and grass-roots change.

4

Stress vulnerability model of serious mental illness

Geoff Brennan

KEY ISSUES

- ◆ Prevalence of serious mental illness
- ◆ Analysis of vulnerability factors
- ◆ Stress and life events
- ◆ Coping: relevance for practitioners

INTRODUCTION

Let us imagine a world in which mental illness is as well defined as a medical condition such as measles or diabetes. A practitioner in this world would have a definitive test for mental illness. More than likely this would involve a superior scan or chemical analysis. It would be evidence-based and valid. We could show people definitive pictures or numbers denoting the definite presence of … something. From this we could accurately diagnose the condition, administer the recommended treatment and, eventually, cure the ailment. If we are all honest, we would all like to live and work in this world – a world of definites.

In this world, how easy it would be to say to an individual 'We know that you have this form of illness but don't worry, take this medication, change your diet, wear this plaster. In a year's time your symptoms will have completely disappeared, and we won't need to see you again' or 'You have schizophrenia type A, which means that you will suffer from voices for several years. We know that medication X will reduce these voices and let you function as normal, but the voices will persist.' No matter how many claims are made that this world is soon to be discovered (and the progress in clarification and diagnosis), all practitioners, clients and carers know that we do not live in this ideal world. Moreover, if we went back and looked closer at the medical world we would find that diagnosing some physical ailments, for example meningitis, is not that clear-cut either. Indeed, many physical illnesses are also influenced by factors discussed in this chapter.

This would appear to be a depressing way to begin an exploration of the manifestation of mental illness and yet the above paragraph highlights the mistakes in thinking that many practitioners make. This mistake is summed up by a desire to make mental illness a disease of the body. The first flaw in this conceptualisation is the misconception that the client, the patient, the sufferer, Mr or Ms X, is a person 'to be cured'. The practitioner's drive to 'cure' is a battle between them and illness. The practitioner, however, is not the person with the illness. Only by considering the person, and what constitutes illness and health for this individual, can we set realistic treatment objectives and measure outcomes.

In order to achieve this we need to reinstate the person within the explanation of serious mental illness. In doing this we should beware of alienating the individuals who manifest symptoms. This is because symptoms are not separate phenomena that manifest themselves in an isolated population. Having said this, the population of individuals diagnosed with serious mental illness do have unique experiences, which should be seen as an aspect of the continuum of human experience. In this case, however, difference does not equate to deviance. Consider the following two descriptions.

Mr A is a schizophrenic, first diagnosed 6 years ago. His first admission involved being arrested by the police and treated under Section 3 of the Mental Health Act. He is now maintained on medication and been well for 2 years.

Mr B is a happily married man with one child. Six years ago he suffered a breakdown following the death of his mother. Only in the past 2 years has Mr B felt that life is worth living again. He works part time and is able to support his family. He is interested in writing about his experiences and is active within his church.

Given that Mr A and Mr B are the same person, it is interesting the differing impressions we get from the short descriptions. The first, Mr A, reduces our understanding and is focused around psychiatric terminology. This results in a distorted picture of who this person is and what his capabilities are. It is what I call 'practitioner speak' and is related to reducing Mr A to the essentials that are of import for the clinical world. If we look closely we will see that the description reduces Mr A to the manifestation itself: 'Mr A is a schizophrenic'. We begin to think of Mr A and others who share such experiences as 'them', the 'other', not like 'us', someone else. This is because all his experiences, as described, are outside our understanding. We do not know what it is like to be labelled 'schizophrenic', to be arrested when experiencing psychotic symptoms, to be detained under the Mental Health Act, or to have 2 years of health after a psychotic relapse.

An example of this reduction of the person can also be explained by the continuing use of the label 'schizophrenic', as described by Haghighat & Littlewood (1995): 'Another important aspect of the semantics of labels relates to adjectives used as nouns. An adjective used as a noun, e.g. a schizophrenic, may rob the individual of his other aspects as it subsumes personhood and agency into illness.' From here it is a short step to thinking of the individual ('the schizophrenic', 'the manic depressive') as less than us, not equal, sub-human, tainted. If we accept this, it is up to us, the 'more able', to dictate to the 'poor sufferer', to take on the burden of care, to alleviate the suffering, to administer our services for the good of the poor afflicted. The reduction of people to stereotypical labels is the cornerstone of all prejudice, as has been shown throughout human history.

So how can practitioners begin the difficult path of addressing treatment of serious mental illness without reducing individuals' personhood or being patronising? How should we begin to conceptualise the process that will best address the challenges that the position of practitioner holds?

There are no definitive answers to these questions but a beginning would be to find a way to view serious mental illness from the individual's point of view. This may be easier said than done. As mentioned, it requires us to view individuals in their unique circumstances without shirking the difficult reality that they are experiencing phenomena we find alien to our own experience. One means of aiding this process is to view the manifestation of the difference – serious mental illness – within the explanatory model of stress vulnerability.

COMPONENTS OF STRESS VULNERABILITY

The concept of stress vulnerability is essentially simple. In it we think of the person's health as influenced by several factors that interact. As the title suggests, it is the interface and relationship between stress and vulnerability that are the main determinants of the model.

To begin with, let's take a brief look at these components.

Stress

Stress is a fairly modern concept, yet has become fully incorporated into our language. It is a word that is used in a myriad situations and has various meanings. The physical and psychological effects of excessive exposure to stress are recognised as anxiety, agitation, insomnia, irritability, low motivation, anger, frustration, poor concentration and difficulties in decision making. In this situation, stress means a force that acts upon the system in such a way as to place it under strain. It is important to remember that stressors can be either negative factors such as boredom and inactivity or pleasant events such as marriage, birth or promotion, as the latter can also put strain on an individual.

Within the stress vulnerability model there is an understanding that stress is a variable that influences the manifestation of symptoms. To understand its impact fully we need to consider the differing forms that stress can take.

Ambient stress

All individuals have stressors in their lives. To live is to be under strain. We are directly aware of this in our own lives. If you stop for a second and begin to think about your own stressors you will realise that there are always things that cause concern. Maybe you haven't paid a bill, your cat/child/partner/plant is ill, your job is not all it could be, you've got a headache, you have to write an essay and are bored reading this chapter. All these things can cause you strain, no matter how small. This type of strain is what constitutes 'ambient stress'. As with vulnerability, these levels can vary from person to person. The ambient stress of junior doctors going through the years of over-work and late hours may be high, while the ambient stress of retired people on a comfortable pension may be quite low. Alternatively, junior doctors may love their job and feel a low level of ambient stress, while retired people may be suffering major ambient stress due to losing self-worth, being under-stimulated, etc. (In addition, retirement itself can be seen as a life event, as we shall see.) As with beauty, stress is in the eye of the beholder.

The emotional atmosphere within families can be a cause of variable ambient stress and has been shown to be influential in people's levels of health. Expressed emotion (or EE) is a means by which the family management of the psychosis can be judged as working to exacerbate symptoms or alleviate them. Families who cope better (and in some cases extremely well) manage to create a climate of tolerance that balances asking too much or too little of the individual with the symptoms and so reduces the latter's ambient stress. These families fall into what is known as the 'low expressed emotion' category. Families who find the illness difficult to accept or adjust to can become critical of the ill person as they are unaware of the effects of the illness or extremely frustrated with the challenges they have to deal with. They can also overcompensate for the illness and can infringe the person's autonomy in an attempt to ensure the person is cared for. These families fall into what is known as the 'high expressed emotion' category and can unwittingly increase the level of ambient everyday stress for the individual (Leff & Vaughn 1985).

The comments above also apply to professionals, as we can increase the ambient stress of our clients if we deal with them in ways that denote criticism of them as people, or overcompensate and patronise them.

Life event stress

All people go through episodes or events that cause specific and high levels of stress. These episodes or events can be recognised as common experiences that most people report as placing them under high stress. Table 4.1 shows a rating for life experiences.

It has been acknowledged that many people who undergo a psychotic experience for the first time have recently experienced a traumatic life event (Ambelas 1987) such as a death in the family or losing their job. What is also recognised is that some people will have short-lived psychotic experiences that are strongly linked to a life event. A good example of this is when people hear the voice of a loved one who has recently died. As we shall see below, this is not necessarily indicative of a psychosis.

Vulnerability

An individual's vulnerability is the disposition of the person to manifesting symptoms of serious mental illness. At present, vulnerability is thought to be dependent on two components (Box 4.1).

Table 4.1 Ranking of life events in order of perceived severity

Rank	Life event
1	Death of a child
2	Death of a husband/wife
3	Being sent to gaol
4	Death of a close family member
5	Serious financial difficulty
6	Miscarriage or stillbirth
7	Court appearance for serious offences
8	Business failure
9	Marital separation due to arguments
10	Unwanted pregnancy
11	Divorced
12	Fired
13	Death of a close friend
14	Serious illness of family member
15	Unemployed for 1 month
16	Serious personal physical illness

Source: With permission from Ambelas (1987)

Box 4.1 Components of vulnerability

Inborn vulnerability
◆ Genetically determined
◆ Reflected in the neurophysiology of the organism

Acquired vulnerability
◆ Specific to individual life experience
◆ Can include: specific disease, perinatal complications, family experience, adolescent peer interactions, previous life events

Source: Adapted from Zubin & Spring (1977)

In other words, our vulnerability is determined by a combination of nature and nurture, as further demonstrated by Figure 4.1.

Within this hypothesis there will be a range of vulnerabilities within the population, with some people having vulnerability factors that place them at high probability of developing symptoms while others will have a low probability, with all levels in between.

One implication of this hypothesis is that it potentially challenges the concept that serious mental illness is confined to those diagnosed with psychosis. As Zubin & Spring (1977), in their seminal article on stress vulnerability with regard to schizophrenia, write: 'whether such vulnerability extends to all of mankind and whether it is the same sort that predisposes an individual to disorders other than schizophrenia remains an open question'. This would appear to be reinforced by the fact that some symptoms that are the cornerstone of diagnostic criteria are found in people who are not diagnosed. If hallucinations are taken as an example, the percentage of the population who report visions or hear voices is greater than that of people diagnosed with a

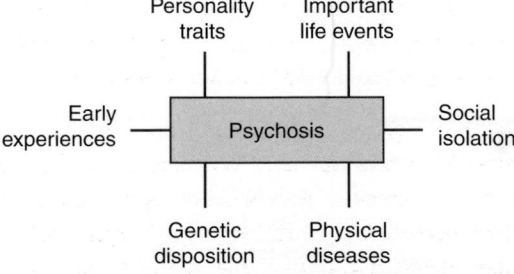

Figure 4.1 Vulnerability to stress. (With permission from Honig 1993.)

serious mental illness (Slade & Bentall 1988). Indeed, when consideration is given to individuals who hear their dead relatives in the early stages of bereavement or those who believe in the power of divine intervention, clairvoyance, telepathy, tarot cards, horoscopes, etc. we can see that one person's 'symptom' is another person's coping strategy, belief system or normal reaction to abnormal events.

This further adds to a deconstruction of our understanding of serious mental illness by means of the diagnostic process alone. Indeed, the stress vulnerability concept suggests that there is the potential for any person to develop and experience transient psychotic symptoms.

MANIFESTATION OF ILLNESS WITHIN THE STRESS VULNERABILITY MODEL

So why don't more people get diagnosed with serious mental illness? Well, there is a wide range of vulnerability factors and stress levels. The more stress people have, the more their health is placed under a strain, and the higher the probability that they will reach a level where the vulnerability will be expressed. Perhaps most people have certain internal and external protective mechanisms to guard them against stress and therefore never reach the level of vulnerability necessary to develop psychosis. Horowitz (1986) has this to say in writing about stress response:

> *Additional evidence regarding the duration of stress responses and the frequency of occurrence of stress symptoms arose from the most deplorable circumstances imaginable. Studies of concentration camp victims indicated that profound and protracted stress may have chronic or permanent effects no matter what the predisposition of the pre-stress personality. This evidence was found in the decades of studying the survivors of the Nazi concentration camps …. Study after study … confirm the occurrence of stress response syndromes, persisting for decades, in major proportions of those populations who survived …. As just one example 99% of the 226 Norwegian survivors of a Nazi concentration camp … had some psychiatric disturbance when intensively surveyed years after their return to normal life.*

Concentration camp survivors must have undergone some of the most stressful experiences known to humans. With regard to this exploration, what is interesting is the conception that victims were not protected by their coping skills or their personality in the face of this overwhelming stress. What is less clear is how many of the 'psychiatric disturbances' noted would be classified as psychotic symptoms. Indeed, Lifton, cited by Horowitz (1986), outlines the experiences of Hiroshima victims who talked of 'pictures in their mind' and 'people walking with their skin peeling off'. These vivid portrayals were still present 17 years after the event. Others who have experienced less famous, but still significant, traumas have described intrusive thoughts, flashbacks, nightmares and depression. From such descriptions it would appear necessary to reconsider further the supposition that psychotic experience is isolated to a few individuals.

Psychosis: a unique experience

What should also be considered is that individuals who describe psychotic symptoms are more vulnerable to stress. These individuals will not have single, isolated experiences that are explainable in reference to recent life events, specific biological changes such as happen through illicit drug use and thyroid gland malfunction, but have a capacity either to experience complex psychotic symptoms for a long period of time or have frequent episodes of recurring symptoms. The differences between the individual who will be diagnosed with a serious mental illness and the individual who will experience specific phenomena such as auditory hallucinations is the basis of psychiatry.

COPING

The discussion so far has perceived the individual as a passive recipient of life's traumas. In reality, of course, the individual has personal attributes that influence their reaction to stressors. This reaction is termed 'coping'.

In common usage, coping seems to imply a positive value judgement (in the same way that 'stress' tends to imply a negative value judgement). This means that the word 'coping' seems to be used in positive instances. In actual fact, there is positive coping and negative coping.

Positive coping is the ability to ameliorate the strain and reduce stressors, whereas negative coping is where the stress or resultant strain is intensified. Often, coping strategies may give an immediate sense of relief but in the long term will result in harm to the individual. These should be considered to be negative coping strategies. An example of this would be an individual who takes street drugs to alleviate symptoms, does experience some relief in the short term but has an increase in symptoms in the long term (De Quardo et al 1994).

Within the stress vulnerability model, coping can influence not only the possible onset of psychotic symptoms but also the course and prognosis of the illness. Some commentators have argued that individuals who develop serious mental illness had limited positive coping skills prior to the illness, but this is a debatable issue. In this regard it would be well to remember the findings from concentration camp victims – not being able to deal with stress in certain circumstances is not only understandable but should be expected.

An individual's coping abilities are affected by many factors, including personality, culture, family experience and education, but it is one of the areas where health professionals can help or hinder individuals. Historically, for example, practitioners were taught and advised to ignore clients when they reported voices and delusions (Hamilton 1984). While the philosophy behind this was non-collusion with symptoms, as this might reinforce them, individuals experienced this attitude as a negation of their experiences. This negation actually increased stress for many.

The notion of not acknowledging the experience appears to relate to the utopian world, previously described, where the aim of treatment is total eradication of symptoms. Subsequently, it was perceived that the manner in which individuals cope with psychosis, irrespective of whether this had a positive or negative effect upon their quality of life, was irrelevant. It is only recently that people have begun to realise that there are more ways to treat and cope with psychosis than medication alone. There is still much to learn from those who experience and cope with psychotic symptoms. Investigations into coping strategies have helped to identify that some people have developed very positive relationships with their voices. As a direct consequence a number of diverse coping strategies have been successfully cultivated. These range from diverting attention from the voices to acknowledging them rather than denying them (for examples see Falloon & Talbot 1981, Tarrier 1987, Carr 1988, Nelson et al 1991). Indeed, the predominant work of Romme & Esher (1993) has helped us to:

◆ uncover the important concept of coping
◆ understand the advantages enjoyed by those who succeed, despite all the odds, in coping well with their experiences, environment and vulnerability.

Coping and prognosis

If we accept that coping can ameliorate the symptoms of mental illness, it would follow that interventions should promote positive coping. A reality is that many individuals find that the illness blocks or hinders effective coping (as will be discussed with regard to negative symptoms). What should also concern us is the possibility that society and, indeed, the mental health system itself, can also block good coping or increase the stress on individuals.

Warner (1994) identifies the following factors that can influence relapse in the individual:

◆ drug use
◆ stressful family environment
◆ labelling and stigma
◆ social isolation or reintegration
◆ social role rehabilitation
◆ patterns of institutional care.

If the above are explored it is possible to question whether the mental health system is effective in reducing the negative aspects of these factors. While drug use and family environment are discussed in later chapters, the other issues remain a constant area of concern. Services do little to address negative stereotypes such as whether clients are employable, have a role in or are perceived as valued members of society. If we take a fresh look at relapse and the so-called 'revolving door client' we may begin to notice that these individuals have the greatest blocks to effective coping. In these cases we need to look for creative means to restore the individual's sense of role. This requires us to do more than alleviate symptoms, but also address political issues such as exclusion from employment, education and indeed all areas of human life.

CONCLUSIONS

Stress vulnerability is a model that has opened up the area of mental illness. It has moved us from seeing individual sufferers as alien to viewing them as people with extraordinary experiences. We must continue to see mental illness as a normal aspect of human experience. The work of the mental health practitioner is to join with individuals who have these extraordinary experiences and reintegrate them and their experiences into society.

 Cross references

All chapters in this first section: give an insight into how stress, life events and coping can influence the manifestation and outcomes for an individual and the family. They should be read prior to or in conjunction with this chapter.

Chapters 7 and 11: from an assessment and intervention standpoint contain references to stress vulnerability; however, it should be pointed out that the content of all of section 2 derives from and is influenced by the model.

References

Ambelas A 1987 Life events and mania: a special relationship? British Journal of Psychiatry 150:135–240

Carr V 1988 Patients' techniques for coping with schizophrenia: an exploratory study. British Journal of Medical Psychology 61:339–352

De Quardo J R, Carpenter C F, Tandon R 1994 Patterns of substance abuse in schizophrenia: nature and significance. Journal of Psychiatric Research 28:267–275

Falloon I R H, Talbot R E 1981 Persistent auditory hallucinations: coping mechanisms and implications for management. Psychological Medicine 11:329–339

Haghighat R, Littlewood, R 1995 What should we call patients with schizophrenia? A sociolinguistic analysis. Psychiatric Bulletin 19:407–410

Hamilton M 1984 Fish's schizophrenia, 3rd edn. Wright, Bristol

Honig A 1993 Medication and hearing voices. In: Romme M, Escher S (eds) Accepting voices. Mind, London, p 237

Horowitz M D 1986 Stress response syndromes. Aronson, Northvale, NJ

Leff J, Vaughn C 1985 Expressed emotion in families. Guilford Press, New York

Nelson H E, Thrasher S, Barnes T R E 1991 Practical ways of alleviating auditory hallucinations. British Medical Journal 302:327

Romme M, Esher S (eds) 1993 Accepting voices. Mind, London

Slade P D, Bentall R P 1988 Sensory deception: a scientific analysis of hallucination. Croom Helm, London

Tarrier N 1987 An investigation of residual psychotic symptoms in discharged schizophrenic patients. British Journal of Clinical Psychology 26:141–143

Warner R 1994 Recovery from schizophrenia: psychiatry and political economy, 2nd edn. Routledge, London

Zubin J, Spring B 1977 Vulnerability: a new view of schizophrenia. Journal of Abnormal Psychology 86:260–266

Annotated further reading

Bentall R 2003 Madness explained: psychosis and human nature. Penguin, Harmondsworth

This book provides a welcome review of the medical model and challenges traditional treatment approaches. It reviews the origins and misunderstandings about psychosis and challenges the reader to radically shift their opinions about the manner in which severe mental illness is managed and perceived.

Kingdon D G, Turkington D 1995 Cognitive behaviour therapy of schizophrenia. Guildford Press, London

Chapters 3 and 4 of this book, 'Vulnerability and life events' and 'Suggestibility', contain a valuable, in-depth summary of the issues raised within this chapter. It is a concise, user-friendly account of manifestation of illness.

5

An introduction to and rationale for psychosocial interventions

Helen Healy, David Reader and Kenny Midence

KEY ISSUES

- ◆ Background to development
- ◆ Overview of psychosocial interventions: cognitive–behavioural and family work approaches
- ◆ Literature review of evidence-based practice
- ◆ Implementation issues

INTRODUCTION

Psychosocial treatments for schizophrenia are not new in the research literature. For example, in terms of behaviour therapy, operant approaches such as token economy programmes were used in the 1960s and 1970s to improve the behaviour of patients in long stay hospitals. However, the evidence suggests that the clinical gains were limited and did not generalise beyond the therapeutic setting and also did not address delusional convictions (Himadi et al 1991). Other psychological treatments for schizophrenia can be traced to early work devoted to studying the impact of the social environment on mental illness. A plethora of early studies focused on the role of the family environment in the maintenance of schizophrenia, which in turn led to the concept of expressed emotion (Brown et al 1972). Family interventions were first developed as a method of reducing levels of expressed emotion among relatives and are now recognised as a significant aspect in the treatment of schizophrenia. This approach marked a paradigmatic shift in the way family members were viewed by clinicians and has led to efforts to improve communication between clinicians and carers. Recent years have seen such cognitive approaches expanded to interest in interventions that combine the principles of cognitive and behavioural approaches.

However, despite all the research available providing evidence of their effectiveness, these approaches are not widely available in routine clinical practice (Slade & Haddock 1996). It is now clear, however, that psychosocial interventions are necessary to help patients cope with their condition and improve their quality of life. These interventions are also beneficial to relatives and are effective in improving the quality of the family environment (Penn & Mueser 1996).

This chapter provides an overview of family interventions and cognitive–behavioural therapy (CBT) for psychotic symptoms. There has been a lot of research and clinical interest in the effectiveness of CBT for patients with psychosis. Unfortunately, the provision of family interventions in routine services has been disappointing, despite vigorous training programmes. Notwithstanding some notable exceptions in the UK, such as Bath (Smith & Velleman 2002) and Somerset (Stanbridge et al 2003), increasing the availability of family work remains a challenge for most service providers. The aim here is not to provide a comprehensive academic review of family interventions and CBT for serious mental illness. Instead, it is to give the reader an overview of the state of research and developments of recent research studies. This chapter also tries to condense the available evidence to help health care professionals get a general outlook of these exciting and promising new approaches. Recommended empirical, theoretical or review papers and books (in asterisks) are provided in the reference section for those readers who want a comprehensive description of the theoretical and empirical research of these interventions.

FAMILY INTERVENTIONS

Early research on expressed emotion (EE) carried out in the last 20 years by researchers in the MRC Social Psychiatry Unit at the Institute of Psychiatry, London, provided evidence of the negative impact of high EE families on the course of schizophrenia. According to Leff & Vaughn (1985), these high EE families not only experienced distress in coping with the condition but they also showed behaviours that were either extremely critical or hostile, or both, and were emotionally overinvolved with the relative with schizophrenia. During this period, the influential vulnerability–stress model proposed by Zubin & Spring (1977) drew attention to the importance of environmental factors, such as the family, on the course and prognosis of schizophrenia. According to this model, exacerbations of a person's symptoms are the product of the interaction between environmental stress and the person's predisposition for the illness. In this way, effective management of environmental stress might reduce the risk of an individual's symptoms re-occurring and, as Tarrier & Barrowclough (1995) say, 'this supposition has been the driving force behind family interventions'.

Hence the development of family intervention programmes to reduce the effects of schizophrenia on patients (e.g. relapse, hospitalisation), to increase patients' social functioning and to reduce family burden and improve the quality of life of sufferers and their families. Family interventions are based on broad psychoeducational and/or behavioural approaches, and research examining the effectiveness of these approaches has been mainly carried out by Falloon and colleagues and Hogarty and colleagues in the USA, and Vaughan and colleagues in Australia. In the UK, research has been conducted by Leff and colleagues in London and Tarrier, Barrowclough and colleagues in Manchester.

What are the components of family intervention?

According to Kavanagh (1992), the components of family intervention include engagement of families, education, communication training, goal setting, problem solving, cognitive–behavioural self-management, increasing family well-being and maintenance of skills. Bellack & Mueser (1993) have suggested that four main aspects of the psychosocial treatment of patients should be emphasised. These are:

◆ the need for a comprehensive and long-term treatment, including drugs
◆ individually tailored treatment programmes
◆ an active participation by patients and relatives
◆ the acknowledgement of patients' cognitive limitations.

Reviews by Lam (1991) and Fadden (1998) have identified common features of successful family interventions, which include the development of a therapeutic alliance between family and therapists, the provision of education and information about the disorder, a behavioural or cognitive–behavioural approach to problems, an emphasis on enhancing skills in problem solving and communication, and promoting activities and interests outside the family. Lam (1991) has also identified three possible mechanisms underlying the better outcome of patients who receive family therapy: lower negative family affect (i.e. EE); improved patient adherence with medication and better patient monitoring by the treatment team.

The techniques involved in family intervention include initial assessment of relatives' and patients' needs, educating families, stress management and coping responses, issues about engaging and maintaining the family involvement, dealing with violence and suicide risk, assessment of psychotic symptoms, and coping strategies (cognitive and behavioural) (Barrowclough & Tarrier 1992). Family intervention by Kuipers et al (1992) includes assessing the relative and their family, engaging the family, education about schizophrenia, improving communication, identification of stressors, setting realistic goals, dealing with emotional issues (e.g. anger, conflict, rejection), dealing with overinvolvement, getting everyone in the family involved, employment, cultural issues, special issues (e.g. substance abuse, suicide, incest) and running a relatives' group.

This approach with single families has been adapted to include multiple families in a group setting. This approach appears to combine the benefits of family work with the experience and advantages of participating in a group, such as mutual support, shared learning and reduced isolation. According to McFarlane and colleagues (1995), multiple family groups can be as effective as family interventions for individual families in reducing relapse rates, although a recent review of family work by Pilling and colleagues (2002) is more cautious about group approaches in this respect. However, on other measures, such as burden and satisfaction, Pilling et al (2002) believe groups can be beneficial and, for particular patient subgroups, such as first-episode psychosis, multiple family groups can contribute to enhanced knowledge and understanding (Mullen et al 2002).

How effective are family interventions?

The positive results of the studies on family interventions have provided strong evidence for the effectiveness of these psychosocial approaches. Overall, research findings indicate that these approaches are more effective than routine treatment, and are beneficial for patients and their relatives. Family interventions are effective in reducing EE in relatives, family burden and relapse rate in patients over 1–2 years, and in improving patients' social functioning, especially when families change from high to low EE. Moreover, long-term family intervention seems to reduce patients' relapse rate, and treatment gains are stable and can be maintained for as long as 2 years. The duration of the treatment is related to the outcome of the intervention, and this means that the longer the treatment the better the outcome; short-term interventions show less beneficial effect on relapse rate. Furthermore, the financial savings to the mental health service in providing family intervention for 9 months has been reported to be as high as 27%, including less social work contact and fewer hospital admissions (Tarrier et al 1991).

Fadden's (1998) review of family interventions showed the effectiveness of these approaches. She points out that 'family interventions have been shown to result in at least a fourfold reduction in relapse rates at one year post intervention, and even though relapse increases in the second year, the rates are still only half what they are when no such intervention is provided'. However, we still do not know which family intervention model provides the best benefits for patients and their families, what aspects of family intervention are most effective, and the characteristics of patients and their families who do not benefit from family intervention. Furthermore, not all families are willing to engage in family intervention. The difficulty in engaging relatives in family work has been investigated by McCreadie et al (1991). In their study, half the families invited to take part refused the treatment (almost half were low EE families), the main reasons given included 'things are fine at the moment', 'it is the patient who needs help, not me' and 'the patient doesn't want anyone else to know he has been ill'. The STEP clinical team in Wales found that 26% of families did not take part in the family intervention (Hughes et al 1996). According to Smith & Birchwood (1990), between 7% and 21% of families tend to refuse family intervention, the number of families withdrawing from treatment ranges between 7% and 14%, and between 8% and 35% of families do not adhere to the treatment.

Implementing family intervention in routine clinical practice

Using family intervention for schizophrenia in routine clinical practice is a difficult task. A number of obstacles to implementation have been identified by follow-up studies of the impact of training programmes (Kavanagh et al 1993, Fadden 1997). These relate mainly to organisational and structural barriers such as failure to provide time for practitioners to carry out family work and receive clinical supervision and difficulties integrating family work with existing clinical responsibilities. To implement family work, service managers need to understand the demands it makes on staff time and provide the conditions to support them (Leff 2000). Hughes et al (1996) have described their experience of providing family work in a management culture of 'benign neglect' and yet they report that the service provided was highly valued by the families themselves. Budd & Hughes (1997) consulted families regarding what they found most helpful in family work and found the following elements emerged: knowledge/understanding of schizophrenia, feeling supported, reassured and encouraged, and having someone to call in emergencies. Families also said that the intervention had helped them to become more tolerant of their relative's behaviour and to improve communication between family members.

In conclusion, there is no doubt that the effectiveness of family interventions is well established. Indeed, Mari & Streiner's (1994) recent meta-analysis of family intervention studies concluded that 'family intervention, as part of a multidimensional approach to care, decreases the frequency of relapse and hospitalisation over periods of 7 months to 2 years. It encourages compliance with medication and may help people stay in employment.' Despite the overwhelming evidence regarding the effectiveness of family intervention, however, Anderson & Adams (1996) have rightly pointed out that this psychosocial intervention is not being used to its full potential in clinical practice. Training is a necessary first step in addressing this problem but until services have structures in place to support family work it seems likely that it will remain difficult to implement.

COGNITIVE–BEHAVIOURAL THERAPY FOR PSYCHOSIS

Cognitive–behavioural therapy is a structured psychological therapy originally applied to the management of depression (Beck et al 1979). According to the cognitive therapy model, behaviour and actions are determined by the way an individual interprets or appraises situations. Cognitive therapy assumes that there is a set of psychological constructs that apply to all persons, including those with and without a psychiatric disorder. The CBT model challenges the 'gap' between psychosis and normality (Chadwick & Lowe 1994). It is generally accepted that 'normal' psychological processes are implicated in the maintenance of specific psychotic symptoms (Buchanan et al 1993, Drury et al 1996). CBT focuses on altering the thoughts, emotions and behaviours of patients by teaching them skills to challenge and modify beliefs about their delusions and hallucinations. The importance of both environmental stress and emotional distress is central to the cognitive–behavioural treatment of psychotic symptoms. Instability in arousal levels and emotional regulation is a typical pathway to exacerbation of psychotic symptoms. CBT aims to reduce the emotional consequences of delusions and to alleviate the consequences of environmental stress through enhanced coping strategies. Haddock & Tarrier (1999) provide a clinical heuristic that describes the factors contributing to psychotic symptoms and in addition provides a framework to guide a CBT model of therapy addressing emotional, behavioural and cognitive consequences of a psychotic episode.

The aim of CBT is to help patients gain knowledge about schizophrenia and its symptoms, to overcome hopelessness, to reduce distress from psychotic symptoms, to reduce dysfunctional emotions and behaviour and to help them analyse and modify dysfunctional beliefs and assumptions (Slade & Haddock 1996). Since the 1970s, researchers have tried to modify psychotic symptoms using cognitive–behavioural techniques including psychoeducation, coping responses, delusional belief modification, relabelling psychotic experiences, dealing with dysfunctional assumptions, and goal setting. Effective treatment, however, may depend on the patient's motivation, the distress associated with positive symptoms, the type and structure of the symptoms and the patient's cognitive deficits (Sellwood et al 1994). The available literature on psychological treatments for positive psychotic symptoms is mainly in the form of individual case studies or a series of case studies, and few large, controlled trials have been compared with traditional or routine treatments. The majority of treatment reports have been on the treatment of hallucinations or delusions, including operant procedures, counterstimulation (e.g. distraction), use of ear plugs, thought stopping, focusing (e.g. content and beliefs about voices) and systematic desensitisation. The treatment interventions of some researchers have focused on particular symptoms rather than addressing all the psychotic symptoms experienced by patients (Bentall et al 1994, Chadwick & Birchwood 1994).

There are various techniques used in CBT, including 'coping strategy enhancement', which is aimed at building on the coping strategies that patients already have when they experience residual symptoms (Tarrier et al 1990, 1993). The procedures to help patients cope with these symptoms include explaining the treatment rationale; describing each psychotic symptom through a structured interview; assessing the frequency, duration, antecedents and consequences; assessing the interference of the symptoms and the patient's beliefs and preoccupation; assessing the coping methods already used by the patients; identifying a target symptom and appropriate coping strategy; practising coping strategy during sessions; homework, and reassessment of the symptoms. Results from case studies suggest that coping strategy enhancement is effective in improving residual auditory hallucinations (Tarrier et al 1990). Coping strategy enhancement and problem solving therapy have also been found to be superior in reducing positive symptoms compared with waiting list controls (Tarrier et al 1993). Bentall et al (1994) have used a different approach to deal with psychotic symptoms by looking at the fundamental cognitive bias underlying hallucinations (i.e. misattribution of internally generated events to an external source). Results of their studies have shown a reduction in the frequency and distress of auditory hallucinations in patients.

The cognitive–behavioural approach for psychosis used by Fowler et al (1995) includes improving coping responses, psychoeducation and belief modification. The main goals include the reduction of the distress and interference that arise from the experience of persistent psychotic symptoms, increasing the patient's understanding of psychotic disorders, fostering motivation to engage in self-regulation behaviour, and reducing the occurrence of dysfunctional emotions and self-defeating behaviour arising from feelings of hopelessness, negative self-image or perceived psychological threat (Kuipers et al 1996). Research is still ongoing, and preliminary results are promising. Haddock & Slade (1996) have maintained that patients' distress is related to their beliefs about the origin and content of their voices. Chadwick & Lowe (1990, 1994) have used non-confrontational verbal challenge and reality testing to reduce delusional beliefs. Delusions are assessed on the basis of the available information, including interpretation of the beliefs, and behavioural experiments to invalidate the delusions. Results suggest that CBT reduces patients' conviction in and preoccupation with delusional beliefs. Moreover, there is evidence that some patients may reject their delusional beliefs completely (Chadwick et al 1994).

Nelson (1997) has provided a comprehensive practical manual to guide clinicians in their work with patients with schizophrenia. This manual provides information about treatment strategies with delusions, including assessment, lessening the impact/distress of delusional ideas, promoting insight, modifying and challenging delusions, and long-term strategies. Treatment strategies with hallucinations include assessment and setting the goals of therapy, practical ways of reducing the voices, promoting insight, CBT with non-psychotic beliefs, disempowering the voices, modifying and challenging the delusional beliefs about the voices, and long-term strategies. However, despite the encouraging findings of these studies, some patients can be reluctant to engage in therapy because of their strong beliefs and feelings about their voices. Fortunately, some researchers have developed a number of techniques to deal with the resistance shown by some patients by looking at the connections between the perceived benevolence or malevolence and resistance and engagement in relation to the voices (Chadwick & Birchwood 1996).

How effective is cognitive–behavioural therapy for psychosis?

Schizophrenia is a progressive debilitating illness characterised by hallucinations, delusions, emotional withdrawal and poor social functioning (Kane & McGlashan 1995). Many patients with schizophrenia have residual psychotic symptoms and impaired social functioning that persists well into adulthood (Bustillo et al 1999). Pharmacological treatments have traditionally been the treatment of choice. However, while the effectiveness of antipsychotic medication has made it central to the treatment of schizophrenia (Schwartz et al 1993), there is increasing knowledge that pharmacological treatment alone is rarely sufficient for optimal outcomes.

There are a number of reasons for this claim. First, the issue of compliance has demonstrated that the social and cognitive context in which pharmacological treatment is delivered has a major impact on its success (Bebbington & Kuipers 1994). There is also evidence to suggest that young people in their first episode are sensitive to both its therapeutic and adverse effects (Remmington et al 1998). Second, the actual effectiveness of antipsychotic medication has been challenged, since up to 40% have a poor response to medication and continue to demonstrate moderate to severe psychotic symptoms (Kane 1996). Furthermore, a recent meta-analysis has suggested that the benefit of new atypical antipsychotics is less than was previously thought (Geddes et al 2000).

A number of systematic reviews and meta-analytical studies of psychological treatments for schizophrenia have been performed over recent years (Marl & Streiner 1994, Mojtabai et al 1998, Adams 2000, Dixon et al 2000). All of the above papers vary in the methodology and focus. Only Gould et al (2001) and Cormac et al (2002) have concentrated on randomised controlled trials of cognitive therapy for schizophrenia. The results of the former study suggest that cognitive interventions are a promising approach for targeting the positive symptoms of persistent delusions and hallucinations in schizophrenia.

For example, Drury et al (1996) demonstrated a high level of engagement using this approach, which they suggested was linked to the clients' feeling that their beliefs were addressed directly and not ignored or dismissed. Unlike a biomedical approach, which tends to focus on the form of psychotic symptoms, CBT addresses content. Psychotic beliefs are not directly challenged (Fowler et al 1995). The aim is to enhance natural coping mechanisms that the patient may already have. During the treatment process the emphasis is on applying rationality to the patient's attitudes and underlying cognitive assumptions. Active problem-solving strategies are promoted that address day-to-day problems, and an attitude of acceptance is fostered towards the patient and the patient's experiences that is maintained throughout the therapy. Hallucinations, delusions, negative symptoms and depression have all been shown to be responsive to CBT (Sensky et al 2000). In addition, Turkington et al (2002) demonstrated that the benefits of CBT translate into community settings in which community psychiatric nurses were trained in this therapy and given weekly supervision. This approach allowed them to engage collaboratively with patients and achieve both significant reductions in overall symptoms and improvement.

Nevertheless, given the diversity of trials exploring the efficacy of CBT for psychosis and increased interest in this approach in recent years, a number of questions remain. How generalisable are the results of studies investigating the efficacy of CBT for psychosis? Are there methodological issues that limit the conclusions drawn from such studies? Finally, how can we combine the results of diverse outcome studies in meaningful ways to draw reliable conclusions about its effects? Healy's (2003) meta-analysis of eight independent, controlled studies involving 888 participants suggests that a cognitive–

behavioural intervention is an effective and promising therapeutic approach in the treatment of psychotic symptoms. Moreover, three of the studies followed patients for up to 9 months. The result of these follow-ups is important given that a primary aim of therapy is to prevent relapse and, if early benefits of treatment can be maintained over time, such psychological treatment should be encouraged and implemented.

One of the studies included in the review did demonstrate that the benefits of CBT can also be implemented in a community setting. Turkington et al (2002) found that, when community trained psychiatric nurses were trained in CBT for psychosis over a 10-day period and given weekly supervision, this intervention was effective in reducing overall symptoms and depression. Levels of insight also improved. Such findings have positive implications for economic evaluations of psychological therapy for psychosis. However, while these results suggest promising effects, a number of questions still need to be addressed. There has been a significant paucity of controlled studies investigating the efficacy of CBT for psychosis. All the trials have been conducted in the UK, whereas none of the recent trials have taken place in the USA. It is uncertain whether the results found would generalise to a different culture such as the USA, with a predominance of many ethnic minorities.

Schizophrenia is associated with a number of cognitive deficits such as difficulty in concentrating, problem solving and other attentional deficits. Such impairments have significant implications for the success of CBT and there has been a long-held view that psychotic patients are not amenable to cognitive therapy. Lack of insight is another reason that is also posited for their failure to engage. The results of other meta-analyses (Gould et al 2001, Cormac et al 2002) clearly demonstrate that this is not the case. For example, Garety et al (1994) found that cognitive variables were not related to treatment response. Nevertheless, given the nature of CBT, a certain degree of insight and willingness to disclose symptoms are necessary prerequisites to engage in it (Chadwick et al 1994). Thus those patients who are more severely deluded and suffering from marked negative symptoms of depression and withdrawal may not benefit from such a psychological approach. This hypothesis is supported by findings from Garety et al (1994), where it was found that a greater insight did predict a better outcome among patients randomised to CBT therapy.

Identification of therapeutically relevant factors is very important in order to be able to implement them in clinical practice. A study by Andres et al (2000) investigated the significance of coping as a therapeutic variable for the outcome of purely psychoeducational and behavioural therapy in schizophrenia. They demonstrated that better outcomes in terms of psychopathology and social outcome was best predicted by the patient's mastery of active problem-focused strategies, levels of cognisance about the disorder and levels of social functioning. While the treatment intervention employed in this study was not CBT per se, such significant predictors of outcome can be readily mapped on to a CBT approach where level of insight, as previously discussed, is an important variable to consider.

A criticism sometimes levelled at a cognitive–behavioural approach to psychosis is that the focus of treatment is typically target symptoms of hallucinations and delusions. Other symptoms, such as affective state and psychosocial functioning, have not been specifically addressed. This issue has been addressed in a recent study by Gumley et al (2003) that looked at CBT for relapse. Significant improvements in two social functioning domains (shopping, managing finances, etc.) and prosocial activities were found. As opposed to using withdrawal- or avoidance-oriented coping with perceived relapses, participants exposed to a psychological intervention appeared to adopt more adaptive coping strategies that enhance social and interpersonal functioning. This represents a further promising role for the efficacy of this treatment approach and should be pursued in future studies. In conclusion, the results from studies on psychotic symptoms have provided strong evidence of the effectiveness of CBT in helping patients to cope with psychotic symptoms (Haddock & Slade 1996). However, some of these benefits may be temporary and patients may need continued intervention to maintain any improvements.

CONCLUDING REMARKS

Considerable progress has been made in the development of psychological treatment for schizophrenia. Traditionally, patients with schizophrenia and their relatives have been rather passive recipients of care delivered by the mental health service. A cognitive–behavioural approach radically changes this dyadic relationship in that both patients and carers become active participants in the management of the psychotic symptoms. The therapy fosters a collaborative relationship and dialogue that affords patients some control over their care management and an opportunity to identify individual relapse signatures. The trials reviewed here provide encouraging results for the efficacy of cognitive–behavioural intervention in the treatment of psychosis. However, many issues remain to be clarified including the identification of the therapeutic processes activated by such treatment interventions. In addition, some trials suffer from a number of methodological limitations, which have been discussed. Future studies should address these issues.

Finally, the Department of Health (1999) now acknowledges the importance of psychological interventions. Clearly there is a need for a new approach to treatment if the needs of individuals with schizophrenia are to be fully met. Such an intervention should also be readily incorporated into the training and subsequently integrated into routine clinical practice.

Cross references

For practical strategies and implementation ideas see:

Chapter 11 Dealing with voices and strange thoughts

Chapter 12 Dealing with blankness and deadness

Chapter 13 Working with families and informal carers

Chapter 18 Integrated approaches to relapse prevention

References

Adams C E 2000 Psychosocial interventions for schizophrenia. Effective health care bulletin. NHS Centre for Reviews and Dissemination, University of York, York

Anderson J, Adams C 1996 Family intervention in schizophrenia. British Medical Journal 313:232–236

Andres K, Pfammtter M, Garst F et al 2000 Effects of coping-oriented group therapy for schizophrenia and schizoaffective patients: a pilot study. Acta Psychiatrica Scandinavica 101:318–322

Barrowclough C, Tarrier N 1992 Families of schizophrenic patients: cognitive behavioural intervention. Chapman & Hall, London

Bebbington P E, Kuipers E 1994 The predictive utility of expressed emotion in schizophrenia. Psychological Medicine 24:707–718

Beck A T, Rush A J, Shaw B, Emory G 1979 Cognitive therapy for depression. Guilford Press, New York

Bellack A S, Mueser K T 1993 Psychosocial treatment for schizophrenia. Schizophrenia Bulletin 19:317–336

Bentall R P, Haddock G, Slade P D 1994 Psychological treatment for auditory hallucinations: from theory to therapy. Behaviour Therapy 25:51–66

Brown G W, Birley J L, Wing J K 1972 Influence of family life on the course of schizophrenic disorders: a replication. British Journal of Psychiatry 121:241–258

Buchanan A, Reed A, Wesself S et al 1993 Acting on delusions 11: the phenomenological correlates of acting on delusions. British Journal of Psychiatry 163:77–81

Budd R, Hughes I 1997 What do relatives of people with schizophrenia find helpful about family intervention? Schizophrenia Bulletin 23:341–347

References (cont'd)

Bustillo, J R, Lauriello, J, Keith, S J 1999 Schizophrenia: improving outcome. Harvard Research Psychiatry 6:229–240

Chadwick P, Birchwood M 1994 The omnipotence of voices. A cognitive approach to auditory hallucinations. British Journal of Psychiatry 164:190–201

Chadwick P, Birchwood M 1996 Cognitive therapy for voices. In: Haddock G, Slade P D (eds) Cognitive-behavioural interventions for psychotic disorders. Routledge, London, pp 71–85

Chadwick P D J, Lowe C F 1990 Measurement and modification of delusional beliefs. Journal of Consulting and Clinical Psychology 58:225–232

Chadwick P D J, Lowe C F 1994 A cognitive approach to measuring and modifying delusions. Behaviour Research and Therapy 32:353–367

Chadwick P D J, Lowe C F, Horne P J, Higson P J 1994 Modifying delusions: the role of empirical testing. Behaviour Therapy 25:35–49

Cormac I, Jones C, Campbell C 2002 Cognitive behaviour therapy for schizophrenia (Cochrane Review). Cochrane Library, issue 2. Update Software, Oxford

Department of Health 1999 National service framework for mental health. Stationery Office, London

Dixon L, Adams C, Luckstead A 2000 Update on family psycho-education for schizophrenia, Schizophrenia Bulletin 26:5–20

Drury V, Birchwood M, Cochrane R, McMillan F 1996 Cognitive therapy and recovery from acute psychosis: a controlled trial. British Journal of Psychiatry 169:593–601

Fadden G 1997 Implementation of family interventions in routine clinical practice following staff training programmes: a major cause for concern. Journal of Mental Health 6:599–612

Fadden G 1998 Family intervention. In: Brooker C, Repper J (eds) Serious mental health problems in the community: policy, practice and research. Baillière Tindall, London, pp 159–183

Fowler D, Garety P A, Kuipers E 1995 Cognitive behaviour therapy for psychosis. John Wiley, Chichester

Garety P A, Kuipers L, Fowler D et al 1994 Cognitive behavioural therapy for drug resistant psychosis. British Journal of Medical Psychology 67:259–271

Geddes J, Freemantle N, Harrison P, Bebbington P 2000 Atypical antipsychotics in the treatment of schizophrenia: systematic overview and meta-regression analysis. British Medical Journal 321:1371–1376

Gould R A, Meuser K T, Bolton E et al 2001 Cognitive therapy for psychosis in schizophrenia : an effect size analysis. Schizophrenia Research 48:335–342

Gumley A, O'Grady M, McNay L et al 2003 Early intervention for relapse in schizophrenia: results of a 12-month randomised controlled trial of cognitive behavioural therapy. Psychological Medicine 33:419–431

Haddock G, Slade P D 1996 Implications for services and future research. In: Haddock G, Slade PD (eds) Cognitive-behavioural interventions for psychotic disorders. Routledge, London, pp 265–275

Haddock G, Tarrier N 1999 Assessment and formulation in the cognitive behavioural treatment of psychosis. In: Tarrier N, Wells A, Haddock G (eds) Treating complex cases: the cognitive behavioural approach. John Wiley, New York

Healy H 2003 Is CBT effective in the treatment of psychosis in adults? A review of recent controlled studies. Unpublished manuscript, University of Wales

References (cont'd)

Himadi B, Osteen F, Kaiser A J, Daniel K 1991 Assessment of delusional beliefs during the modification of delusional verbalisations. Behaviour Residual Treatment 6:356–366

Hughes I, Hailwood R, Abbati-Yeoman J, Budd R 1996 Developing a family intervention service for serious mental illness: clinical observations and experiences. Journal of Mental Health 5:145–159

Kane J M 1996 Treatment resistant schizophrenic patients. Journal of Clinical Psychiatry 57(suppl 9):35–40

Kane J M, McGlashan T H 1995 Treatment of schizophrenia. Lancet 346:820–825

Kavanagh D J 1992 Family intervention for schizophrenia. In: Kavanagh D J (ed) Schizophrenia: an overview and practical handbook. Chapman & Hall, London, pp 407–423

Kavanagh D J, Piatkowska O, Clark D et al 1993 Application of cognitive behavioural family intervention for schizophrenia in multidisciplinary teams: what can the matter be? Australian Psychologist 28:181–188

Kuipers E, Garety P, Fowler D 1996 An outcome study of cognitive–behavioural treatment for psychosis. In: Haddock G, Slade P D (eds) Cognitive–behavioural interventions for psychotic disorders. Routledge, London, pp 116–136

Kuipers L, Leff J, Lam D 1992 Family work for schizophrenia: a practical guide. Gaskell, London

Lam D 1991 Psychosocial family intervention in schizophrenia: a review of empirical studies. Psychological Medicine 21:423–441

Leff J 2000 Family work for schizophrenia: practical application. Acta Psychiatrica Scandinavica 102(suppl 407):78–82

Leff J, Vaughn C 1985 Expressed emotion in families: its significance for mental illness. Guilford Press, New York

McCreadie R, Phillips K, Harvey J et al 1991 The Nithsdale schizophrenia surveys. VIII: Do relatives want family intervention, and does it help? British Journal of Psychiatry 158:110–113

McFarlane W R, Lukens E, Link B et al 1995 Multiple family groups and psychoeducation in the treatment of schizophrenia. Archives of General Psychiatry 52:679–687

Mari J J, Streiner D 1994 An overview of family interventions and relapse on schizophrenia: meta-analyses of research findings. Psychological Medicine 24:565–578

Mojtabai R, Nicholson R A, Carpenter B N 1998 Role of prosocial treatments in the management of schizophrenia: a meta-analytical review of controlled outcome studies. Schizophrenia Bulletin 24:569–587

Mullen A, Murray L, Happell B 2002 Multiple family group interventions in first episode psychosis: enhancing knowledge and understanding. International Journal of Mental Health Nursing 11:225–232

Nelson H 1997 Cognitive behavioural therapy with schizophrenia. Stanley Thornes, Cheltenham

Penn D L, Mueser K T 1996 Research update on the psychosocial treatment of schizophrenia. American Journal of Psychiatry 153:607–617

References (cont'd)

Pilling S, Bebbington P, Kuipers E et al 2002 Psychological treatments in schizophrenia 1: meta-analyses of family intervention and cognitive behaviour therapy. Psychological Medicine 32:763–782

Rector N A, Beck A T 2001 Cognitive behavioural therapy for schizophrenia: an empirical review. Journal of Nervous and Mental Diseases 189:278–287

Remmington G, Kapur S, Zipursky R B 1998 Pharmaco-therapy of first episode schizophrenia. British Journal of Psychiatry 172(suppl 33):66–70

Schwartz B J, Cecil A, Iqbal N 1993 Psychosocial treatments of schizophrenia. Psychiatric Annals 23:216–221

Sellwood W, Haddock G, Tarrier N, Yusupoff L 1994 Advances in the psychological management of positive symptoms of schizophrenia. International Review of Psychiatry 6:201–215

Sensky T, Turkington D, Kingdon D et al 2000 A randomised controlled trial of cognitive–behavioural therapy for persistent symptoms in schizophrenia resistant to medication. Archives of General Psychiatry 57:165–172

Slade P D, Haddock G 1996 A historical overview of psychological treatments for psychotic symptoms. In: Haddock G, Slade P D (eds) Cognitive-behavioural interventions for psychotic disorders. Routledge, London, pp 28–44

Smith G, Velleman R 2002 Maintaining a family work for psychosis service by recognising and addressing the barriers to implementation. Journal of Mental Health 11:471–479

Smith J, Birchwood M 1990 Relatives and patients as partners in the management of schizophrenia: the development of a service model. British Journal of Psychiatry 156:654–660

Stanbridge R I, Burbach F R, Lucas A S, Carter K 2003 A study of families' satisfaction with a family interventions in psychosis service in Somerset. Journal of Family Therapy 25:181–204

Tarrier N, Barrowclough C 1995 Family interventions in schizophrenia and their long-term outcomes. International Journal of Mental Health 24:38–53

Tarrier N, Harwood S, Yusopoff L et al 1990 Coping strategy enhancement (CSE): a method of treating residual schizophrenic symptoms. Bchavioural Psychotherapy 18.283–293

Tarrier N, Lowson K, Barrowclough C 1991 Some aspects of family interventions in schizophrenia. II: financial considerations. British Journal of Psychiatry 159:481–484

Tarrier N, Beckett R, Harwood S et al 1993 A trial of two cognitive–behavioural methods of treating drug-resistant residual psychotic symptoms in schizophrenic patients, I: outcome. British Journal of Psychiatry 162:524–532

Turkington D, Kingdon D, Turner T 2002 Effectiveness of a brief cognitive behavioural therapy intervention in the treatment of schizophrenia. British Journal of Psychiatry 180:523–527

Zubin J, Spring B 1977 Vulnerability: a new view of schizophrenia. Journal of Abnormal Psychology 86:103–126

Annotated further reading

Bentall R 2003 Madness explained: psychosis and human nature. Penguin, Harmondsworth

This book provides a welcome review of the medical model and challenges traditional treatment approaches. It reviews the origins and misunderstandings about psychosis and challenges the reader to radically shift their opinions about the manner in which severe mental illness is managed and perceived.

Kingdon D G, Turkington D 1995 Cognitive behaviour therapy of schizophrenia. Guildford Press, London

Chapters 3 and 4 of this book, 'Vulnerability and life events' and 'Suggestibility', contain a valuable, in-depth summary of the issues raised within this chapter. It is a concise, user-friendly account of manifestation of illness.

Section 2

2

Engaging, assessing and formulating care

6

Building relationships: lessons to be learnt

Catherine Gamble

KEY ISSUES

◆ Engagement and the development of positive, therapeutic relationships
◆ Rogerian principles: qualities and characteristics
◆ Core elements of relationship building
◆ Lessons learnt from clinical examples
◆ Practical recommendations

'SCHIZOPHRENIA INVITED YOU IN – WE DIDN'T'

Mental health professionals should never presume that service users and their families want us in their lives. The statement 'Schizophrenia invited you in – we didn't' was made by a mother during a routine family visit. It was not a criticism and was not heard as such, but it served as a timely reminder that mental health professionals constantly tread a fine line. Indeed, by their very nature mental health practices can unwittingly be interfering and invasive. Fortunately, the changing context of mental health care delivery has enabled service users and families to become central to service delivery. This helps to reduce the 'Us and Them' element of mental health care. This 'working in partnership' paradigm shift reinforces the importance of 'learning together'. Central to this process is the relationship between professionals and services users; positive working alliances with each other are therefore crucial. The challenge for mental health professionals working in this reformed National Health Service is how to listen, value and respect the wishes and views of service users and their significant others (Stuart 1999).

The aim of this chapter is to examine the qualities and characteristics required to achieve this goal. Through lessons learnt from first-hand observations and accounts, it will go on to explore the process of relationship building and provide some practical advice and strategies to aid the development of positive therapeutic relationships.

QUALITIES REQUIRED BY PRACTITIONERS

Throughout any mental health practitioner's training and working life, reference will be made to the sort of personal qualities that are required to build relationships with clients, their families and carers. Little emphasis, however, is laid on the development of these attributes during pre- and postregistration education for mental health professionals (McQueen 2000). From the literature it is clear that, in order for any intervention to be successful, clients need to feel safe to disclose important and often distressing information (Romme & Escher 2000) Therefore, the relationship between themselves and the practitioner has to be based upon non-judgemental support, honesty, warmth and therapeutic hope. In this way, clients are more likely to achieve their personal aspirations and develop methods to manage and live with their mental health problem. They will feel reassured that their experiences and needs will be taken seriously (Sainsbury Centre 1998). The qualities required to aid this process range from having a considerable degree of sensitivity, knowledge and expertise (Perkins & Repper 1996) to being self aware, approachable, purposeful, flexible and ordinary. Indeed, having the ability to be a companion with a sense of fair play and humanity is what matters, as these qualities can be extraordinarily effective in helping clients find a sense of affinity with professionals (Taylor 1994). The effectiveness of such characteristics in helping clients learn and achieve their personal goals remains difficult to define, especially when much of the literature focuses upon the implementation of detailed interventions or approaches and not the process of their delivery (Repper 2002); nevertheless, as counterintuitive skills have long been recognised to be necessary to work successfully with this client group and achieve positive therapy outcomes (Tuma et al 1978, Blaauw & Emmelkamp 1994), it is important to consider how these qualities should be applied in routine clinical practice.

ROGERIAN PRINCIPLES

Carl Rogers (1983) promoted the client-centred hypotheses that are now considered essential to the development and sustainability of therapeutic relationships. The guiding 'rogerian' principles are:

◆ *Empathetic understanding*, which is sensitivity to others' feelings

- *Genuineness*, which is reflected in an open, honest, hopeful approach
- *Unconditional positive regard*, which is accomplished by accepting that all individuals are entitled to respect and care.

Rogers (1983) believes that exposure to such attributes produces learning, or changes, in people. That is, they begin to perceive themselves differently, accept their feelings more readily, become more accepting of others, more self-confident and self-directing. Thus they are more able to change behaviours and adopt realistic goals. Gamble and Curthroys (2004) recognise that the promotion of these attributes provides common ground regardless of which treatment philosophy or affiliated school of thought is adopted. Indeed, at the core of any contemporary practice is the recognition that people are unique, that irrespective of their diagnosis they are able to collaborate, and that no positive outcome will be achieved if these principles are not adhered to or utilised by practitioners. Such qualities can be developed over time, using communication and observation skills. However, as highlighted by McQueen (2000), after qualifying some practitioners have limited opportunity to refine or revisit these skills.

Empathetic understanding

Empathetic understanding is displayed through the manner in which we treat and portray ourselves to others. In many instances, this is acquired through observation and listening to other's experiences. Indeed, to hear effectively professionals need to stop speaking, and listen. An opportunity is then afforded to give attention to what the other person is saying. Listening, therefore, is an art that involves intelligent concentration, summarising what is said without changing the meaning of the words and paying attention to the context as well as content (Bostrom 1997). This can sometimes be difficult to achieve when working in busy, under-resourced clinical settings. To guide you through the art of listening and methods to overcome potential barriers, Table 6.1 suggests some strategies.

Undertaking formal assessment processes and balancing note taking with personalised interaction (Table 6.1) is another skill that needs careful consideration. Formal methods of enquiry can aid practitioners to gather objectively important information about service-users' prevailing needs (see Chapter 8). Nevertheless, until recently assessment tools have not been routinely used or valued by practitioners, as they have been negatively perceived as cumbersome barriers that reduce the likelihood of therapeutic alliances being developed and do not readily lend themselves to measuring process outcomes (Repper & Brooker 1997). However, Rose's (2001) service users study identified that 17–36% felt their needs had not been assessed properly and an even higher proportion (30–79%) reported that their strengths, abilities and interests had

Table 6.1 Strategies for effective listening

The art of listening involves four Cs	Potential barriers	Methods of overcoming barriers
Considering situations in which you may find it difficult to concentrate	Interruptions. Noisy external exchanges. When there is more than one item on the agenda or someone going over the allocated time. Client's current symptoms may be too troublesome and distracting for them. TV and radio on	Plan for and report your unavailability. Put a 'Do Not Disturb' sign up for the duration of the meeting. Challenge interruptions if they are made. Set an agenda and a realistic time frame; adhere to them. Assess how the client feels; is this the right time and place to be meeting? Negotiate where and when would be more appropriate and/or turn off the telephone/mobile, TV, radio
Collating methods to facilitate being a 'better listener'	Not planning for the interaction and missing valuable cues. Others not agreeing to formal approach. Tape recording and/or note taking perceived to be journalistic rather than therapeutic. Clients and/or carers will be suspicious, won't they?	Discuss your interaction with another experienced member of the team. Plan how to structure and evaluate the session. Balance note taking with personalised interaction. Adhere to trust and/or university guidelines, so as not to breach local confidentiality guidelines. Provide a rationale for note taking and/or audiotaping. No harm in just asking and gaining consent to audiotaping. Challenge own and others' assumptions
Constructing a rationale for why you can't always listen	Being occupied by all the above and other clinical responsibilities	Being honest. Acknowledging distractions and reporting other items on the agenda. Recognising inability to time-manage
Consolidating what you will do with the information	Information obtained challenges others' perceptions. Being unable to objectively document or report on what you have learnt. Other members of the team don't want to acknowledge and there is no forum for feedback	Listen attentively. Reflect and summarise. Encourage others to listen to client's and/or carer's viewpoint. Document what you have learnt in the case notes. Disseminate to other 'listeners', such as the client, their carers and others on the team. Attend the next possible clinical review meeting to feed back

Source: adapted from Norman & Ryrie (2004), p 270

not been taken into account. In the light of these findings, it would be imprudent to suggest that formal assessment methodologies are sufficient in gaining deeper, empathetic understanding of clients' experiences and their reactions to interventions. There is clearly a need to augment these methodologies with qualitative ones; indeed, Strauss (1994) concludes that 'the subjective in all its aspects is an essential part of our data'. Feedback from a service user who employed such an approach with a student undertaking psychosocial interventions training reinforces this:

> *To be honest, I didn't really know about formal assessments until my CPN and I went through some – I have been receiving mental health treatment for 4 years and never knew anything like this existed – I don't think I could have hacked it when I was really tormented with voices, but going through the paperwork afterwards made sense – it was actually reassuring and gave us something concrete to discuss and focus on. In fact, even my Mum was pleased 'cos it was the first time anyone had made notes and really taken an interest!*

Such feedback is reassuring; however, it is important to highlight that, while this service user was pleased with the outcome, others may not appreciate a formal approach in the first instance. Indeed, even the aforementioned service user reported being uncertain as to whether it would have been appropriate when 'I was really tormented with voices'. Therefore, to promote empathetic understanding practitioners need to be:

◆ able to judge the timing and pace of meetings and assessment processes and tailor-make appropriate, realistic, achievable interventions (Addis & Gamble 2004)
◆ realistic about the nature of change – for example some people's goal may just be to maintain their functioning, others may wish to return to work, while others may find suggestions about improving their quality of life overwhelming (Repper 2002)
◆ mindful that understanding the client's experience/s strengths, aspirations and wishes is only gained over time
◆ objective listeners who don't contaminate what they hear with their own hypotheses, thoughts and ideas
◆ attentive to the fact that being 'nice' does not equate to the aforementioned definition of empathetic understanding – service users want and need more than placating platitudes.

Genuineness

'Genuineness', as defined by Rogers (1983), is reflected in being open and having an honest, hopeful approach. If practitioners were routinely following the principles of recovery and social inclusion as described in Chapter 3 it would be possible to conclude that 'genuineness' was occurring on a daily basis. However, all too frequently in the clinical area, professionals can be heard to make 'non-genuine', sweeping generalisations about clients and their needs, such as:

1. 'Oh yes, him again. Send him straight to the ward, we know all about him – we've treated him before.'
2. 'The fact is that, despite every effort being made, he refuses to take medication, so what do you expect?'
3. 'This is the third time she's been in this year and it's only July! What she really needs to do is to leave her boyfriend – he's a nightmare and makes her condition worse, but there's no telling her.'
4. 'No, there is no point organising that for him, we tried it before and he said he couldn't be bothered – don't you remember?'
5. 'We've dealt with cases like this on numerous occasions – what we need to do is review the treatment again. Get him back on depot medication and then get the social worker involved to sort out his housing.'
6. 'Don't you realise how difficult it is for your family to cope with your behaviour?'

How do you react to statements like these? Suggesting possible solutions is easier to write than to put into practice. However, the first step to promote 'genuineness' and hopefulness is to challenge our assumptions, understand the reason for them and consider why they are made in the first place. For example, in statement 1 there is an assumption that a person never changes. Clearly, this is not the case, as the recovery process is uniquely individualised and not static. Indeed, Reeves (2000, p.334) acknowledges that 'as the person grows and achieves his/her goals and dreams the person may feel that even greater levels of recovery and understanding of themselves has been achieved'; therefore the idea that people should always be treated the same way despite what may have happened between admissions is highly disputable.

Statements 2, 3 and 4 give the impression that clients wilfully contribute to their condition. These examples present clients as being themselves part of the problem, and they are not perceived as having the ability or desire to contribute to possible solutions. Indeed, these statements are an illustration of how medically orientated services understand problems, i.e. attention is paid only to how individuals are behaving to aid compliance and control symptoms, and little is directed towards helping resolve what may be happening in these people's social networks (Reeves 2002). In statement 5 the client is removed from the decision making process altogether and the issues are reduced to practical problems, with treatment being decided *for* him, rather than *with* him. The practitioner is also making assumptions about another professional's role and this further reduces the possibilities of collaboration.

Statement 6 is a direct criticism and also patronising. It induces guilt and makes the assumption that the remark will stop the behaviour. This is never the case. In fact, assistance from friends, families and peers is generally more acceptable to service users than professional help (Repper & Perkins 2003). Yet, paradoxically, little or no attempt is made to acknowledge this role or consistently involve family or friends in the treatment that individuals receive (Gamble & Curthroys 2004).

If, at this point, you are thinking 'I've made those types of statement' – good, we all have. We all make such comments without thinking of their consequences. No one is perfect. It is a fact of life that we will not get on with everyone we come into contact with. But we should try to avoid writing off individuals for this reason alone. If a relationship has been established for some time, it may be initially difficult to change entrenched interaction patterns. Nevertheless, it is important to realise the need for change and it is worth assessing and continually re-evaluating your ability to promote 'genuineness' and hopefulness. To enhance this process, begin by asking yourself: 'When was the last time I thought or said something positive about the clients I am working with?' An important technique is to reframe client behaviour and interactions positively. In other words, we need to have the ability to redirect or change the perception of a situation and place it in another more appropriate context.

Begin, then, by being open to new concepts and ideas – think about your clients, how you perceive them and the work you are doing together. In other words, try to stop viewing clients as a problem and start seeing them as people facing issues that are currently affecting their dreams and aspirations. In summary, to promote 'genuineness' practitioners need to:

- ◆ adopt positive, hopeful, non-blaming attitudes
- ◆ recognise that an individual's choice is of paramount importance
- ◆ be able to formulate agreed, flexible, realistic plans of care that incorporate and work with the person's social networks
- ◆ remember that no one knows more about their illness than those who are experiencing it; a diagnosis of schizophrenia or other severe mental illness does not indicate mental incapacity
- ◆ reflect upon how their actions are perceived by service users
- ◆ value, respect and make use of the strengths, skills, coping mechanisms and support networks that the individual already has.

Unconditional positive regard

'Unconditional positive regard' is accomplished by accepting that *all* individuals are entitled to respect and care. This has many facets – too numerous to mention in this chapter – but to promote this philosophy both on an individual basis and on mental health services generally, there is an overwhelming need to:

◆ challenge exclusive practices, negative assumptions and attitudes – see Chapter 3
◆ celebrate and work with diversity and difference – see Chapters 19 and 3
◆ consider the ethical implications of our actions – see Chapter 20.

Additionally, to ensure that positive relationships are formed with service users and their significant others, it is important to raise another issue that can potentially affect unconditional positive regard being achieved.

Confidentiality: knowing what information to share and when

If all individuals are entitled to respect and care, service users, family and friends must be involved. Yet, as highlighted previously, little or no attempt is consistently made to acknowledge or include them. Families and friends all too often report that, when they contact services to ascertain how to support their significant other, they are brushed off with inconclusive proclamations such as 'Oh yes, her care coordinator should be able to help, but unfortunately he's not around at the moment; I'll leave a note to let him know you called' or 'Sorry, I can't go into any depth, you're not a relative and anyway I am not really the right person to clarify that for you'. After being exposed to such responses, it is not surprising that some families and friends are left bewildered and uncertain about how their needs will be addressed and by whom. There are many reasons for this, some of which are discussed in Chapters 2 and 5. Another, from a professional's perspective, is the prevailing dilemma of knowing how and when to share exactly what information.

Undoubtedly some professionals feel concerned about unearthing family problems that could intensify workload responsibilities, or they do not wish the inclusion of family and friends to breach client confidentiality (Faddon & Birchwood 2002, Furlong & Leggatt 1996). In this instance, are rights of the individual more important than those of their family and friends? Many practitioners would accept the client's right to privacy. However, in the author's experience it is rare for clients to turn everyone away and maintain this standpoint once they begin to recover. Therefore, it is important to review who will be taking an active caring role, offer general information and creatively consider how best to offer support in the interim.

In summary, to promote 'unconditional positive regard' practitioners need to:

◆ develop a positive attitude to the inclusion of family and friends

- review and discuss policies and procedures regarding information sharing and confidentiality issues with service users and their significant others
- explain the terms of engagement at the onset of client–practitioner contact and specify what kinds of contact will be made and how (Furlong & Leggatt 1996)
- ensure that, as relationships develop between clients and their practitioners, significant others are not excluded.

CONCLUSION

Throughout this manual, numerous practical strategies will be described to help practitioners engage and work with service users who experience serious mental health problems. Building relationships with service users and their significant others can sometimes be a difficult task and may take a considerable amount of time. This chapter has argued that the identified methods will be effective only if practitioners are prepared to reassess their communication skills, assumptions, attitudes and beliefs. All too often, professionals make sweeping generalisations about clients and have inappropriate expectations of what can and cannot be achieved. Putting these ideas into practice will be an ongoing challenge, especially if the practitioner is working in isolation, does not have access to an appropriate clinical supervisor, or is surrounded by team members who are unwilling to change or reflect upon their behaviour or assumptions. Nevertheless, whatever the circumstances, we have a professional responsibility to ensure that everyone who uses mental health services is treated fairly by objective, knowledgeable mental health professionals who are prepared routinely to use rogerian principles.

Cross references

For additional practical strategies and ideas see:

Chapter 2 Inside caring in mental health.

Chapter 3 Social inclusion

It should be pointed out that all of Section 2 requires practitioners to use rogerian principles.

References

Addis J, Gamble C 2004 Assertive outreach nurses' experience of engagement. Journal of Psychiatric and Mental Health Nursing 11:452–460

Blaauw E, Emmelkamp P M G 1994 The therapeutic relationship: a study on the value of the therapist client rating scale. Behavioural and Cognitive Psychotherapy 22:25–35

Bostrom R N 1997 The process of listening. In: Hargie O (ed) The handbook of communication skills, 2nd edn. Routledge, London

Faddon G, Birchwood M 2002 British models for expanding family psychosocial education in routine practice. In: Lefley H P, Johnson D L (eds) Family interventions in mental illness – international perspectives. Praeger, Westport, CT

Furlong M, Leggart M 1996 Reconciling the patient's right to confidentiality and the family's need to know. Australian and New Zealand Journal of Psychiatry 30:614–622

Gamble C, Curthroys J 2004 Psychosocial interventions. In: Norman I J, Ryrie I (eds) The art and science of mental health nursing: a textbook of principles and practice. Open University Press, Buckingham

McQueen A 2000 Nurse–patient relationships and partnership in hospital care. Journal of Clinical Nursing 9:723–731

Norman I J, Ryrie I (eds) 2004 The art and science of mental health nursing: a textbook of principles and practice. Open University Press, Buckingham

Perkins R, Repper J 1996 Working alongside people with long term mental health problems. Chapman & Hall, London

Reeves A 2000 Creative journeys of recovery: a survivor perspective. In: Birchwood M, Jackson C, Fowler D (eds) Early intervention in psychosis: a guide to concepts, evidence and interventions. John Wiley, Chichester

Repper J 2002 The helping relationship. In: Harris N, Williams S, Bradshaw T (eds) Psychosocial interventions for people with schizophrenia: a guide for mental health workers. Palgrave Macmillan, Basingstoke

Repper J, Brooker C 1997 Difficulties in the measurement of outcome in people who have serious mental health problems. Journal of Advanced Nursing 27:75–82

Repper J, Perkins R 2003 Social inclusion and recovery: a model for mental health practice. Baillière Tindall, London

Rogers C 1983 Freedom to learn for the 80s. Merrill, Columbus, OH

Romme M, Escher S 2000 Making sense of voices: a guide for mental health professionals working with voice hearers. Mind Publications, London

Rose D 2001 Users' voices. The perspectives of mental health service users on community and hospital care. Sainsbury Centre for Mental Health, London

Sainsbury Centre 1998 Keys to engagement. Sainsbury Centre for Mental Health, London

Strauss J S 1994 The person with schizophrenia as a person. II: approaches to the subjective and complex. British Journal of Psychiatry 164(suppl 23):103–107

Stuart G 1999 Government wants patient partnerships to be integral part of NHS. British Medical Journal 319:788

Taylor B 1994 Being human: ordinariness in nursing. Churchill Livingstone, New York

Tuma A H, May P R A, Yale C, Forsythe A B 1978 Therapists' characteristics and the outcome of treatment in schizophrenia. Archives of General Psychiatry 35:81–85

Annotated further reading

Perkins R, Repper J 1996 Working alongside people with long term mental health problems. Chapman & Hall, London

The title of this book clearly reflects its content. It provides an informative, thought-provoking explanation about how to work positively with people who experience long-term mental health problems. The authors address how to enhance collaborative working relationships so that a greater understanding of clients' personal needs can be achieved. In doing so, the text is refreshingly controversial. It explores the attitudes and assumptions professionals often make about people who have a serious mental health problem, by challenging the notion that clients are unable to control their own lives or take an active role in treatment and service provision.

7

Severe mental illness: symptoms, signs and diagnosis

Tom KJ Craig

KEY ISSUES

◆ What is meant by serious mental illness
◆ The importance of distinguishing the form from the content of mental state
◆ Symptoms of serious mental illness: definitions and useful questions for eliciting these
◆ Signs of severe mental illness: the assessment of appearance, speech and behaviour
◆ Putting signs and symptoms together: the principles of diagnostic classification

INTRODUCTION

This chapter describes the phenomenology of severe mental illness, starting with definitions of abnormal experiences and closing with a brief overview of current diagnostic guidelines for schizophrenia and the major affective disorders. It is aimed at non-medical members of the multidisciplinary team who need to carry out front-line assessments and to undertake sophisticated psychosocial interventions that call for precision in assessing the abnormal experiences of their clients.

Consider, for example, the assessment of a young man who has been referred with a 3-month history of anxiety and depression during his first term at university. The assessment proceeds slowly as his account is vague and rambling. He says that he has always been a loner who has difficulty making friends. He has not settled into university life and has fallen out with another student after complaining about a radio that was playing all night. He has subsequently heard this student referring to him as a 'poofter', although the student denied having said any such thing. The noises continue to keep him awake and he is convinced that this is deliberate. The more he thinks about it, the more certain he is that something unpleasant is going on, involving spreading rumours about his sexuality to other students, who are now avoiding him.

The questions asked by the assessor from this point on are crucial. One might be dealing with a shy young man with a rather prickly, sensitive personality who has been unlucky enough to have been placed next door to an extroverted insomniac. But it is also possible that his story reflects an altogether more sinister process. Schizophrenia, arguably the most serious mental illness, may begin in just this way – anxiety and perplexity associated with vague persecutory ideas. While the first explanation might be resolved by a change in residence and his shyness helped by counselling, this is unlikely to be enough for a major mental illness. Equally, one would not wish to recommend drug treatment without first obtaining more definite evidence of mental illness. But how to continue? What questions are most helpful? What answers should we look for?

AN ORGANISATIONAL FRAMEWORK FOR ASSESSMENT

Mental disorders affect an individual's cognitive processes, their beliefs, perceptions and outward behaviour. Many of the phenomena lie on a continuum that includes everyday experiences, making it quite difficult to decide when an experience should be labelled abnormal. A useful rule of thumb is that experiences are likely to be abnormal when they are involuntary, out of proportion to any situation that precipitated them and cannot be turned off or greatly reduced by conscious effort. They are usually distressing to the sufferer or their response to the experiences may be distressing to others.

A fundamental principle in describing and classifying these abnormal experiences is the distinction of form from content. *Content* refers to what a person describes as their mental experience. It is unique to the individual and influenced by previous experiences and the culture and society in which they dwell. *Form*, on the other hand, is a codified description of the common threads of these experiences that are recognisable across individuals. For example, consider two young men, both of whom are suffering from schizophrenia. One, in a small village in upper Egypt, states that he is possessed by

a djinn that has resisted all efforts at exorcism. As evidence for this possession, he says that the djinn is able to take over his will and can cause him to
shout out even when he tries to keep silent. At times he hears the djinn
laughing at him and passing rude remarks about his appearance. The other
young man has spent all his life in London. He also believes his will has been
replaced by an alien power but attributes this to a microchip that has been
implanted in his ear while he was asleep. This chip receives signals from a
computer some miles away and the controllers can make him shout out when

Table 7.1 Overview of a schema for the assessment of mental state

Topic	Subjective experience (symptoms, complaints)	Observed behaviour (signs)
Mood (affect)	**Tension:** Worry, nervous tension, muscular tension, tiredness, restlessness	Tense, fidgety, pacing
	Anxiety: Free floating anxiety, anxious foreboding, panic attacks and phobic avoidance	Anxious tense appearance, sweaty, shaky, shallow rapid breathing
	Irritability	Irritability/impatience
	Depression: Loss of interests, tedium vitae, hopelessness, suicide, guilt, self-deprecation	Sad expression, tearful, frozen gloom
	Elation: Expansive mood, excitement, grandiose thoughts	Euphoria, excitement, irritation/hostility Perplexity Incongruity Blunting or flattening Suspiciousness
Body functions	**Sleep problems:** Delayed sleep, early waking, middle insomnia **Appetite and weight change** **Altered levels of activity:** Subjective slowing or excitement	Psychomotor retardation, excitement, stupor
Thinking	Thought flow and structure, thought echo, withdrawal, loud thoughts Thought content (delusions) Replacement of the 'will'	Incoherence, neologisms, thought blocking, etc.
Perception	Heightened/diminished perception Depersonalisation/derealisation Hallucinations	Behaves as though hallucinating
Cognition	Orientation, concentration, memory	Consciousness, orientation, concentration, memory

he tries to keep silent. They often laugh at his reactions to their torments. They also pass disparaging remarks about the clothes he is wearing and his personal hygiene. While the specific *content* of the experiences of these two men clearly reflects their different social origins, the *form* of the experience is similar – both report that their will has been replaced by an alien power and both hear voices that comment on their actions.

A basic schema outlining the form of common mental symptoms and observed behaviour is given in Table 7.1. The framework is a useful starting point for a discussion of the assessment of an individual's mental state.

1. Assessing mood

This is often an early step in the assessment, although it is usual to refine initial impressions as the interview proceeds.

Tension symptoms:

Questions include:

- ◆ Have there been times lately when you have been worried, tense or anxious?
- ◆ Have you had difficulty relaxing?
- ◆ Have you been very tired and exhausted for no particular reason?

This first group of symptoms includes complaints of worry, apprehension, restlessness, muscular tension, irritability and excessive tiredness or fatigue. These occur on a continuum with normality, can occur singly or with each other and are seen in most disorders. Although they are non-specific, they are good indicators of the severity of distress.

Anxiety with autonomic nervous system arousal

Questions include:

- ◆ Have there been times lately when you have been very panicky or frightened?
- ◆ Do you ever get fearful that something terrible is about to happen?
- ◆ Have you ever been so frightened you simply had to stop what you were doing?

If any of these are endorsed:

- ◆ When you have felt like that, did you also have palpitations/butterflies in your stomach/sweating/giddiness/difficulty breathing?

As with symptoms of tension, just about everyone will have been anxious at some time. It is pathological when it is out of proportion to the circumstances that provoked it and when it persists against all efforts at self-control for hours at a time. While anxiety is often triggered by a worrying thought or by some phobic situation, it can also arise out of the blue (*free-floating anxiety*) or be caused by an apprehension that something dreadful is about to happen (*anxious foreboding*). *Panic attacks* are discrete episodes of marked fearfulness, beginning abruptly and rising rapidly to a crescendo that may last up to an hour, after which the anxiety gradually abates, leaving the sufferer feeling exhausted, drained and shaky. The attacks may be associated with escape responses, as in, for example, the agoraphobic who rushes out of a super-market or off a crowded bus. Common generalised phobias, which result in significant social impairment, include agoraphobia and social phobia.

Depression

Questions include:

- ◆ Have you been depressed or low-spirited?
- ◆ Have you lost interest in work/hobbies/seeing friends/your appearance?
- ◆ How do you see the future? Has life ever seemed not worth living?
- ◆ What opinion do you have of yourself compared to others?
- ◆ Have you been feeling particularly guilty or blaming yourself at all?
- ◆ Do you get the feeling that others are blaming you for things?

The complaint of depressed mood can have many different expressions, e.g. sadness, low spirits, gloom or an incapacity to enjoy anything. Tearfulness may be a clue to severity but very severe depression may also be a frozen misery that is subjectively beyond tears. A reduction in the usual reactivity of mood to day-to-day events is a fairly good guide to severity. When the mood is very low, the sufferer's mind will be almost totally absorbed by gloomy topics. The *syndrome* of depression will typically also include non-specific 'tension' symptoms as well as poor concentration, sleep disturbance, appetite disturbance and loss of interests. In addition there may be a loss of hope for the future that may extend to a feeling that life holds nothing of interest and little to live for (*tedium vitae*) and even to suicidal thoughts or acts. The depressed mood may show a characteristic diurnal variation, being worst during the early part of the day. Depressed people lose confidence in their day-to-day dealings with other people, withdraw from social contact and feel inferior or worthless (*self-depreciation*). Feelings of lassitude and general ill health can result in *hypochondriacal preoccupations* with some imagined and often fearful physical disease. *Pathological guilt* refers to over-concern with actions that most people would not take very seriously. The sufferer recognises that this guilt is exaggerated but cannot help feeling it all the same. This symptom can intensify to the point where individuals blame themselves for almost everything that goes wrong. A similar experience is that of *guilty ideas of reference* in which sufferers feel that they are accused of some blameworthy act, which they may not actually have committed.

Elation

Questions include:

◆ Have there been times when you felt particularly cheerful without any reason?
◆ Have you felt very full of energy or full of exciting ideas?
◆ Have you felt especially healthy?
◆ Have you any special talents or abilities?

The person with a pathologically *elevated mood* is euphoric and elated, excited, irritable and impatient with those around, who seem slower in their bodies and wits than themselves. When euphoric, the mood often has an infectious quality. Linked with these changes in mood are various alterations in speech and motor activity that can be observed in the assessment. The sufferer is typically over-talkative and difficult to interrupt. Concentration is often objectively impaired, yet sufferers experience the opposite, feeling themselves to be full of exciting ideas and of above average ability and intelligence. Self-esteem is exaggerated and they may be excessively optimistic about the future, feeling that nothing can stand in their way. There may be marked *motor overactivity* with a decreased need for sleep and increased sexual drive. Reckless actions are common – inappropriate shopping sprees, reckless driving, quarrels and generally foolish behaviour that are out of character. The changes in mood and activity may also be linked to *grandiose beliefs* – for example, that the sufferer is of extraordinarily high intellect or is a gifted inventor.

2. Assessing thought processes

Questions include:

◆ Can you think clearly? Have you any difficulty concentrating?
◆ Is there any interference with your thinking?

Difficulties concentrating, making decisions and feeling muddled are common accompaniments of most mental disorders. In addition to these very non-specific experiences, there are others that are rarer and traditionally linked more closely to specific mental conditions.

Obsessional ruminations and compulsions

Questions include:

- ◆ Do you have to keep checking things you know you have already done?
- ◆ Do you have to spend a lot of time on personal cleanliness?
- ◆ Do you get awful thoughts coming into your mind even when you try to keep them out?

These are experienced as the patient's own thoughts yet are intrusive, unwanted and irresistible or incapable of being stopped for any length of time. The intrusive thoughts may lead to compulsive rituals involving checking, counting or cleaning. *Obsessional incompleteness* involves the intrusive need to get everything right before a task can be considered complete. Sufferers may, for example, rehearse an event in their mind over and over again in order to convince themselves that they can remember every detail.

Many other symptoms can easily be confused with obsessions. For example, neglect of everyday tasks while brooding over unhappy events may be mistaken for obsessional incompleteness, and hypochondriacal fears of contracting a disease may be confused with the obsessional fear of contamination. The experience of the intrusion of the unwanted thoughts against conscious resistance, coupled with the awareness that the thoughts are their own, are the key features for distinguishing obsessional ruminations. Even when resistance has waned after years of struggle, the patient seldom forgets the power of their initial reaction.

Abnormalities in the possession of thought

These include a variety of experiences through which individuals come to believe that the innermost secret workings of their mind are accessible to outsiders. These experiences are usually indicative of a psychotic illness, although they can occur fleetingly in healthy people and may be induced through certain activities linked to religious rituals, sleep deprivation, physical ill health or substance use.

- ◆ **Thought echo**: Do you ever hear your thoughts repeated or echoed?

Sufferers experience an immediate repetition of their last thought. They are aware that it is their own thoughts that are echoed but are unable to control the experience.

- ◆ **Thought broadcasting**: Have you ever heard your thoughts spoken aloud, so that someone standing nearby could hear them?

With this symptom, the usually silent process of thinking is experienced 'aloud' so that someone standing nearby would be able to hear the thoughts. Sometimes this is elaborated so that the person feels that others can hear his thoughts even when they are not in the same room. The experience of hearing thoughts aloud differs from auditory hallucinations in that the sufferer is aware he is 'hearing' his own thoughts. Both thought echo and loud thoughts differ from the ruminations seen in obsessional disorders in the relative lack of consistency or theme to the content of the thoughts and by the fact that obsessional ruminations do not have the 'aloud' quality.

◆ **Thought insertion**: Are thoughts put into your mind that are not your own?

Here there is the loss of the normal sense of ownership of thoughts. This experience is almost always accompanied by a delusional explanation; for example, that the thoughts have been placed there by telepathy or X-rays. The quality of 'alienness' is crucial. These thoughts are not simply unwanted, as might be the case with, say, a wicked thought that is 'blamed' on the devil or an intrusive obsessional rumination where the person acknowledges ownership of the thoughts even if they blame some outside influence for leading them to think that way.

◆ **Thought block and withdrawal**: Do your thoughts ever stop abruptly so that there are none left in your mind? Are your thoughts ever taken out of your head, as though some outside force were removing them?

The sufferer experiences a sudden stoppage of all thoughts. The experience is passive but abrupt. Thoughts were flowing quite freely before and there is no sense of the individual searching for their thoughts as, for example, happens when one loses one's train of thought at times of stress. In thought withdrawal, the experience is elaborated by a delusion that the thoughts have been withdrawn by someone or something. The experience goes beyond the simple delusion that thoughts are being read in that the client experiences the physical removal of their thoughts.

◆ **Abnormalities in the possession of a 'will'**: Do you feel under the control of some force or power as though you were a robot or a zombie without a will of your own...does this ever make your movements without your willing it or use your voice or your handwriting?

This is perhaps the most dramatic of all symptoms of severe mental illness and also one of the most difficult to elucidate accurately. The essential element is that the sufferer's will is taken over or replaced by some external force or agency and that this is not under the sufferer's control. There are dozens of different ways this may be experienced; for example, the replacement of handwriting, voice, bodily movements and decision making (will). Sufferers often believe they are victims of possession, having been turned into a zombie or puppet of the higher being or force. This is a very different experience from believing that one's life is determined by fate or that God ultimately controls everything. It is not that one's choices are constrained but rather that one has no capacity to choose at all, that any feeling of personal intention has been replaced by the alien will. The only 'normal' situation in which this is seen may be in socially sanctioned trance states – e.g. the automatic writing reported by some spiritualists or the shaman who induces a possession state to communicate with the gods.

Abnormalities in the content of thought (delusions)

A delusion is a belief that is held with absolute and compelling conviction, is not amenable to modification by experience or argument, is largely idiosyncratic, impossible, incredible or false and is described clearly by the sufferer and not simply assented to following a leading question. The idiosyncratic nature of delusional beliefs helps to distinguish delusions from eccentric beliefs that are part of belonging to a particular religious, political or other social group (e.g. accounts of alien abduction).

Delusions are typically subclassified according to their basis in abnormal mood (e.g. delusions concerning sinfulness, catastrophe or guilt in severe depression and grandeur in mania). Such delusions are said to be '*mood congruent*', in contrast to '*incongruent*' delusions, which have no such basis and are thought to be more typical of schizophrenia.

Some commonly encountered delusions include:

◆ Delusions of *reference* in which sufferers are convinced that people are saying things with a double meaning or that items in newspapers, on the TV or in advertisements refer to themselves and that people are tracking them, spying on them or checking up on them in some way.
◆ In delusions of *misidentification*, innocent bystanders seem to be members of the Mafia or the secret police; doctors and nurses are impostors, and even the sufferer's family or friends have been replaced by look-alikes (*Capgras syndrome*).
◆ *Delusions of persecution* are perhaps the most commonly encountered delusions and involve someone or some organisation on a campaign to harm, defame or destroy the sufferer.

Other fairly common delusions include *grandiose identity* (belief that the sufferer is of royal blood, Christ, etc.); *grandiose ability* (chosen for a special mission in life; a mathematical genius, etc.); *guilt, catastrophe, depersonalisation* and *hypochondriacal delusions.*

Some delusions appear as primary experiences in themselves. Their content cannot be explained by other delusions and seems to arise from some very ordinary perception. For example, one patient had a sudden insight that he was God when a traffic light turned from amber to green; another 'knew' the devil was inside his daughter at the instant a flash of lightening reflected in her eyes. These experiences are called *primary delusions* and are thought to be strongly suggestive of schizophrenia. They sometimes occur after a period of perplexity in which the sufferer is vaguely aware that something strange is going on – familiar surroundings seem changed in some way, there is an ominous or threatening atmosphere (*delusional mood*).

3. Assessing perceptions

Questions include:

◆ Is there anything unusual about the way things sound, or look, or smell, or taste?

Perceptual experiences can be diminished, heightened or distorted by severe mental illnesses.

Altered perceptions

Diminished perceptions include the subjective experience of sounds being dull, colours lifeless and tastes bland. *Heightened perceptions* include sounds that are unnaturally clear, a vivid intensity of colours and an intrusive perception of patterns in everyday objects.

Hallucinations

Questions include:

◆ Do you ever hear noises or voices when there is no one around to explain it?
◆ What does the voice say?
◆ Do you ever hear several voices talking about you?
◆ Does the voice(s) comment on what you are doing?
◆ Do they speak directly to you? Give you orders?
◆ Do you ever have visions or see things that others cannot see?
◆ Do you ever notice smells that other people seem not to notice?

Hallucinations are false perceptions in the sense that there is usually no adequate external stimulus to account for the experience. However, some may be triggered, as, for example, the young man who heard the police talking about him while listening to a record. Hallucinations can occur in any sense (hearing, smell, touch, etc.) Hallucinations do not necessarily imply mental illness. For example, fleeting hallucinations are fairly common following bereavement. Those affected see the lost person in some familiar setting (e.g. sitting in their favourite chair), may hear the loved one saying some familiar phrase, feel a comforting pat on the shoulder or catch a whiff of a familiar scent.

Pathological hallucinations are typically grouped according to the sensory modality affected – auditory, visual, tactile, gustatory (taste) and olfactory. They may be highly invasive, frequent and interfere with virtually all normal function or may occur largely in the background with little apparent impact on ordinary functioning.

Auditory hallucinations may involve noises such as the sound of an engine running, electrical hums or rumbling. There may be voices speaking directly to the sufferer (*second person auditory hallucinations*) or talking about the sufferer, either commenting on his behaviour, what he is wearing, etc., or having a conversation with another 'voice' (*third person auditory hallucinations*). The nature of the 'voice' may be congruent with mood, for example tending to be deprecatory with depressive delusions (e.g. 'you are a sinner and will burn in Hell').

Visual hallucinations may be fleeting and fragmentary (e.g. flashes of light), formed objects or even vivid and complex scenes. Visual hallucinations are particularly associated with organic brain diseases such as temporal lobe epilepsy and delirium but also occur in schizophrenia and other functional psychoses.

Olfactory hallucinations include simple hallucinations of perfume or burning and others with delusional elaboration, such as the patient who can smell the poison gas pumped into the room by his persecutors.

Tactile hallucinations include feelings of touch as well as of more noxious insertions of wires or needles into the body.

Gustatory hallucinations include tastes of poison in food. For example, one man claimed to be able to distinguish two varieties of cyanide in the food at a local café – one the 'usual' cyanide poison and the other a special ingredient put in the food by the hospital and designed to be helpful in building a resistance to the toxic effects of the former.

4. Assessing appearance, speech and behaviour

In addition to the multitude of mental experiences that people with severe mental illness may report to the interviewer, their behaviour as described by someone who knows them well or as manifest during the interview also holds important information.

General appearance

This concerns fairly obvious abnormalities – poor self-care, bizarre appearance and dress, and evidence of self-neglect or injury. More specific abnormalities include the presence of *mannerisms, posturing* and *stereotypies.* Mannerisms are odd stylised movements that suggest a special meaning or purpose (e.g. saluting, twirling); posturing is the assumption of an uncomfortable posture for hours at a time and stereotypies are repetitive movements such as rocking, nodding and grimacing. There may also be one or more *inappropriate behaviours,* e.g. giggling, behaving as if hallucinating, acting in an exaggerated, embarrassing or irreverent manner.

Observed abnormalities in speech/thinking

In addition to non-specific changes to the tone, pitch and volume of speech, a number of changes are characteristically associated with severe mental illness. These include *pressure of speech* (a rush of words that can only be interrupted with difficulty), *flight of ideas* (the patient skips from topic to topic with frequent punning and sound associations, although the logic of the associations is usually apparent), *rambling* in a vague and muddled way, *perseveration* (in which a particular theme is repeated over and over so as to be meaningless) and frank *incoherence* (there being no logical connections between one part of a sentence and another – e.g. 'I've seen the end of the circles of the moon through the miracle working of the prophets'). *Poverty of speech* describes a severe form of rambling in that the patient speaks freely but so vaguely that no information is conveyed. This differs from restricted quantity of speech when the patient repeatedly fails to answer at all, requiring repeated prompting, in an extreme form ending in mutism.

Observed abnormalities of affect

This includes observed anxiety, depression, elation and hostile irritability or suspiciousness at interview. More difficult states to identify reliably include *perplexity,* in which patients look puzzled and cannot provide adequate explanations for their abnormal experiences. *Lability of mood* describes frequent and abrupt changes in mood – i.e. at one moment fearful, at the next elated and at another tearful. *Blunted (flattened) affect* involves a global reduction in the usual emotional expressions seen in social interactions. There is little facial expression and speech is flat and emotionless. Apparently distressing topics may be discussed with indifference. *Incongruous affect* refers to a state where the range of emotional expression is normal or even increased but in the opposite direction to that expected (e.g. laughter on hearing distressing news or when discussing a sad event).

Objective orientation, concentration and memory

Finally, it is customary to check out the important cognitive functions of orientation, concentration and memory. Can the respondent account for themselves and are they aware of where they are and the date? Is concentration (typically assessed by counting backwards from 100 in steps of 7) and short-term memory (tested by recall of a fictitious name and address at 5 minutes) intact? Any suggestion of impairments in these areas would call for a more specialised assessment that is beyond the scope of this chapter (but see Kopelman 1994 for an excellent review).

DIAGNOSIS: THE 'TOP-DOWN' APPROACH:

Up to this point we have provided working definitions of the common symptoms of severe mental illness and some suggested questions for accessing these. The next step involves an exploration of how these symptoms cluster together and an outline of modern clinical diagnostic systems as they apply to the functional psychoses. The approach favoured has been described as the 'empirical' approach to diagnosis. It begins with the astute observation that certain complaints that are deviations from normal functioning tend to occur in a pattern that is recognisable between sufferers and over time. These patterns, borrowing from medical roots, are often referred to as 'diagnoses', even though it is accepted that the conditions they describe may not represent diseases in the usual biological model of medicine.

All diagnostic systems in current use have to cope with three facts:

1. A small number of disorders are known to be the result of brain injury or disease.
2. People suffering from these organic brain disorders can experience any of the symptoms described earlier. So people with temporal lobe epilepsy may experience auditory hallucinations, brain tumours may present with symptoms that are entirely indistinguishable from schizophrenia and some people in the early stages of dementia may experience severe depression.
3. Similarly, many symptoms, including hallucinations, thought disorder and delusions, can be caused by the ingestion of psychoactive substances.

All classification systems, therefore, distinguish 'organic' and 'functional' disorders and are arranged hierarchically so that it is only possible to end up with a label of, say, schizophrenia after organic brain disease has been excluded. Many classification systems also apply these hierarchical rules to distinguish functional psychoses from neurotic disorders. The term 'psychotic' is used as a shorthand expression for a disorder in which people's capacity to recognise reality, their thinking processes, judgement and communications are seriously impaired, together with the presence of delusions and hallucinations. For example, schizophrenia takes precedence in diagnosis over bipolar psychoses if criteria for both are present, and affective psychoses in turn take precedence over simple depression and anxiety. Thus each disorder tends to manifest the symptoms of those lower down the hierarchy but not higher up (Foulds 1965, Sturt 1981).

With the exception of the handful of conditions for which a cause is known, most classification systems are descriptive and reflect a consensus between experts as to which symptoms and signs should be put together under one diagnostic grouping. The ICD-10 Classification of Mental and Behavioural Disorders (ICD-10 1992), for example, brought together experts from around the world in order to identify those aspects of mental disorders that were commonly encountered across cultures and for which some consensus could be obtained. The broad result of their deliberations is outlined in Box 7.1. These broad categories are further broken down into a large number of separate conditions, each of which is defined in terms of the commonly encountered symptoms, typical course and cause of the disorder if this is known. Two of these broad categories are of particular concern to this chapter.

Box 7.1 ICD-10 classification of mental and behavioural disorders	
F00–F09	Organic mental disorders (dementia, delirium, organic amnesia)
F10–F19	Psychoactive substance use (intoxication, harmful use, dependency, withdrawal)
F20–F29	Schizophrenia, schizotypal and delusional disorders
F30–F39	Mood (affective) disorders
F40–F48	Neurotic, stress related and somatoform disorders (phobic disorder, OCD, stress reactions, somatoform disorder)
F50–F59	Behavioural syndromes (eating disorder, sleep disorder, sexual dysfunction)
F60–F69	Disorders of adult personality
F70–F79	Mental retardation
F80–F89	Disorders of psychological development (speech disorders, autism)
F90–F98	Behavioural disorders in childhood (hyperkinetic disorder, conduct disorder, emotional disorder, tics, etc.)
F99	Mental disorder not classified elsewhere

Schizophrenia, schizotypal and delusional disorders

Schizophrenia

The concept of schizophrenia owes much to two psychiatrists working at the turn of the 20th century. Emil Kraepelin (1896) noticed the characteristic disturbances in thinking and behaviour that typify the disorder that he labelled 'dementia praecox'. He went on to distinguish this disorder from others that had recurring or periodic episodes involving mania and depression. His view of the disorder was a generally gloomy one; he saw it as having clear biological origins and an almost universally deteriorating course. Few psychiatrists have found the course quite as gloomy as suggested by Kraepelin, although the underlying beliefs in a largely incurable and progressive disease continues to influence classification systems to this day.

Eugen Bleuler introduced the term 'schizophrenia' in 1911 to describe a disorder that encompassed most of the features of Kraepelin's dementia praecox together with some important additional observations. Bleuler maintained the separation from manic depressive psychosis but pointed out that affective symptoms (particularly depression) could also occur in schizophrenia. His concept was based on the identification of a small number of primary symptoms that occurred in all cases. The most important of these were a form of thought disorder (loosening of associations), an autistic withdrawal from reality, ambivalence and incongruous or restricted emotional expression. He regarded hallucinations and delusions as secondary to these primary defects. He had a more optimistic view of the outcome of the illness that partially reflected the tendency of his diagnostic approach to include a broader range of conditions but also may well have reflected a genuine improvement in the outcome of the disorder in Switzerland at that time.

Most modern approaches to the diagnosis of schizophrenia can be traced to one or both of these 'founding fathers' with variations in the way symptoms are packaged together. A possibly helpful distinction has been to distinguish 'positive' and 'negative' symptoms of the illness. Another German psychiatrist, Kurt Schneider (1959), is responsible for what has come to be the definitive list of positive symptoms. These 'symptoms of the first rank' include abnormalities in the possession of thoughts (loud thoughts, thought echo, withdrawal, broadcast, insertion or alien thoughts); auditory hallucinations in the 'third person'; passivity experiences; delusional mood and delusional perception. They carry no special theoretical or prognostic significance but most psychiatrists will diagnose schizophrenia when several of these symptoms are present together and there is no organic brain disease or recent history of drug abuse to explain them. Negative symptoms include apathy, social withdrawal, flattening and narrowing of affect, and poverty of content and production of thought and speech. Negative symptoms are particularly important markers of prognosis, those in whom negative symptoms are prominent tending to do badly in terms of future social function and adjustment. Environmental conditions of understimulation appear to amplify the manifestation of negative symptoms while overstimulation can trigger positive symptoms.

The ICD-10 diagnostic criteria for schizophrenia are set out in Box 7.2. The diagnosis is characterised by distortions in thinking and perception and by inappropriate or blunted affect. Characteristically, the individual's sense of self is eroded so that they come to believe that their most intimate thoughts and feelings are known by others, while mysterious forces seem to be able to influence their actions. Hallucinations are common and perception is usually disturbed in other ways. Thinking becomes vague and obscure and speech may be incomprehensible. Breaks in the train of thought are common and thoughts may appear to be withdrawn by some outside agency. Mood is typically shallow, incongruous or blunted. The onset may be sudden but is

---

Box 7.2 ICD-10 classification of mental and behavioural disorders: schizophrenia

Any one of (a) to (d) or any two of (e) to (h) for 1 month or more, on most days and not due to organic brain disease or alcohol or drug intoxication, dependence or withdrawal.

a. Thought echo, insertion, withdrawal or broadcasting

b. Delusions of control, influence or passivity, clearly referred to body or limb movements or specific thoughts, actions or sensations; delusional perception

c. Third person auditory hallucinations, either as running commentary on actions or discussing the patient among themselves

d. Persistent delusions that are culturally inappropriate and completely impossible

e. Persistent hallucinations when accompanied by fleeing or half-formed delusions without clear affective content, or by persistent overvalued ideas or when occurring every day for weeks or months on end

f. Breaks or interpolations in the train of thought, incoherence, irrelevant speech or neologisms

g. Catatonic behaviour

h. 'Negative' symptoms of apathy, paucity of speech and blunting or incongruity of affect, usually resulting in social withdrawal; not due to depression or neuroleptic medication.

more typically gradual, with the slow emergence of odd ideas and behaviour. The course of the condition is variable.

Subtypes of the disorder are widely recognised. The most common are as follows.

1. **Paranoid**: the clinical picture is dominated by stable persecutory delusions and hallucinations (usually auditory) with only minor changes in affect, volition and speech. Negative symptoms may be present but do not dominate the clinical picture.

2. **Hebephrenic**: affective symptoms are the most prominent with only fleeting or fragmentary hallucinations and delusions. Behaviour is often irresponsible and unpredictable and mannerisms are common. The mood is often shallow or incongruous, accompanied by giggling or self-absorbed smiling, grimaces and vague hypochondriacal complaints. Thought is disorganised and speech rambling and incoherent. 'Negative' symptoms of blunted affect and loss of volition are prominent. This form of schizophrenia usually starts between the ages of 15 and 25 years and tends to have a poor prognosis because the loss of drive leaves the patient aimless and devoid of purpose in life.

3. **Catatonic**: psychomotor symptoms dominate the clinical picture. The patient may alternate between the extremes of excitement and stupor, and adopt constrained attitudes and postures that are maintained for hours at a time. Other features, of negativism, rigidity, waxy flexibility and command automatism may also be present. Catatonia is now very rarely seen in Western industrialised society. This has led some to speculate that catatonic symptoms are a somatic expression of delusions of possession, symbolic thinking and fear, much as bodily symptoms of hysteria are conversion symptoms for anxiety. Both catatonia and hysteria have receded in the West as the population has developed a capacity for expressing emotions in psychological rather than purely bodily terms.

Persistent delusional disorders

Sometimes the only abnormality encountered comprises a long-standing delusion or set of related delusions that are not congruent with any obvious mood disorder. Often these are persecutory but they may also involve jealousy, be hypochondriacal, or comprise beliefs that parts of the body are misshapen or give off an unpleasant smell. The content of the delusion can often be related to the individual's life situation. Depression may be present intermittently and a few cases develop limited olfactory or tactile hallucinations. However, more classical schizophrenic symptoms such as marked blunting of affect or the experience of passivity symptoms are not seen. Onset is commonly in middle age (except for beliefs about having a misshapen body, which tend to begin in early adult life). The ICD-10 diagnostic criteria require symptoms to be present for at least 3 months in the absence of brain disease and clear schizophrenic symptoms.

Acute, transient psychotic disorders

These are among the most controversial disorders, not least because it is not at all clear where these end and schizophrenia begins. The ICD-10 recommends restricting the use of this category to disorders that have an abrupt onset (within 2 weeks) and where there is a typical syndrome and an associated acute stress. There are said to be two typical syndromes. In the first, hallucinations, delusions and perceptual disturbances are marked but highly changeable from day to day and even hour to hour. Emotional turmoil with intense but transient feelings of elation, irritability and anxiety is common. Complete recovery usually occurs within a couple of months. In the second syndrome, the picture is that of schizophrenia, with relatively stable symptoms but with an explosive onset and a very short course with recovery occurring within a month of onset. The validity of these syndromes as separate diagnoses is hotly disputed. It is likely, for example, that they represent one end of the spectrum of schizophrenic disorder or some variant of an affective psychosis or, possibly, of an unrecognised complication of illicit drug use.

Schizoaffective disorder

The concurrence of both typical schizophrenic and affective symptoms is well recognised and presents a challenge to all diagnostic systems. In ICD-10, this is classified in the same broad group as schizophrenia. The affective symptoms can be either depressive or manic in nature. The diagnosis should only be made when the schizophrenic and affective symptoms are prominent within the same episode of illness, either simultaneously or within a few days of each other and not for cases where the client has experienced schizophrenic symptoms and mood symptoms in quite separate episodes of illness. Other systems, such as the American DSM-IV (1994), categorise these disorders separately from both schizophrenia and mood disorders.

Mood (affective) disorders: depression, mania and bipolar disorders

The ICD-10 approach to the classification of mood disorders is shown in Figure 7.1. The fundamental disturbance for all these disorders is a change in mood, which may be to depression or to elation. The mood change is accompanied by changes in level of activity and interests, most other symptoms being secondary to these. The disorders tend to be recurrent, the onset of individual episodes typically being triggered by stressful circumstances.

Manic Episode

	Lower	Hypomania
Severity	⇓	Mania
	Higher	Mania with psychotic symptoms

Depressive episode

Mild (somatic symptoms)

Moderate (somatic symptoms

Severe (psychotic symptoms)

Recurrent Depressive disorder

Bipolar affective disorder

Current manic episode

Current episode depression (somatic or psychotic features)

Persistent mood disorder

Cyclothymia

Dysthymia

Figure 7.1 ICD-10 classification of mood (affective) disorders.

Depressive episode

The client reports low mood, a loss of energy and a reduction in the capacity to enjoy their usual pursuits and activities. There seems to be little point in the future, a desire to die or the contemplation of suicide. The low mood tends to persist, with little change from day to day, and is unresponsive to circumstances. Concentration is impaired and marked tiredness may be common even after slight effort. Appetite is usually disturbed (typically a loss of appetite), as is sleep. The sufferer often feels a sense of failure, worthlessness or guilt.

The ICD-10 takes a rather complex approach to the classification of depression based on symptom patterns and the longitudinal course of the disorder (Box 7.3). Depressive episodes are classified as mild, moderate or severe depending on the number of symptoms and their intensity. Episodes may be further subclassified according to the presence of the 'somatic syndrome' and whether psychotic symptoms are also present.

Severe depressive episodes are characterised by marked distress and agitation, and feelings of guilt and hopelessness, often with suicidal thoughts. Somatic symptoms are always present. Some will experience delusions of guilt, catastrophe or nihilism and auditory or visual hallucinations, hearing,

> **Box 7.3** ICD-10 and depressive episodes
>
> **Core symptoms**
> a. Depressed mood
> b. Loss of interest and enjoyment
> c. Decreased energy or increased fatigability
> d. Reduced concentration and attention
> e. Reduced self-esteem and self-confidence
> f. Ideas of guilt and unworthiness (even in a mild type of episode)
> g. Bleak and pessimistic view of the future
> h. Ideas or acts of self-harm or suicide
> i. Sleep disturbance
> j. Change in appetite and corresponding weight change
>
> **Severity classification**
> ◆ Duration must persist for at least 2 weeks
> ◆ Core symptoms
>   ● mild   at least two of a–c plus at least one of d–j
>   ● moderate   at least two of a–c plus at least three of d–j
>   ● severe   all three from a–c plus at least four of d–j
> ◆ Somatic syndrome – at least four of:
>   ● marked loss of interest/pleasure
>   ● lack of emotional reactions to events
>   ● waking in the morning 2 or more hours before usual time
>   ● depression worse in the morning
>   ● marked psychomotor retardation or agitation
>   ● weight loss of 5% or more body weight in previous month
>   ● marked loss of libido
> ◆ Psychotic symptoms – mood-congruent delusions and hallucinations.

for example, the screams of sufferers in hell or smelling their own body decaying.

The former distinction between neurotic and endogenous depression has been largely abandoned in favour of the view that these represent variations in the severity of disorder and the presence of co-morbid anxiety, and that both types are frequently seen at different times in the same client.

Mania

In a manic episode the client is euphoric, with grandiose ideas and excitement. The elation is accompanied by increased energy, overactivity, pressure of speech and a decreased need for sleep. Self-esteem is inflated, with feelings of improved mental and physical well being. Normal social inhibitions are lost so that sufferers may be over-familiar, intrusive and boorish. They may embark on extravagant schemes, spend money unwisely or display other immoderate behaviour. Heightened perceptions such as seeing colours more vividly are common. As the severity worsens, the client may become angry, intrusive and sexually disinhibited.

When psychotic symptoms occur, these are typically congruent with the prevailing mood. So, for example, the sufferer may claim to have special powers, to be related to royalty or to be God. The pressure of speech may be so great as to make speech unintelligible. Motor excitement may result in profound self-neglect and dangerous states of dehydration and self-neglect.

Mania with psychotic symptoms can be very difficult to distinguish from schizophrenia, the delusions, hallucinations and apparent thought disorder obscuring the underlying change in mood. The distinguishing feature is most often the history of the illness, whether previous episodes of mood disorder have occurred and how the current episode began. The difficulty in diagnosis largely explained the large differences in the 1960s in the observed rates of schizophrenia between America and the UK. It has been suggested that the failure to recognise core symptoms of mania and to wrongly attribute these to schizophrenia is still a problem where ethnic minority groups are concerned.

Bipolar affective disorder

In the ICD-10 classification, this term is applied to those who have experienced at least two episodes of mood disturbance, at least one of which was mania. The ICD-10 subclassifies each episode according to whether the current episode involves mania, depression or both together, the severity of the mood disorder and whether psychotic symptoms are present. Some clinicians distinguish two subtypes of bipolar disorder, referring to type I disorder, for the classic picture of episodes of major depression and episodes of mania, and type II disorder, in which there are episodes of depression and hypomanic symptoms but the latter are never sufficient to meet the criteria for full-blown mania. In both types, recovery occurs to a greater or lesser extent between episodes. The frequency of episodes and remissions is variable between sufferers, although there is a tendency for the remissions to get shorter as time passes.

Persistent mood disorders

Two disorders are recognised. First is *cyclothymia*, in which the sufferer reports a protracted period of unstable mood, lasting at least 2 years and involving multiple episodes of depression and hypomania that were not sufficiently severe to meet criteria for a manic or a depressive episode alone. The disorder is frequently found in relatives of those who have a bipolar affective disorder and some go on to develop this condition eventually. In *dysthymia* the sufferer reports a chronic low-grade depression that does not currently meet criteria for a depressive episode. It is not unusual for this to appear as a prolonged 'tail end' of an earlier depressive episode. To meet ICD-10 criteria, the disorder must have lasted for 2 years with no periods of hypomania and no recoveries longer than a week or two. In earlier classifications, this disorder was commonly referred to as 'neurotic depression' or as a depressive personality disorder. It is not unusual for clients with dysthymia to experience additional episodes of more severe depression, resulting in a so-called 'double depression'.

Co-morbid substance use or 'dual diagnosis'

Since the first edition of this book was produced there has been growing concern about the increase in prevalence of substance use disorder (SUD) in people suffering from severe mental disorders such as schizophrenia and bipolar disorder. People suffering from severe mental disorders seem to be more sensitive to the effects of psychoactive substances as relatively low doses exacerbate the symptoms of their illness and very few can sustain even moderate use without negative consequences. Relapse rates are higher, as are a plethora of social problems linked to poor outcome, including financial and housing difficulties, medication non-compliance, legal problems, violence, depression and suicide. Recent studies in the UK and in North America suggest that as many as a third of people suffering from psychotic disorders are also abusing alcohol or illicit drugs. As in the general population, drug use is more likely in young single men, those with a history of conduct disorder and those of lower educational attainment. Alcohol, cannabis and cocaine are the most common substances and, just as in the general population, their use tends to be a social behaviour. Indeed it may be that the network of users and pushers provides what there is of a social network for some clients. The notion that drug use is a form of self-medication for side effects or for managing illness has only weak support in the literature. Users more commonly report taking substances to combat loneliness, boredom and as a recreational pastime, just as do other substance users who do not suffer from a mental illness.

Screening for co-morbid substance use is critical as it tends to be played down or denied. Clinicians in all mental health settings should ask all clients about substance use and be particularly vigilant when assessing social problems that may have a basis in SUD. People are sometimes more willing to acknowledge past use while playing down current use and the effects of use on their lives. The assessment of SUD involves establishing the quantity of the substance consumed, whether there are features of dependence and the social and medical consequences of consumption. The severity of dependence on a substance is a combination of the strength of the desire to take the substance, the extent to which getting it has become a priority in the client's life; increased tolerance (requiring more or stronger substances to get the same effect) and withdrawal symptoms. These withdrawal symptoms vary across drugs but often include anxiety, depression and sleep disturbance that are relieved by further substance use.

CONCLUSIONS

The diagnostic categories outlined in the last section represent the current consensus of how abnormal mental experiences should be grouped together. These will certainly be modified and eventually abandoned as the biological, psychological and social processes that underpin mental illness are elucidated. In fact, none of the psychoses have ever clearly been demonstrated to be a disease entity in the sense that all sufferers with the particular condition share all the features. But by these criteria, few conditions in medicine qualify. For example, even simple infectious diseases fail in the sense that not everyone who is infected with the same bacillus experiences the same symptoms, course or outcome, while many different infections share common symptoms. For much of medicine the resolution of this conundrum has only followed greater understanding of the basic biological processes that are disturbed by disease and how a particular disturbance leads to specific symptoms. For mental disorders, the equivalent step is now under way with increasingly successful efforts to link the experience of specific symptoms to neuropsychological processes and changes in brain structure. New classifications will eventually emerge from this research but in the meantime, the simple descriptive approach continues to be an essential underpinning of everyday clinical practice.

Cross references

Chapter 4 should be read prior to exploring diagnosis, as stress vulnerability complements this chapter.

References

Bleuler E 1911 Dementia praecox or the group of schizophrenias. International Universities Press, New York

DSM-IV 1994 Diagnostic and statistical manual of mental disorders, 4th edn. American Psychiatric Association, Washington, DC

Foulds G A 1965 Personality and personal illness. Tavistock, London

ICD-10 1992 Classification of mental and behavioural disorders. World Health Organization, Geneva

Kopelman M D 1994 Structured psychiatric interview: assessment of the cognitive state. British Journal of Hospital Medicine 52:277–281

Kraepelin E 1896 Dementia praecox. In: Cutting J, Shepherd M (eds) The clinical roots of the schizophrenia concept. Cambridge University Press, Cambridge, pp 15–24

Schneider K 1959 Clinical psychopathology (trans M W Hamilton). Grune & Stratton, New York

Sturt E 1981 Hierarchical patterns in the distribution of psychiatric symptoms. Psychological Medicine 11:783–794

Annotated further reading

American Psychiatric Association 1992 Diagnostic and statistical manual of mental disorders, 4th edn (DSM-IV). American Psychiatric Association, Washington DC

A comprehensive description of all mental illness from the perspective of American psychiatrists.

Gelder M, Gath D, Mayou R 1989 Oxford textbook of psychiatry, 2nd edn. Oxford University Press, Oxford

One of the leading textbooks of psychiatry. Useful as a reference source to current thinking about mental illness and disorder.

World Health Organization 1992 ICD-10 Classification of mental and behavioural disorders. World Health Organization, Geneva

The internationally agreed definitions of mental illness and disorder. Similar to DSM-IV in approach. Contains helpful descriptions of all the common disorders and should be widely available in most clinical settings.

Kopelman M D 1994 Structured psychiatric interview: assessment of the cognitive state. British Journal of Hospital Medicine 52:277–281

An introduction to clinical tests for the cognitive and memory impairments that accompany organic brain disease. Describes how to carry out both the common tests of memory and concentration as well as some more specialised tests of parietal and frontal lobe disorder.

Mueser K T, Tarrier N 1998 Handbook of social functioning in schizophrenia. Allyn & Bacon, Boston, MA

Multi-author textbook that includes descriptions and examples of the assessment of social function and disability.

Bentall R P 2003 Madness explained: psychosis and human nature. Penguin, Harmondsworth

A recent very readable and thought-provoking challenge to the diagnostic paradigm.

8

Assessments: a rationale for choosing and using

Catherine Gamble and Geoff Brennan

KEY ISSUES

- ◆ Systematic assessment: a rationale
- ◆ Core elements of information gathering
- ◆ Standardised tools glossary
- ◆ Implementation of assessment date: practical guide

INTRODUCTION

The outcome-orientated assessment process is about doing the right thing in the right way at the right time for the client; in combination with clinical expertise and client preferences it involves making sure that the care offered is based on sound evidence. In 1995, the Department of Health discovered that standards of care and provision of service for people who experience serious mental health problems were inadequate. Quality assessment began to be recognised as the cornerstone of effective interventions, indicating directions for treatment at point of contact and a baseline to judge the effect of these interventions. The philosophy of measuring health and social functioning is now heralded as a major aspect of clinical practice (National Institute for Clinical Excellence 2002). However, despite recognising the value and importance of systematic assessment processes, most practitioners are unfamiliar with global needs and more symptom- or need-specific assessments, which leaves them uncertain about how to undertake this task (Dickerson 1997), and/or once an assessment process has been conducted there remains a lack of consensus about how it should be used to plan individual treatment strategies or influence multidisciplinary decision making.

This chapter seeks to address this issue by:

◆ presenting a rationale for undertaking an agreed systematic assessment
◆ outlining the core elements of the information-gathering process
◆ providing a practical guide to choosing and using relevant assessments and outlining standardised tools via a glossary
◆ considering practical strategies to aid interpretation and effective implementation of assessment data.

A RATIONALE FOR UNDERTAKING A SYSTEMATIC ASSESSMENT

Richards and McDonald (1990) argued that 'Any treatment plan is only as good as the information it is based upon'. While meaningful and accurate assessment is essential for all disorders, it is particularly important if an individual's needs are highly complex. The purposes of assessment include:

◆ judging and understanding levels of need
◆ planning programmes of care and observing progress over time
◆ planning service provision and conducting research.

While all the above are interconnected, their focus and use are different. The expansion of each item below highlights this:

Judging and understanding individual levels of need

Ascertaining the individual level of need helps to fulfil the following:

◆ reaching a diagnosis of the main issues/problems
◆ determining the most appropriate interventions
◆ determining individual strengths, abilities and wishes
◆ understanding the culture, family system and social networks.

This is the most recognised focus for practitioners yet it is often carried out with little or no scientific rigour. Assessing need relies on accurate observation and on the use of sound, practical interviewing and rating procedures. It is no longer acceptable to 'think' an intervention is appropriate – we should know and be able to provide evidence to this effect. Indeed, in order to do this thoroughly it is important to incorporate and have an understanding of clients' cultural (see Chapter 19), psychological and biological vulnerabilities, their background, upbringing, social supports and past and current experiences of treatment. The process should also include reviewing their current mental state, mood and level of risk. In this way, assessment procedures will become recognised as an objective, therapeutic way of getting to know the client (Lam et al 1999).

Planning a programme of care and observing progress over time

This aspect of care delivery is particularly important as it helps practitioners and clients demonstrate whether or not interventions are effective. Indeed the process can be likened to pre- and post research studies. Here, a baseline is taken prior to intervention and subsequently reassessed to measure any changes that have taken place. We need to be careful in these situations that we do not confuse change with improvement and that prescribed interventions are not seen to occur within a vacuum. The individual will experience and be subject to many other variables that affect health outcomes – life effects, family environments, drug use, etc. (Repper and Brooker 1998). Nevertheless, a systematic assessment procedure does help to construct a tentative prognostic statement regarding the probability of the success of interventions. The process of setting a baseline and then evaluating change can be carried out using either standard assessment tools or clients' own assessment of their problems and progress. The common feature of both standard tools and client's own assessments is that they encourage a formalised measure of problems or needs. Such measures facilitate a more robust, scientific method of setting baselines and monitoring change occurring for both the individual and their family.

Planning service provision and conducting research

The above have focused on the rationale for undertaking assessments with individuals. However, the process can also help practitioners and their organisations to audit need within whole populations. Reliable, valid instruments help to ascertain need and the subsequent allocation of resources. Indeed they can also help to highlight service user satisfaction and plan for any shortfall in service provision (Lelliot et al 2003). For example, when making the transition from hospital- to community-based care there is a need to collect some basic but extremely important data, such as the length of time people have been in hospital, the levels of dependency, mental and physical disabilities and community provision. Again, as with individual assessment, population need should be continually evaluated to ensure that service provision adapts to any change in need.

Research is an integral part of clinical work, although most people do not recognise it. This is possibly because 'research' is perceived to be the domain of academics who arrive in the clinical area asking to interview staff or clients. Not all practitioners carry out formal research work, so it is seen as elusive, exclusive and outside normal everyday practice. In this instance, however, 'research' should be reframed as a process of 'gathering evidence to facilitate understanding and enhance decision-making'. Within this reframe, it is possible to deduce that all the aforementioned is, in fact, 'research'.

Outlining the core elements of the information-gathering process

The gathering of information should be conducted in a systematic way and comprises a number of core elements. The first step is to gather information from all reliable sources. The procedure which is standard practice in cognitive–behavioural work should elicit the following:

1. *History of psychiatric disorder and past physical history*
   ◆ Family and social background
   ◆ Relevant chronological details of the individual's past treatment, contact with services and risk levels
   ◆ Current medication and its side effects.
2. *Current financial, social functioning and environmental factors.* Particular attention should be paid to the duration and stability of personal relationships and employment, since they have prognostic implications.
3. *The psychiatric diagnosis and current symptoms* should be noted and, more importantly, the degree to which these may influence behaviour. This is of particular relevance because behaviour rather than symptoms is a decisive factor in community survival.
4. Information should be sought that may help to estimate the person's insight into their difficulties.

A summary of what has been learnt can then be encapsulated in a life chart, which:

◆ enables the client to put the illness into personal context
◆ identifies how life experiences and events link to stresses and highlights if there is a pattern
◆ examines responses to treatment over a longer time perspective
◆ provides useful evidence to weigh up the pros and cons of taking medication (Lam et al 1999).

To effectively achieve the above, rather than merely reading old medical notes, it is highly advisable that much, if not all, of the aforementioned process is conducted with the client and their significant others. Indeed, Nelson (1998) recommends meeting before reading medical notes, for the following reasons:

◆ Rather than gaining one narrow professional view it allows you to get a clearer three-dimensional picture of how things seem to client and carer

> **Box 8.1** Summary of areas to be assessed prior to developing a treatment plan
>
> ◆ Risk
> ◆ Physical and mental health status
> ◆ Social needs and functioning
> ◆ Symptomatology and coping skills
> ◆ Quality of life and its effects on others
> ◆ Housing and money
> ◆ Social support
> ◆ Medicine and its effects
> ◆ Work skills and meaningful daily activity

◆ It prevents you from prejudging the issues
◆ It will help you to be more empathetic and ask the appropriate questions naturally
◆ If a person cannot recall some of their experiences and symptoms you can genuinely offer to look in the notes and find out for them.

Box 8.1 covers the core elements that should be considered for assessment.

A PRACTICAL GUIDE TO CHOOSING AND USING STANDARDISED ASSESSMENT TOOLS

Assessment is a complex process, especially when one considers the number of conflicting interests of the various stakeholders involved in care. Therefore we need to be clear about why a particular tool is chosen and be able to present a rationale as to who it is for and what purpose it serves.

The general principles surrounding this issue are:

1. Practitioners should be wary of only choosing and using one type of assessment method. Indeed, one alone is not sufficiently sensitive to assess all aspects of a client's needs. As an example of this, during the process of preparing for a care programme meeting, a practitioner filling in a CPA form asks a client if they have any unmet needs. When the client replies 'Everything is OK' it is reported that all needs have been met. In this instance, a formalised, thorough needs assessment would have to be completed for this statement to be correct.

2. Only valid and reliable methods that are sensitive to change should be used. A scale may be used or frequently referred to in professional journals but it should not be assumed that it is therefore reliable or valid. When

choosing a particular tool, practitioners should ascertain whether it is pertinent, easy to follow and user-friendly. When a tool does not appear to be applicable or relevant to the practice setting, some practitioners have a tendency to cut corners and make modifications. A possible example of this is when an acute ward team tries to adapt a tool designed for use in community settings. Modifying tools can bring the validity and reliability of the instrument, and the results the practitioner identifies, into question. Any modifications should be made on the basis of careful rationale and in consultation with recognised experts in the area. When in doubt as to whether the aforementioned has occurred it is highly advisable to undertake a literature search, read the literature and examine the original evidence.

As mentioned previously, we need to be able to clarify why we are assessing and what purpose the process serves. This is particularly relevant if the assessor is not in a position to act on information gathered. An example would be when we are assessing the side effects of medication and are not able to adapt the medication regime. In this situation we should ask ourselves: Do all relevant parties know that the assessment procedure is taking place? To carry out a side effects assessment without informing medical staff of the concerns that lead to this is not good practice. They may feel coerced into making treatment changes before they feel it is appropriate, or they might have wished to carry out the assessment themselves.

Box 8.2 Questions to ask before commencing an assessment procedure

◆ Am I the best person to carry this out? – if so, why?

◆ Do I have an ulterior motive? – is this assessment in the client's and/or their carers' best interest or has the need been identified by someone else?

◆ Has the assessment been carried out already? – if so, what is the benefit of a new or different assessment and who is it for?

◆ Have I chosen the correct battery of tools or am I making presumptions?

◆ Will the results have implications for another practitioner?

◆ Who else will be informed of the assessment process and the results?

◆ How can I translate what I have learnt to the wider care team and in which format or forum should this occur?

◆ What immediate feedback should I give and how do I summarise this for client and carer?

◆ Are there any subsequent assessments I may need to undertake as a consequence of this initial process? – if so, when should I do it and how do I inform the client that this may happen?

When you can answer the questions in Box 8.2 to your own satisfaction you are ready to formulate a rationale for your client and the care team. The assessment flow chart (algorithm) for people with a psychosis, adapted by Wilcox (2004) from the first edition of this book, is intended to guide practitioners through an overall assessment process.

USE OF THE ASSESSMENT ALGORITHM

The flowchart (Fig. 8.1) **gives** a rough guide to processing assessment in six key areas:

◆ needs
◆ symptomatology
◆ informal carers
◆ structured activity
◆ relapse prevention
◆ carer and user expectations of services.

The flowchart breaks the possible assessment tools down into two categories:

◆ **global**: these are assessments that give an overall view of the area being assessed
◆ **clarifying**: these are assessments that focus on specific aspects, identified from global assessments.

Table 8.2 provides a brief glossary of assessment tools. Table 8.3 provides a 'good practice guide' that identifies a standardised time frame and rationale for assessment completion (Wilcox 2004). The glossary contains additional tools to the flow chart that may be useful to practitioners and clients. Neither the flowchart, the time frame or the glossary should be thought of as a definite prescription. They are simply a guide to thinking and processing.

CARER ASSESSMENT

There is at present some debate as to the assumptions underpinning carer assessment. Early assessment concerned itself with the concept of 'carer burden'. Carer burden assumes that the experience of caregiving is a negative one and, therefore, the assessments looked for areas of difficulty in the caregiving relationship, carer coping and carer health. Practitioners working in the field have realised that the assumption of caregiving as being exclusively negative needs to be challenged. This is not to say that an individual informal carer may not find the experience a negative one but rather that practitioners should not automatically assume that all carers will find caregiving a burden.

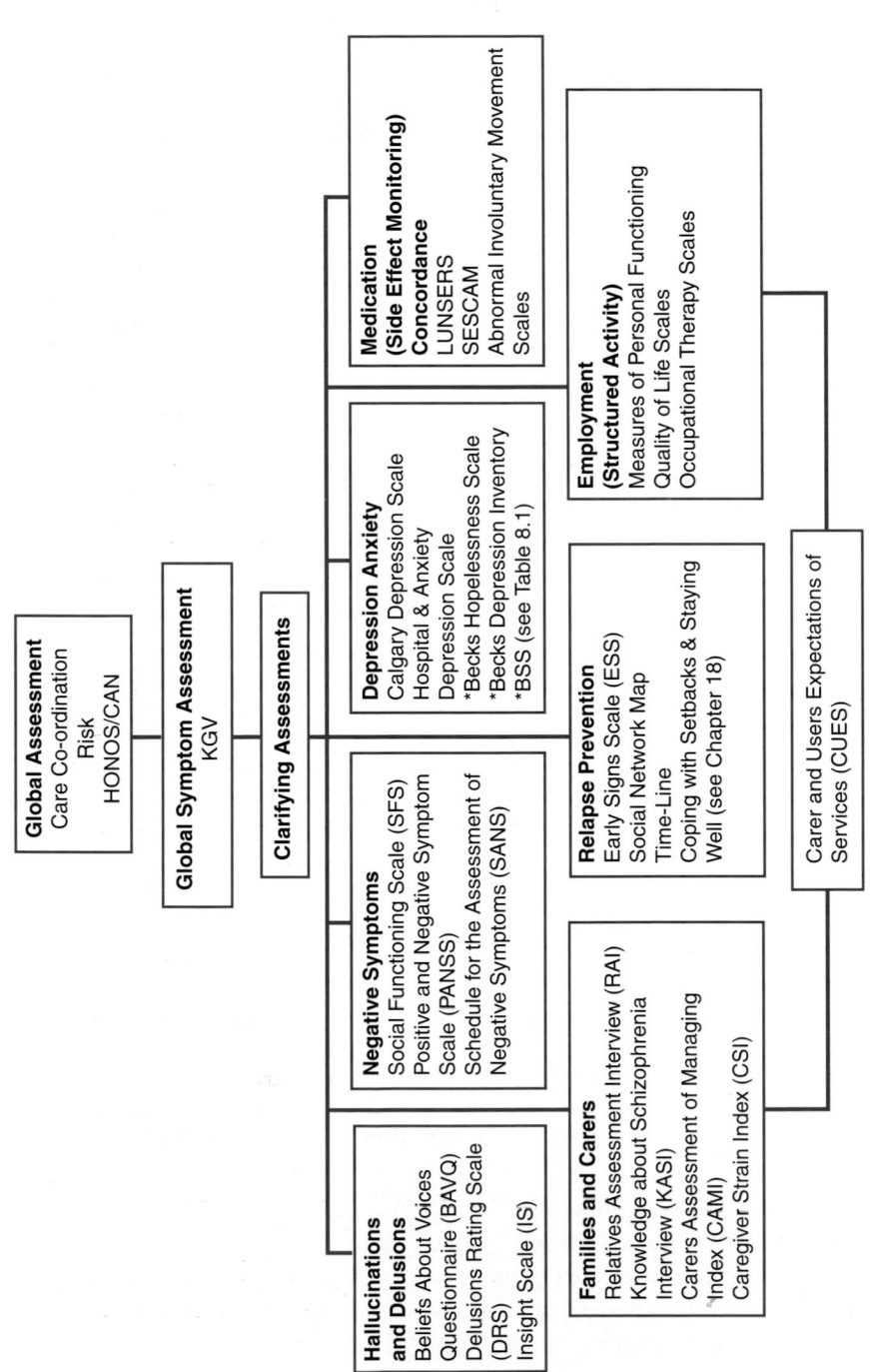

Figure 8.1 Assessment flow chart (algorithm) for people with a psychosis

Table 8.1 A glossary of standardised assessment scales

Assessing	Abbreviation	Suggested scales/tools
Anxiety	BAI	*Beck Anxiety Inventory.* Beck A T, Steer R A 1990 Manual for Beck Anxiety Inventory. Psychological Corporation, San Antonio, TX
	FQ	*Fear Questionnaire.* 16-item scale that rates on a Likert scale, 0 (would not avoid it) to 8 (always avoid it), how much a person avoids certain situations. Can be used as a self-report instrument or when practitioners wish to assess clients' fears re travelling alone or going into crowded shops. Marks I M 1997 Living with fear: understanding and coping with anxiety. McGraw-Hill, Cambridge
Carers	CSI	*Caregiver Strain Index.* Assesses strain using a simple questionnaire. 13 predetermined questions answered as yes or no by interviewee. Has the benefit of being simple and quick, although crude. Robinson B C 1983 Validation of a caregiver strain index. Journal of Gerontology 38:344–348
	CAMI	*Carers' Assessment of Managing Index.* Assesses coping styles and management of stress by questionnaire. Carers are given examples of coping strategies and asked if they use these and if they are effective. Important in that it assumes that carers have coping strategies that can be enhanced. Nolan et al (1995) Carers' Assessment of Managing Index (CAMI): an approach to assessment with family carers. British Journal of Adult/Elderly Care Quarterly 4:822–826
	CUES	*Carers' and Users' Expectations of Services.* Comprehensive questionnaire, which addresses areas such as how to get help, information about care workers, information about the illness, involvement in planning of treatment, relationships, well being, risk and safety. Can be used as a supplement to others described or as a stand-alone, to facilitate discussion and as a baseline to direct intervention. Lelliot P, Beevor A, Hogman G et al 2003 Carers' and users' expectations of services – carer version: a new instrument to support the assessment of carers of people with a severe mental illness. Journal of Mental Health 12:143–152

Table 8.1 A glossary of standardised assessment scales (*cont'd*)

Assessing	Abbreviation	Suggested scales/tools
	ECI	*Experience of Caregiving Inventory.* Assessment of both burden and coping. 66 questions covering ten areas. Eight areas described as 'negative'; two described as 'positive': Negative – difficult behaviours; negative symptoms; stigma; problems with services; effects on family; need to backup; dependency and loss. Positive – positive personal experiences; good relationships with patients. Note that areas such as stigma and relationship with care team are covered. Szmukler G I, Burgess P, Hermann H et al 1996 Caring for relatives with serious mental illness: the development of the Experience of Caregiving Inventory. Society for Psychiatry and Psychiatric Epidemiology 31:137–148
	KASI	*Knowledge About Schizophrenia Interview.* Assesses and evaluates relatives' knowledge, beliefs and attitudes about six broad aspects of schizophrenia: diagnosis; symptomatology; aetiology; medication; prognosis; management. Barrowclough C, Tarrier N 1995 Families of schizophrenic patients: cognitive behavioural intervention. Chapman & Hall, London (see Ch. 13)
	RAI	*Relatives Assessment Interview.* Based on the Camberwell Family Interview but modified for clinical use. Aims to obtain essential information that helps to direct family intervention work. Covers seven main areas, summarised as: client's family background and contact time; chronological history of the illness; current problems/symptoms; irritability; relatives' relationship with client; effects of the illness on relatives. Barrowclough C, Tarrier N 1995 Families of schizophrenic patients: cognitive behavioural intervention. Chapman & Hall, London (see Ch. 13)
	RAISSE	*Relatives Assessment Interview for Schizophrenia in a Secure Environment.* Adaptation of RAI for a secure environment. Assessment based on a semi-structured interview, three areas covered: schizophrenia; admission; visits. While not as robustly researched for validity as other assessments, has been constructed by experts in this area who have tested it in the field. McKeown

Table 8.1 A glossary of standardised assessment scales (*cont'd*)

Assessing	Abbreviation	Suggested scales/tools
		M, McCann G A 1995 A schedule for assessing relatives: the relatives assessment interview for schizophrenia in a secure environment (RAISSE). Psychiatric Care 2:84–88
Depression	BDI	*Beck Depression Inventory.* Beck A T, Ward C H, Mendelson M et al 1961 An inventory for measuring depression. Archives of General Psychiatry 4:561–571
	CDS	*Calgary Depression Scale.* A nine-item structured interview scale developed to assess depression in schizophrenia sufferers. Addington D, Addington J, Maticka-Tyndale E 1993 Assessing depression in schizophrenia: the Calgary Depression Scale. British Journal of Psychiatry Supplement 22:39–44
Delusions	DRS	*Delusions Rating Scale* (Haddock G 1994). Structured interview designed to elicit details regarding different delusional beliefs. Consists of six items which range from the amount of preoccupation to the intensity of distress and disruption. The Delusions Rating scale. Unpublished scale, University of Manchester
	IS	*Insight Scale.* Self-report instrument. Consists of eight statements (four negative and four positive). Clients can agree, disagree or be unsure. Statements include the need for medication; the need to see a doctor; illness recognition, and relabelling of psychotic experiences. Birchwood M, Smith J, Drury V et al 1994 A self report Insight Scale for psychosis: reliability, validity and sensitivity to change. Acta Psychiatrica Scandinavica 89:62–67
Early signs of relapse	ESS	*Early Signs Scale.* Describes problems and complaints people sometimes have prior to relapse. It contains 34 items that describe feelings and behaviours that can occur prior to relapse. Each item is rated on a 0 (not a problem) to 3 (marked problem) scale. Birchwood M, Smith J, Macmillan F et al 1989 Predicting relapse in schizophrenia: the development and implementation of an early signs monitoring system using patients and families as observers. Psychological Medicine 19:649–656

Table 8.1 A glossary of standardised assessment scales (*cont'd*)

Assessing	Abbreviation	Suggested scales/tools
Global Need	CPA	*The Care Programme Approach*. Provides for the continuity of care and accountability for clients and the managing agency. Department of Health 1990 The Care Programme Approach for people with a mental illness referred to specialist psychiatric services. Joint health/social services circular HC(90)23/LASSL(90)11. HMSO, London
	CAN	*Camberwell Assessment of Need*. Rates met and unmet service needs. Phelan M, Slade M, Thornicroft G et al 1995 The Camberwell Assessment of Need: the validity and reliability of an instrument to assess the needs of people with severe mental illness. British Journal of Psychiatry 167:589–595
	GHQ	*General Health Questionnaire*. Measures neurotic symptoms. To ensure that this instrument is not used inappropriately it is not in the public domain. Goldberg D, Williams P 1988 A user's guide to the General Health Questionnaire. NFER-Nelson, Windsor
	HoNOS	*Health of the Nation Outcome Scale*. 12-item health and social functioning scale. Measures risk behaviours, physical problems, deterioration and/or improvement in symptoms and social functioning. Can be completed by the care team and/or the individual practitioner. Wing J, Curtis R, Beevor A 1995 Measurement for mental health: Health of the Nation Outcome Scales. Royal College of Psychiatrists Research Unit, London:33–46
	SFS	*Social Functioning Scale*. Assesses aspects of day-to-day social functioning that are adversely affected by clients' mental health difficulties. It covers seven main areas of social functioning, eg. social engagement; interpersonal behaviour; independence in living skills (competence and performance). It can provide a guide to goals and interventions, as well as measuring progress and outcome. Birchwood M, Smith J, Cochrane R 1990 The Social Functioning Scale: the development and validation of a new scale of social adjustment for use in family interventions programmes with schizophrenic patients. British Journal of Psychiatry 157:853–859

Table 8.1 A glossary of standardised assessment scales (*cont'd*)

Assessing	Abbreviation	Suggested scales/tools
	WSAR	*Work and Social Adjustment Ratings*. Marks I M, Bird J, Brown M, Ghosh A 1986 Behavioural psychotherapy: Maudsley pocket book of clinical management. Wright, Bristol
Hallucinations	BVQ	*Beliefs About Voices Questionnaire*. Chadwick P, Birchwood M 1995 The omnipotence of voices. II: the Beliefs About Voices Questionnaire (BAVQ). British Journal of Psychiatry 166:733–776
	HRS	*Auditory Hallucinations Rating Scale*. Haddock G 1994 An 11 item checklist for auditory hallucinations. Assesses distress control and belief re origin of voices in addition to how client experiences voices. Unpublished scale, University of Manchester
Medication: side effects	LUNSERS	*Liverpool University Neuroleptic Side Effect Rating Scale*. Enables clients to rate their own side effects. A simple measure that covers 51 side effects, ten of which are red herrings, such as hair loss. Day J C 1995 A self rating scale for measuring neuroleptic side effects: validation in a group of schizophrenic patients. British Journal of Psychiatry 166:650–653
	SESCAM	SESCAM combines both the clinician's and the client's assessment of signs and symptoms of abnormal movements and other common side effects. Most importantly, it finishes with two global questions that explore the client's opinion of their medication (which essentially opens the dialogue for joint decision-making on medication treatment). Bennett J, Done J, Harrison-Read P, Hunt B 1995 A rating scale/checklist for the assessment of the side-effects of antipsychotic drugs. In: Brooker C, White E (eds) Community psychiatric nursing: a research perspective, vol 3. Chapman & Hall, London, pp 1–19.
	AIMS	*Abnormal Involuntary Movement Scale*. Commonly used tool that provides a comprehensive assessment of involuntary movements of different body sites. Guy W 1976 ECDEU assessment manual for psychopharmacology, revised edn. US Department of Health, Education and Welfare, Washington DC.

Table 8.1 A glossary of standardised assessment scales *(cont'd)*

Assessing	Abbreviation	Suggested scales/tools
Substance abuse	CMRS	*Case Managers Rating Scale.* Contains a five-point scale with each point operationally defined in terms of levels of substance abuse and their biopsychosocial consequences (see Ch. 14). Drake R, Noordsy F 1994 Cases management for people with coexisting severe mental disorder and substance use disorder. Psychiatric Annals 24:427–431
	LDQ	*Leeds Dependence Questionnaire.* Designed to detect and rate the severity of illicit substance abuse. Contains ten items rated on a four-point scale (see Ch. 14). Raistrick D, Bradshaw J, Tober G et al 1994 Development of the Leeds Dependence Questionnaire (LDQ): a questionnaire to measure alcohol and opiate dependence in the context of a treatment evaluation package. Addiction 89:563–572
	MAST	*Michigan Alcoholism Screening Test.* Designed to detect problematic alcohol use by rating its effect on an individual's psychical and social circumstances (see Ch. 14). Selzer M 1971 The Michigan Alcoholism Screening Test: the quest for a new diagnostic instrument. American Journal of Psychiatry 127:1653–1658
Suicidality risk	BHS	*Beck Hopelessness Scale.* Beck A T, Steer R A 1988 Manual for Beck Hopelessness Scale. Psychological Corporation, San Antonio, TX
	BSS	*Beck Scale for Suicide Ideation.* Beck A T, Steer R A 1993 The Beck Scale for Suicide Ideation. Psychological Corporation, San Antonio, TX
Symptoms	BPRS	*Brief Psychiatric Rating Scale.* Well-validated measure of general psychiatric symptoms. Originally contained 16 items, nine scored on verbal responses (somatic concerns, anxiety, guilt, grandiosity, depressive mood, hostility, suspiciousness, hallucinatory behaviour and unusual thoughts), the other seven on observation at time of interview. Scoring is on a Likert scale from 1 (not present) to 7 (extremely severe). Developed by Overall J E, Gorham D R 1962 The Brief Psychiatric Rating Scale. Psychological Reports 10:799–812

Table 8.1 A glossary of standardised assessment scales (*cont'd*)

Assessing	Abbreviation	Suggested scales/tools
	KGV	*Manchester Symptom Severity Scale.* A simplified version of the BPRS. It has recently been radically revised by Stuart Lancashire at the Institute of Psychiatry. It is a semi-structured psychiatric assessment tool that uses a phenomenological battery of questions. It identifies the type and severity of psychiatric symptoms and contains 12 items. The first five are rated on verbal responses, the remainder are rated on observation at interview. Krawiecka M, Goldberg D, Vaughn M 1977 A standardised psychiatric assessment scale for rating chronic psychotic patients. Acta Psychiatrica Scandinavica 55:299–308
	PANSS	*Positive and Negative Syndrome Scale.* 30-item scale for practitioners. Seven items address negative symptoms and seven positive symptoms. The remaining 16 focus on general psychopathology. Some items are based on interview, others on observation. Each item is rated using a Likert scale (0–6 with 6 most severe). Kay S R, Fiszebein A, Opler L A 1987 Positive and Negative Syndrome Scale. Schizophrenia Bulletin 13:261–276
	SANS	*Schedule for the Assessment of Negative Symptoms.* Assesses 20 of the negative symptoms: affective flattening, alogia, avolition/apathy, anhedonia/asociality and attention. Symptoms are rated on a 0–5 scale of increasing severity. Andreasen N 1982 Negative symptoms In schizophrenia: definition and reliability. Archives of General Psychiatry 39:784–788

These instruments are not in the public domain. Some organisations and institutions have a licence to use them for clinical practice and research purposes. This should be clarified prior to use. If not, they can be purchased from the Psychological Corporation, San Antonio, TX, USA.

Table 8.2 A good practice guide and time frame

Standard	Rationale
A KGV(M) Symptom Scale will be completed as soon as therapeutically possible (not exceeding 8 weeks) following acceptance of a service user on to a clinician's caseload and repeated when necessary (but not exceeding 6 months between assessments)	A KGV assessment provides a global measure of common psychiatric symptoms (feelings/thoughts) experienced with a psychosis. The framework ensures that important questions are asked and a consistent measure of symptoms is provided. The KGV is a valid tool with high interrater reliability. A 6-monthly assessment provides a progress benchmark for evaluation of interventions
Clarifying assessments will be completed as soon as is therapeutically possible and repeated when necessary (but not exceeding 6 months between assessments)	Clarifying assessments outlined in the algorithm (Fig. 8.1) provide a measure of specific symptoms identified in the KGV. A 6-monthly assessment provides a progress benchmark for evaluation of interventions or in the initial assessment and formulation
A Time Line will be formulated with the service user as soon as is therapeutically possible and updated prior to each care coordination review	A Time Line provides a chronological account of life experiences and psychiatric events. It enables a collaborative and shared picture of the service user's life history in relation to their psychiatric episodes to be easily constructed. The process of developing a Time Line aids engagement, assists in the therapeutic process of psychoeducation, facilitates the understanding of the Stress Vulnerability Model, helps develop a normalising rationale and assists in organising relapse prevention strategies
A Social Network Map will be formulated with the service user and updated when necessary and before each care coordination review	Developing a Social Network Map is a graphical exercise between service user and clinician to map out people the service user has contact with, including frequency and relationship quality. Doing so enables the identification of relationships and social networks

Table 8.2 A good practice guide and time frame (*cont'd*)

Standard	Rationale
A Liverpool University Neuroleptic Side Effect Rating Scale (LUNSERS) should be completed for anyone receiving antipsychotic medication and should be repeated where necessary and before each care coordination review	Neuroleptic medication is an important intervention in the treatment of psychosis. Despite the clear benefits of medication, service users can experience adverse side effects that are not only distressing but are also a main reason for not taking medication, which often contributes to a relapse. The LUNSERS is a valid and reliable self-rating scale for the measurement of neuroleptic side effects, which can lead to an effective management of these side effects, improve concordance, reduce relapse events and improve quality of life for the service user
Once the assessments have been completed an Outline Formulation should be developed with the service user and recorded in the case notes	A formulation is important in providing a picture or overall map of the individual's situation. Issues and problems can be prioritised and a plan of intervention devised. Formulations help relate theory to practice, e.g. Stress Vulnerability Model, CBT and family interventions
Coping with setbacks and staying well. Each service user will have a detailed Relapse Prevention Plan including the identification of relapse indicators (early warning signs) and an agreed current management plan	Each relapse in psychosis brings increased likelihood of future relapse, residual symptoms and accelerates social disability. Service users can experience prodromal symptoms prior to a relapse that may be particular to that individual. By recognising these symptoms and responding quickly, effectively and appropriately the risks associated with relapse can be greatly reduced
Families and carers will be offered information, advice and psychoeducation regarding psychosis, PSI, medication management, symptom management and relapse prevention strategies (see Ch. 13 for more detail)	The important role of families and carers cannot be underestimated. To enable them to fulfil this role effectively they need to be informed and supported

Table 8.2 A good practice guide and time frame (*cont'd*)

Standard	Rationale
Families and carers should be offered opportunities to have their needs assessed and the relevant care plans developed	Providing the relevant information/ education and level of support may help reduce carer burden, thereby helping to improve the service user's quality of life, support and clinical outcomes (recovery)
Care coordinators will facilitate the opportunity for the service user to explore, develop and engage in structured activity and work experience	The ability and opportunity to engage in structured purposeful activity and occupation plays a crucial role in relapse prevention but also develops the person's confidence, raises self-esteem and reduces social isolation, which helps improve clinical outcome and enhance quality of life

The danger here is that, if we assume that carers are burdened and only ask about negative aspects, we will invariably create a bias. An assumption that closely follows the burden assumption is that carers are unable to cope. Many carers cope well and create environments in which not only is the client valued and respected but carers themselves are able to maintain their health and remain in control of very difficult situations.

Newer assessment tools have attempted to address some of these issues by assessing positive attributes within the caregiving relationship. The introduction of the positive aspects tends to be called 'coping' rather than 'burden'. Any assessor undertaking informal carer assessment needs to be aware of their own assumptions as to the caregiving role and not dismiss, reduce or ignore any positive coping or attitude expressed by informal carers as these aspects are crucial in understanding the balance between the burden informal carers face and the personal strengths they can marshal to help them cope. In many ways, this topic mirrors the strengths versus deficit debate within client assessments where some assessments assume that a person will be disabled and handicapped by illness and therefore find this to be the case, whereas other assessments assume that clients will have a range of strengths they can use to control the illness. In this case also, assessors need to be cautious that the tool they use and the assumptions they have do not introduce a bias. (For more strategies re carers' needs and involvement in care, see Chapters 2, 13 and 18.)

PRACTICAL STRATEGIES TO AID INTERPRETATION AND EFFECTIVE IMPLEMENTATION OF ASSESSMENT DATA

One of the main issues for practitioners is what to do with the information once it has been obtained. All too often, practitioners encourage relatives and clients to undertake and complete assessments. However, once this procedure has occurred, the majority of the information gets filed into medical notes and is rarely referred to or looked at again. This can be very frustrating and can lead to the perception that a rigorous assessment process is a waste of time for all concerned. Therefore, practitioners need to present a clear rationale and be able to demonstrate that assessments are not paperwork exercises that are just about statistics. Indeed, they can in fact play a useful part in care, as results from well-constructed scales can be discussed with clients and carers and incorporated into empowering, needs-led treatment plans.

To successfully achieve this it is important to become familiar with the tools and manuals (e.g. administration and scoring). In this way you will be in a better position to value the assessment procedure and understand the reasons for conducting it. A thorough assessment process can be a rewarding experience for the client, the carer and the practitioner. It can empower all concerned. In many instances, clinicians who do not routinely complete formalised assessments have reported being amazed and slightly ashamed by how little they knew and how much clients have been willing to tell them. Such positive experiences have been achieved because the aforementioned practitioners have 'owned' and familiarised themselves with a battery of assessment tools and have been able to wisely interpret the data they have obtained. For example:

> *Over the last couple of weeks, we have completed a number of assessments. One helped us to identify what needs you have generally (HoNOS), and some of the symptoms you are currently experiencing (KGV). The third one gave me an idea of how you and your family are coping at the moment (RAI). I know this seemed like a long process, but I was keen to obtain as clear a picture as possible. The overall process has helped us identify that you have numerous coping strategies and strengths. For example, if we look at your social functioning (SFS), it shows us that you cook, clean, take care of your home and personal appearance and you have a large, supportive social network. Your sister and Dad also reported that they feel you are coping very well. However, one area that the process has illuminated is that*

you wish to be more independent. Should we therefore think about how to address the difficulty you identified about using public transport and going out alone?

It is important to know how to feed back information to the client and informal carer and not to overload them. Indeed, the example above illustrates that is not necessary to flood clients. Information obtained from baseline assessments can be gradually fed back and used on other occasions as and when the need arises.

Not being over-zealous is something that is learned over time. The assessment process should be regarded as a therapeutic intervention. What may be tolerable for one client will not be for another and all practitioners should strive to ensure that the overall process is flexible and tailor-made to suit individuals. There will be cases when clients do not wish to participate. There are numerous reasons for taking this stance, such as lack of rapport, language (i.e. does not speak fluent English), literacy skills, past experiences and/or practitioners making assumptions or jumping to the intervention stage before really identifying what the real need is for the client. Having said this, clients come to services for specific interventions; for example, for help with completing Disability Living Allowance forms and housing. In this situation it is advisable to assist the client to achieve these aims. This engages them and shows that their needs will be addressed. Further assessment can then take place naturally; for example, in the above situation, saying to the client 'Now we have done this – should we check if you have any other unmet needs?'

CONCLUSION

Assessments are an integral part of any practitioner's work. In practice, clients and their carers complain that they repeat the same information over and over again. This indicates that practitioners do not follow a structured process that leads naturally on to intervention. This chapter should guide and clarify the process. The overall aim of assessment is as much to engage clients in the process of treatment as it is to identify their needs and problems. It cannot be emphasised enough that old-fashioned qualities, such as respect, empathy, politeness, punctuality and genuine concern can help to create collaboration and understanding.

Cross references

For additional practical strategies and further implementation ideas see:

Chapter 9 Consolidating the assessment process

Chapter 10 Assessing risk

Chapter 19 Cultural issues

References

Dickerson F B 1997 Assessing clinical outcomes: the community functioning of persons with serious mental illness. Psychiatric Service 48:897–902

Lam D H, Jones S, Haywood P, Bright J A 1999 Cognitive therapy for bipolar disorder: a therapist's guide to concepts, methods and practice. Wiley, London

Lelliot P, Beevor A, Hogman G et al 2003 Carers' and users' expectations of services – carer version: a new instrument to support the assessment of carers of people with a severe mental illness. Journal of Mental Health 12:143–152

Nelson H 1998 Cognitive behavioural therapy with schizophrenia: a practical manual. Stanley Thornes, Cheltenham

National Institute for Clinical Excellence 2002 Clinical Guideline 1. Schizophrenia: core interventions in the treatment and management of schizophrenia in primary and secondary care. NICE, London

Repper J, Brooker C 1998 Difficulties in the measurement of outcome in people who have serious mental health problems. Journal of Advanced Nursing 27:75–82

Richards D, McDonald B 1990 Behavioural psychotherapy: a pocket book for nurses. Heinemann, Oxford

Wilcox A 2004 Clinical governance lead. Newcastle, North Tyneside and Northumberland Mental Health NHS Trust, Newcastle upon Tyne

Annotated further reading

Harris N, Williams S, Bradshaw T 2002 Psychosocial interventions for people with schizophrenia: a practical guide for mental health workers. Palgrave, Basingstoke

Chapter 8, by Julie Everitt and Ronald Siddle on the assessment and therapeutic interventions with positive psychotic symptoms, complements this chapter.

9

Consolidating the assessment process: the semi-structured interview

Jayne Fox and Catherine Gamble

KEY ISSUES

◆ Formulating assessment process
◆ Introduction to semi-structured interview strategy
◆ Problem and goal statement formulation
◆ Clinical case examples

INTRODUCTION

The previous chapter highlighted how to choose and use appropriate assessments. Through this process it was possible to identify that an accurate assessment of the client's main problems is an essential requirement prior to the application of any intervention. Indeed, in cognitive–behavioural terms this provides the foundation on which collaborative, therapeutic interventions are formulated and built. Furthermore, in almost all cases, a large part of any assessment process requires the practitioner to help the individual learn how to identify and work on specific areas of need, so they are more able to monitor their progress in achieving lifestyle adjustments.

By introducing the semi-structured interview technique, this chapter aims to demonstrate how the assessment process can be consolidated and funnelled down to formulate a clear statement or hypothesis, so that Measurable, Achievable, Realistic, Specific (MARS) goals and plans of care can be developed.

THE SEMI-STRUCTURED INTERVIEW

This type of interview is commonly associated with cognitive–behavioural approaches; its simple principles, format and aims make it relatively easy to apply as it involves dealing with the client's thoughts, feelings and behaviours at the time (Clinton & Nelson 1996). In addition, it provides a framework for the total assessment as it can function to establish rapport and gain knowledge of characteristic patterns of living and coping behaviours (McFarland & Thomas 1990, Farrington & Telford 1996). When considering problems associated with serious mental illness, Birchwood & Tarrier (1992) postulated that 'a thorough assessment of the patient's symptomatology and coping skills should be covered through a semi-structured interview'. It is important that the assessor appreciates the client's understanding of their problems or difficulties. While it may be more straightforward to plan interventions according to 'textbook' procedures, this does not necessarily lead to a successful outcome. Anecdotal evidence suggests that, far too often, clients with serious mental illness feel uninvolved in their care as it does not reflect their personal needs or aspirations.

In light of this, the semi-structured interview is a sensible choice to consolidate the assessment process. However, the reader must understand that, while the interview gives a clear overall picture of the individual's main problems or difficulties, the assessor will need to complement this process with other tools designed to elicit specific information.

Beginning the process

Prior to outlining the structure of this interview it is important to understand some of the underlying principles associated with this approach.

1. Be pragmatic

The assessor should approach the interview with a clear outcome in mind. The intention is to establish what problems currently cause this individual difficulty in their day-to-day life and what the implications or consequences of this are. In short, emphasis is placed on practical consequences of problems rather than why they exist or how they began.

2. Expectation

Richards & McDonald (1990) argued that 'clients will have expectations of us, but they will also be influenced by what we expect from them'. In light of this

It is important to demonstrate positive assumptions about the client. These can be summarised as:

◆ This person will be responsive to the help that is offered and they will be working with you in a partnership that allows them to have control and take responsibility
◆ This person tries to cope with the problems they have and they are real problems that do not exist merely because the individual is not trying to help themselves
◆ This person is honest and is telling the truth about their problems. Spending time trying to prove that the client is not being honest about their problems is pointless and potentially damaging to the therapeutic relationship, and contradicts the underlying principles of this procedure (see Ch. 6).

Questioning style

The main aim of this interview is to allow the client an opportunity to describe their problem as they experience it. This information is then formulated into a short sentence, known as a problem statement. Once this is completed the client is able to identify their own goals, describing what they wish to achieve or work towards. Examples of these goals will be described later in this chapter.

The primary role of the assessor in this process is to enable the individual to 'tell their story' by asking a series of questions, beginning with simple open-ended questions and then clinching specific details by asking closed questions. This is known as the funnelling technique (Fig. 9.1).

By applying this approach to questioning throughout the semi-structured interview a clear and accurate definition of the main problem is established. Note how in the example in Figure 9.1 the questions begin by being open and then, based upon information given in responses, become more specific and details are gathered. An outline of the interview format containing information from a client assessed by one of the authors is described below. In addition, examples are also given of how questions could be formulated. To enhance the process you should be mindful of the suggestions given in Box 9.1.

Introduction

'Over the last few weeks we have conducted a number of assessments; these have identified numerous strengths, and your needs as being (see p. 129) ...

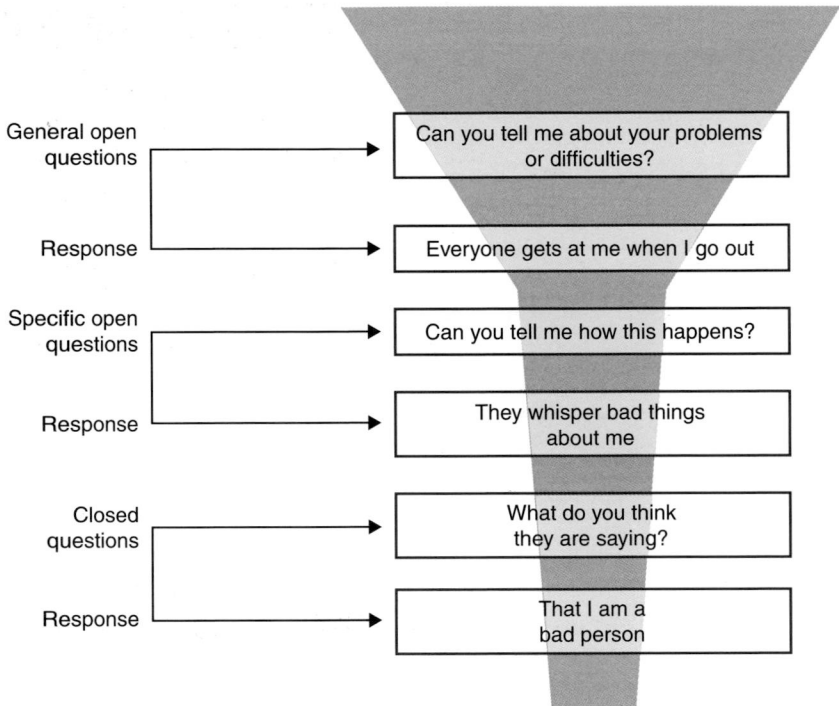

Figure 9.1 The funnelling technique

and currently you are experiencing the following problems with .... By gathering this information I have been able to deduce that we should be thinking of working on the following' (list the main priority areas).

Interview format

1. The five 'Ws'

Once the client has chosen the specific area they wish to work on, the next part of the process (prompted by questions What? When? Where? With? and Why?) allows them to begin describing their problem in more detail, in their own words. In addition, any patterns or predictors of the problem can also be established. Once this is completed you should have a fairly detailed description of the main problem, as the client perceives it (Table 9.1).

2. FIND

Once the initial details of the problem have been described it is now time to funnel down and gather some more specific information (Table 9.2). This

> **Box 9.1** Top tips for successful implementation
>
> ◆ Establish mutually agreed boundaries at the beginning. For example, introducing yourself and your role, the purpose of the interview, agenda and time frames and the possibility of potential or actual distractions.
>
> ◆ Encourage the client to expand on information by asking the question – Is there anything you would like to add?
>
> ◆ Keep questions simple, avoid asking double barrel questions and allow the client time to answer.
>
> ◆ Avoid using jargon. If possible, try and use similar language to that of the client.
>
> ◆ Recap information to gain clarity and more detail. This is also a good strategy to use when the interview loses its flow.
>
> ◆ Take written notes. It is hard to remember information unless you write it down. Most clients will not object but remember to ask permission and keep note taking discreet.
>
> ◆ Do not be afraid to revisit the process as this will help to clinch information that previously may have got missed (Romme & Esher 2000)

helps build a clearer picture of the problem and how it impacts upon the client's day-to-day life.

3. A behavioural analysis

Arguably the most central and perhaps important part of this interview, a behavioural analysis allows the individual to describe their problem in three parts. If this part of the interview is fully completed it will prove to be useful when planning interventions as it draws out strategies that are used to help cope with the impact of the problem. In addition, the individual's emotional experience of the problem can be captured during this part of the interview by applying a three-systems analysis (Richards & McDonald 1990).

An example of a behavioural analysis is as follows:

Antecedent: 'What happens before, or what triggers the problem?'
Response: 'When I am getting ready to go to the day centre. I begin to feel scared.'

If necessary, further understanding can be clinched by asking the client to return to the last time they had this experience and then to recall their feelings, thoughts and behaviour before, during and after it, using an ABC (Antecedents, Behaviours, Consequences) analysis. An example is given in Table 9.3.

Table 9.1 The five 'Ws'

Question	Response
What: what do you see as being your main problem?	Every time I go out people talk about me. They make fun and try to stop me from doing things.
When: when is the problem worst?	Its bad at night time, when it starts to get dark.
When is the problem better/does the problem improve?	In the mornings it's better, because I can see better.
Where: Where/in what situations is the problem most difficult?	At the day centre they talk about me and I don't like it there.
Are there any places/situations where the problem is better?	At home my brother talks to me and this helps.
With: Are there any people who help you with the problem?	My brother helps and so does my mum; they try to understand.
Are there any people who hinder you or make things worse?	The day centre people upset me – they make things worse for me.
Why/consequences: what do you think causes/maintains the problems?	People don't like me – the world is a bad place sometimes and is full of bad people.

NB The 'why' question may elicit delusional thinking in some clients; treat this with as much respect as you would any other question. It should therefore only be asked with caution, as some clients find it very difficult to answer – it can be as overwhelming as being asked 'Why are you mad?' – 'Because aliens stole my soul, they keep hassling me and I don't know why they have picked me … I must be very evil.'

Table 9.2 Funnelling down (FIND)

Question	Response
Frequency: How often does the problem you have described occur?	Every day, except Sunday. On Sundays I can stay at home and read my magazines.
Intensity: How intense do you feel as a result (on a scale of 0–100)?	At the day centre it's really bad, about 100% bad I would say.
Number: Are there any patterns or particular times it occurs?	On Tuesdays, the manager is always there and it happens a lot but I can't remember exactly.
Duration: How long does it last?	Ages – a long time. About 2 hours.

Table 9.3 An ABC analysis

'So I can get a better understanding of your experiences, it would be useful if we looked back at the last time ... occurred'			
	Antecedents	During	**Consequences**	**With whom/ where**
Physical things you noticed: e.g. sweaty palms, knotty feeling in stomach			
Behaviour/s you noticed: e.g. avoiding going out, avoiding people			
Cognition – things you found yourself thinking: e.g. 'I can't do this'			

4. The impact of the problem

The next part of the interview involves questions designed to elicit the impact and consequences of the problem (Table 9.4). While some of this information may already have been gathered, it is important to clarify the information as this will form part of the overall problem definition and will also act as a springboard to meaningful goals.

PROBLEMS AND GOALS

Capturing the interview information

Once all the information has been gathered, it is then summarised into a short, structured sentence known as a problem statement. In addition, the client is asked to describe the things they wish to work towards that, when achieved, would indicate that the impact or severity of the problem had reduced. These are known as goal statements. This is an important process, as the semi-structured interview provides a wealth of information that, while useful, can be hard to evaluate. Summarising in this way allows the health professional and the client to objectively evaluate the ongoing severity of the problem and how close they are to achieving the agreed goals.

The following guide can be used to establish meaningful problem and goal statements.

Table 9.4 Impact and consequences

Question	Response
Behavioural excesses: what things do you do more of because of the problem?	I stay at home more often. I sleep a lot and watch TV
Deficits: What things do you do less of because of the problem?	I don't see my friends or go out with my brother any more.
Modifiers: Is there anything that you do to help?	I get my mum to come out with me. Sometimes I walk around with my hands over my face or close my eyes.
Onset: When did it begin? Anything significant happen?	When I was at school, the others in my class used to say things about me.
Fluctuations: Has it got better at all?	At Christmas after I came home from hospital it was OK. They stopped talking about me.
Has it got worse at all?	It gets worse every day.
Past treatment: Describe any past treatment you have had. Did it help?	Tablets, which I hate. They make my mouth dry. Mum says they help and so does the doctor but I hate them.
Impact: How would you sum up the impact this problem has on your lifestyle?	It makes me scared all the time. Because I am scared I don't see my friends. I am lonely.
Motivation: Are there any things you would like to do that this problem currently prevents?	Go to the pub with my friends. Try and get back to college.

Problem statements

Problem statements should focus directly on difficulties that:

◆ have been identified by the client during the semi-structured interview
◆ have been written, whenever possible in the client's own words; this helps reduce the use of jargon and provides meaning for the client
◆ describe the problem in observable behaviours – for example, Michael described feeling afraid and was encouraged to say how this affected the way he behaved, thus transferring 'feeling afraid' into 'avoiding going to the day centre'
◆ indicate the impact and consequences the problem has on the client's lifestyle.

As described above, each problem statement should include an accurate description of the current presenting problem, its immediate impact and subsequent consequences.

Goal statements

Goal statements should:

◆ describe what the client would like to achieve in relation to the identified problem
◆ describe a behaviour that, when consistently implemented, would indicate a reduction in problem severity
◆ where possible, describe a positive change to be worked towards as opposed to simply stopping certain behaviours; for example, during interview Michael described using alcohol as a way of blocking out his voices, although this led to additional problems; it was important when formulating goals with Michael that they were aimed at achieving alternative coping strategies, such as listening to music, as opposed to solely refraining from alcohol consumption
◆ be reflective of something that the client wishes (and can be realistically expected) to achieve
◆ indicate how frequently and for how long the behaviour would be sustained; this helps to ensure some permanency, as opposed to 'one-off' goal achievement.

Table 9.5 demonstrates a guide that can be used to help with formulating problem and goal statements.

A good start when writing the problem statement with a client is to ask them to try and sum up in one sentence what they believe their problem is.

Table 9.5 A guide to problem statements and goal statements

| **Problem statement guide** | | |
Problem definition	**Impact**	**Consequences**
Avoids going out. Believes others say bad things.	Stays at home in bedroom.	Feels lonely and isolated.

| **Goal statement guide** | | | |
The behaviour	**Conditions**	**Frequency**	**Duration**
Attend day centre	Go to groups	Three times per week	12 hours

As they talk through it, you could fill in the boxes and pull together a statement. This should then be read back to the client to ensure that it fulfils the check list.

The same can be applied to goals except you could ask the client to think of something they would like to work towards which this problem currently prevents.

Measuring problems and goals

Increasingly, health professionals are being asked to demonstrate the effectiveness of their interventions and subsequently the use of clinical measures to monitor treatment outcomes are becoming more routine and popular with clients, as systematic reviews conducted at baseline, mid- and postintervention provide overt evidence that change can occur. Indeed, Marks (1986) argued that the evaluation of any treatment requires some predetermined criteria for outcome and suggests that problems and goals can be measured using a 0 to 8-point scale.

Boxes 9.2 and 9.3 show example problem and goal statements, along with the rating scale.

Problems and goals should be rated to give a baseline rating and then reassessed at intervals prearranged by the client and assessor. It is important that the client understands what and why they are rating; this is best achieved by either asking them to read or reading to them the sentence

---

Box 9.2 Problem statement

Avoidance of going out because I believe others say bad things about me leading to staying at home resulting in being lonely.

Rating scale
This problem interferes with my daily activities:

0 ——— 1 ——— 2 ——— 3 ——— 4 ——— 5 ——— 6 ——— 7 ——— 8

Does not   Slight   Definite   Often   Severe

    Assess

Date

Client

Assessor

directly above the rating scale shown in Box 9.3. Both the client and the assessor should rate the problem and goals as this helps demonstrate mutual and equal commitment. In addition it gives focus to feedback at subsequent sessions.

Top tips for are listed in Box 9.4.

Box 9.3 Goal statement

To attend the day centre, and to go to the groups, remaining 2 hours three times weekly.

Rating scale
My progress towards achieving this goal:

0 ——— 1 ——— 2 ——— 3 ——— 4 ——— 5 ——— 6 ——— 7 ——— 8

Complete success   75%   50%   25%   No success

    Assess

Date

Client

Assessor

Box 9.4 Top tips for problem and goals formulation

◆ Do not write problem and goal statements for the client – this defeats the object and contradicts the philosophy of this process. It is more appropriate to work with the client to help them achieve this.

◆ Be flexible: while it is desirable that the statements follow the suggested format, adherence to this should not take precedence over a statement that has meaning to the client.

◆ Be prepared to compromise – remember, these are the client's goals, not yours.

◆ Do not consider the goal statement to be complete until you have discussed with the client a step-by-step plan on how to achieve it and reviewed the potential pitfalls they may encounter – if this feels overwhelming at this stage, it is highly unlikely that the goal will be achieved, so you need to return to an earlier stage in the formulation of the goal.

References

Birchwood M, Tarrier N 1992 Psychological management of schizophrenia. Wiley, Chichester

Clinton M, Nelson S 1996 Mental health and nursing practice. Prentice-Hall, Sydney

Farrington A, Telford A 1996 Naming the problem: assessment and formulation. In: Marshall S, Turnbull J (eds) Cognitive behavioural therapy: an introduction to theory and practice. Baillière Tindall, London

Marks I 1986 The Maudsley handbook of behavioural psychotherapy. Croom Helm, London

McFarland G K, Thomas M D 1990 Psychiatric mental health nursing: application of the nursing process. Lippincott, London

Richards D, McDonald B 1990 Behavioural psychotherapy: a pocket book for nurses. Heinemann, Oxford

Romme M, Esher S 2000 Making sense of voices. Mind Publications, London

Annotated reading

Fowler F, Garety P, Kuipers E 1995 Cognitive behaviour therapy for psychosis: theory and practice. John Wiley, Chichester.

Chapter 10 covers getting started, engagement and assessment and provides a pragmatic step-by-step guide to how to assess clients' needs and problems.

Marshall S, Turnbull J 1996 Cognitive behavioural therapy: an introduction to theory and practice. Baillière Tindall, London.

A simple, structured format provides the reader with a clear overview of cognitive–behavioural therapy and how its principles can be applied in practice.

10

Assessing risk

Nigel Wellman

KEY ISSUES

- ◆ The nature of risk
- ◆ Principles of risk assessment
- ◆ The process of risk assessment
- ◆ Assessments of suicide risk
- ◆ Assessment for risk of violence
- ◆ The process of risk management
- ◆ Practical strategies

INTRODUCTION AND BACKGROUND

Risk is the probability of something happening. In clinical use, the term is normally applied to the probability of something harmful or undesirable happening to a patient or something harmful or undesirable being done by a patient to others. Risk assessment is the process of assessing the likelihood of a harmful event occurring and of estimating the likely impact on the patient, carers, staff and others (the general public, the care providing organisation, etc.) should that event occur. People with serious mental health problems are at increased risk of a number of different types of harm compared to the general population (Appleby et al 2001), so risk assessment and management is a core and integral part of their care.

The political background to risk assessment and risk management in health and social care is one in which there have recently been several significant policy developments that bear directly on clinical practice. These developments include the establishment in 1996 of the National Confidential Inquiry into Suicide and Homicides by People with Mental Illness. This inquiry has produced a number of recommendations for improving practice and providing safer services based on an ongoing analysis of information from all UK suicides and homicides involving people with mental health problems (Appleby et al 2001). Also significant has been the launch by the UK government of the *Saving Lives: Our Healthier Nation* strategy in 1999 (Department of Health 1999a), which included a target to reduce suicides by 20% by 2010. Another highly significant event was the launch in 1999 of the National Service Framework (NSF) for mental health in England (Department of Health 1999b). The NSF included seven standards for mental health care, two of which bear directly on risk assessment and management: NSF Standard 4, which stipulates that all patients on the enhanced level of the Care Programme Approach (Department of Health 1990), i.e. patients with serious mental illnesses/complex needs, must have a risk management plan as well as an aftercare plan, and NSF Standard 7, which relates to suicide prevention and staff competencies in assessing and managing suicidal risk.

Most recently, the UK government has published the national suicide prevention strategy for England (Department of Health 2002). The national suicide prevention strategy includes an implementation plan with a number of goals of direct relevance to all health and social care practitioners, especially those working with people with serious mental health problems. These goals include the reduction in suicide in key high-risk groups, such as people who are in contact with or who have recently been in contact with mental health services and reducing the number of suicides in the year following acts of deliberate self-harm.

THE NATURE OF RISK

The first thing and most basic thing to understand about risk is that by its nature it is dynamic and constantly changing (Carson 1997). To illustrate this point, imagine a patient with an established bipolar disorder who is recovering from a serious depressive episode and has recently been discharged from hospital. When you see him, the patient appears stable and to be doing well. Imagine then, a couple of days later, the effect on this patient of being told that he is going to be being sacked from his job because of the amount of sick leave he has taken, which immediately prompts his disaffected partner to walk out, declaring that their relationship is over and that she is never coming back, resulting in the return of intense suicidal thoughts and feelings.

It is also important to understand at the outset that risk assessment is concerned with probabilities and not with certainty and that risk can be managed but not eliminated. Risk assessment is a skill that needs to be learned, practised and refined. Clinical risk can take many forms. These forms include danger to the self through self-harm or suicide, through self-neglect, through exploitation (including financial and sexual exploitation by others), through deterioration from lack of treatment or poor treatment, or poor compliance with treatment, and through behaviours that may be offensive or provocative to others, provoking them to violence. Additional to risks to the self, danger to others may arise through verbal, physical and sexual assault, homicide, arson, the emotional, financial or sexual exploitation of others and the abuse or neglect of children or dependent adults.

The comprehensive and systematic assessment of risk provides a basis for clinical decision-making. Risk assessment is concerned not simply with the factors about the individual but also with the circumstances in which that individual lives and moves and with that unique individual's perception of their circumstances. All these factors are dynamic and subject to change so that some types of risk will fluctuate while others may remain relatively static. Clinical risk assessment therefore deals with the probability of events occurring and needs to address the types of harm and the severity of harm that might occur, as well as the likelihood of their occurrence.

Clinical risk assessment informs the decisions that clinical staff make regarding the relative merits of different treatment options. Treatment options may be selected to minimise certain types of risk. For instance, the use of 'depot' long-acting, injectable, antipsychotic medication may reduce the risk of relapse/deterioration in psychosis. Relapse often occurs because of poor adherence to prescribed drug regimes and, in the case of someone who has acted on paranoid delusions and attacked other people, the fact this person is in receipt of regular medication that controls their delusions is likely to reduce the risk to others. However, like all possible treatment options, the use of depot medication itself brings risks, which may include both physical risks (e.g. side-effects) and psychological risks. There are absolutely no physical, psychological or psychosocial approaches that are free of risk. No matter how well intentioned and how well delivered, all health interventions retain the possibility of causing harm. The selection of treatment options thus always involves weighing up the possible benefits of the treatment or intervention against the risks and disadvantages of that approach for the individual patient concerned. Despite the fact that there are no treatments that are entirely free of risk, a vast amount of available evidence demonstrates that the effective treatment of symptoms reduces all types of clinical risk in people with serious mental health problems.

The example given above illustrates the point that risk assessment is integral to all aspects of clinical care and is concerned with threats to health as well as threats to life. It is also important to remember that the clinician also has a duty to consider risks that may exist not only to their individual patient but also to each patient's carers, family and friends, as well as professional staff, members of the general public and others whom they may encounter in their communities. Clinicians often struggle with issues such as

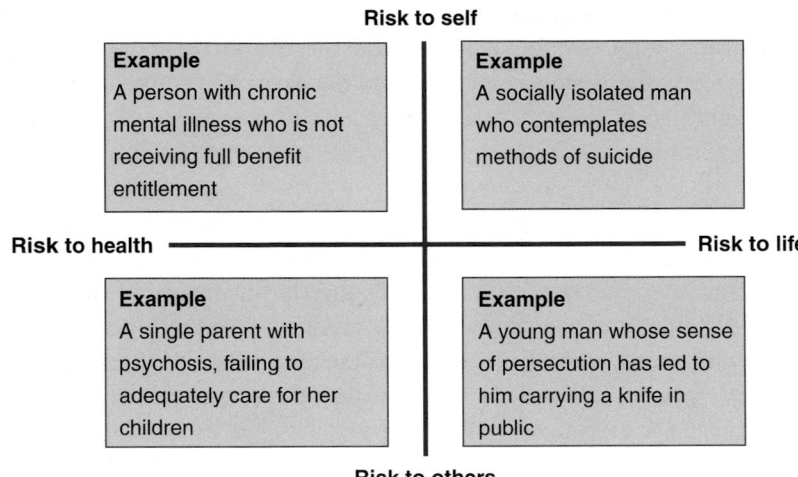

Risk to self

Risk to health ——————————————————— **Risk to life**

Risk to others

Figure 10.1 The scope of clinical risk assessment

the balance between the rights of the individual and the rights of the community at large, but it is undeniable that clinicians have a duty to take all reasonable steps to protect the public from harm and that this duty to protect the public may at times override the clinician's duty of confidentiality to an individual patient. The element that delineates the scope of clinical risk assessment can be understood by viewing them as two continua crossed as axes (Fig. 10.1). This figure helps illustrate the continuity of risk assessment with other areas of patient assessment continually undertaken by health and social care staff in the course of their normal duties.

PRINCIPLES OF RISK ASSESSMENT

Throughout most of the last century the approaches to risk assessment that were predominant in clinical practice relied principally on the judgement of clinicians. From the 1970s onwards, growing research evidence began to cast doubt on the reliability of this approach and seemed to demonstrate that, faced with a particular scenario, individual clinicians might differ greatly in their assessment of risk and that, at worst, their predictions might be little better than chance, especially in relation to risk of violence (Monaghan 1981, 1988). In contrast with clinical prediction, actuarial methods seemed to be more reliable at predicting future untoward events (Grove & Meehl 1996, Kraemer et al 1997). These methods make use of statistical predictions of the likelihood of particular patients performing acts of self-harm or violence, etc. on the basis of the analysis of statistical data about known associations between patient characteristics (e.g. diagnosis, age, gender, clinical history) and self-harm or violence, drawn from databases of recorded patient populations. However, many of these studies overlook the fact that clinicians do not just attempt to predict risk but also have a duty to manage identified risks in order to prevent harm and thus render their own predictions of future harm invalid (Hart 1998, Doyle & Dolan 2002). An example of this would be that if you become aware that a patient you are working with has become very depressed and in your judgement is likely to make a serious attempt to commit suicide in the near future, then your duty of care to that patient dictates that you must intervene to try and prevent their suicide.

Several authors have more recently described approaches to the assessment of risk that seek to systematically combine clinical and actuarial approaches to assessing and managing clinical risk (Hart 1998, Douglas et al 1999, Doyle & Dolan 2002). These approaches attempt to structure clinical judgement so that assessments of risk utilise both actuarial risk data and the clinicians' knowledge of their patients' current state and circumstances so that they are facilitated to make evidence-based, consistent, systematic and reliable assessments of risk. Clinicians constantly assess risk in their normal day-to-day work. Almost all health and social care provider organisations in the UK now use formal written risk assessment tools to help structure the judgement of individual clinicians, but Figure 10.2 illustrates the fact that risk assessment takes place in many clinical settings and that meetings in which formal tools are used represent just one part of the continuum of assessment.

Whenever risk is being assessed and whatever type of risk is being assessed certain key principles apply: these are listed in Box 10.1.

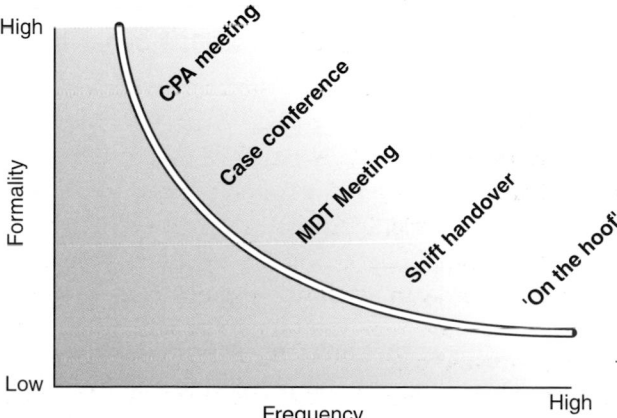

Figure 10.2 The risk assessment continuum (Simpson, in preparation)

Box 10.1 Principles of risk assessment

◆ Risk is complex and should be assessed in a structured and comprehensive manner, using validated clinical instruments where appropriate

◆ Risk assessment is concerned with probabilities rather than certainties

◆ Risk assessment should wherever possible involve the patient and be completed with due tact, although without detracting from the rigour of the assessment

◆ Risk assessment should ideally be undertaken by the clinical team, or at the least be reviewed by the team, rather than depending solely on the judgement of a lone worker

◆ Risk is dynamic and constantly changing, so risk assessments must be subject to review at regular intervals and whenever the condition or circumstances of the patient change significantly

◆ Risk assessment depends crucially on the quality of the information available, so multiple and independent sources of information must be actively sought out

◆ Past behaviour remains the strongest predictor of future behaviour so full review of a patient's history is a vital component of the risk assessment process

Risk assessment tools

As mentioned above, most UK health and social care providers have now adopted the use of structured risk assessment tools designed to aid the clinician in assessing clinical risk. Typically, in addition to recording basic demographic and patient details these tools subdivide risk into different categories of risk:

◆ risk of non-accidental self-harm/suicide
◆ risk of being abused/exploited
◆ risk to others (e.g. staff, carers, family, other clients)
◆ risk to children
◆ risk of relapse or deterioration
◆ risk of absconding or non-engagement with services.

Under each of these headings the clinician will be asked to record the nature, severity and immediacy of the risk and perhaps to rate the risk on a five- or ten-point scale while being presented with a list of factors known to increase that particular type of risk. These forms generally also include space for a risk management plan, based on the completed assessment, which identifies the individuals responsible for completing each part of the plan and includes boxes for recording who has been consulted about the plan (clients, carers), review dates, signatures, etc.

The aim of using tools such as that described above is to ensure that assessments are structured, systematic and comprehensive so that they cover all likely areas of risk, with the assessor being presented with reminders of actuarial risk indicators while completing the assessment. When well executed, these tools genuinely aid clinical risk assessment while avoiding the pitfalls of some of the 'tick-box' risk-scoring tools, which often prove dangerous in practice because their use may replace rather than aid judgement. This means that clinicians may be lulled into a false sense of security when patients attain only low scores on the scales, while actually presenting with high risks in certain specific areas that the scales fail to detect.

There are a very large number of structured instruments in use, which have been designed for assessing many aspects of risk, including risk of self-harm, suicide and violence. Many of these scales require training but some have achieved fairly widespread acceptance. Many of these scales are useful as adjuncts to a comprehensive clinical assessment that gives due weight to the patient's current mental state, recent history and stated intentions. One of the benefits that these scales may bring is the provision of more comprehensive data about particular areas, such as a patient's feelings of hopelessness (Beck et al 1974, 1985) or reasons for living (Linehan et al 1983), than might normally be attained through either a clinical interview or the use of a standard risk assessment tool.

Interpersonal processes

It is possible to complete a risk assessment without the patient being present or without the knowledge or cooperation of the patient. In cases such as that of an aggressive and uncooperative patient who is being involuntarily admitted to a psychiatric intensive care unit, it may be reasonable and even essential to complete the assessment without the patient's cooperation. In these cases, the risk assessment will rely on documented clinical history and on information about recent events, which will be obtained from informants such as relatives, friends, carers, the patient's GP, staff in the Accident and Emergency Department or the police. Ideally, however, risk assessment will involve the active and collaborative exploration of the patient's thoughts, feelings and current circumstances.

Conducting an initial risk assessment will be one of the first tasks that a worker will do with a new patient, and a skilled clinician will have learned to cover these areas sensitively but comprehensively and will be able to use the information gathered to help plan the patient's future care with them. Some workers worry about conducting risk assessments with patients with whom they have yet to form a strong therapeutic alliance, because they fear upsetting the patient and also fear that the patient will not be able to trust them enough to discuss personal and distressing information. It is certainly true that sensitivity is called for in handling these topics and also that, as clinicians build their relationship with their patients, those patients may reveal more about themselves and may well feel more comfortable in discussing sensitive topics. A possible downside of this may be loss of rigour in future risk assessments, where clinicians downplay real risks to third parties for fear of offending the patient or patients conceal information for fear of disappointing or shocking clinicians whom they feel have invested time and hope in them.

Conducting a risk assessment with a patient will inevitably involve discussing issues that will be sensitive for or possibly provocative to that patient and may involve probing difficult and painful areas of that person's life. When carrying out this work, then, it is vital to employ supportive and empathetic approaches, using open questions and active listening skills, and to offer support and help in managing any distress that is generated by the process.

History and situational factors

A vast amount of research evidence supports the view that past behaviour is the strongest single predictor of future behaviour (Beauford et al 1997, King et al 2001) in most areas of life. The use of the patient's personal and clinical history is central to many areas of clinical practice, including risk assessment, so that a recent history of deliberate self-harm signals a higher risk of future self-harm and suicide, a history of sexual offending against children signals an elevated risk of future offending and a history of violence towards healthcare staff signals an elevated risk of similar violence in the future. The careful analysis of each patient's history will also often help the clinician to understand the occurrence of previous untoward events and thus provide information that should help in the prevention of similar events in the future, or at least mitigate their impact.

Knowledge of the detail of a patient's history will also obviously help the clinician to discriminate long-term enduring risk traits, such as Patient A's persisting sexual interest in young children or Patient B's tendency to react with violence when feeling threatened, from situational circumstances that interact with these long-term persistent traits to increase the risk of untoward events occurring. Examples of such situational circumstances would be Patient A being asked to babysit for a friend who has young children or Patient B losing his accommodation and moving in with his highly critical and over-involved parents and beginning to use alcohol to excess.

However, there are real limits to the usefulness of history because people are constantly changing and being challenged, disturbed or tempted by new situations. This means that the fact that someone has never attempted suicide before is absolutely no guarantee that they will not do so in future, and similarly with violence and other harmful behaviours.

All histories are limited and partial. Some histories, including histories from patients and others, may be given with the deliberate intention of creating a particular and possibly misleading impression. This means that it is important to obtain independent accounts of events from different sources. This is particularly important when it is felt that a patient may represent a high risk to themselves or others either in the short, medium or long term, and failure to do so could expose the individual practitioner or their employer to accusations of negligence, as could failure to record and share this information with colleagues and appropriate others and to take appropriate action to mitigate detected risks.

Figure 10.2 suggests that low-frequency but more formal meetings such as CPA meetings and multidisciplinary team meetings may represent ideal opportunities to exchange information, to ensure that assessments are comprehensive and to discuss and update risk assessments. This is particularly true of CPA meetings, where, in addition to the patient and the clinicians immediately involved in their care, others involved in that person's care may be present, including the GP, relatives, housing officers, community support workers, probation workers and others. The sharing of information between different agencies and parties often raises concern over confidentiality; however, all health and social care provider organisations should have local confidentiality and information-sharing policies and protocols compliant with the Department of Health's 1996 guidance on these matters.

In all cases, the clinician's common law duty of confidentiality is overridden in situations where maintaining confidentiality would put individuals or groups at grave risk of harm. When such worries arise, the workers concerned should immediately share their anxieties with their managers and with other relevant members of the multidisciplinary team, agree the actions to be taken, carry out these actions and carefully record all aspects of this process.

Ongoing assessment and management of risk

Given that risk is variable and dynamic, and that long standing characteristics interact with changing circumstances, it follows that risk assessments will remain valid only for limited periods of time and will be invalidated by any significant changes in an individual's health, beliefs or circumstances. Risk assessments, then, are the first stage of an ongoing process of risk management (Keirle 1997).

ASSESSING RISK IN CLINICAL PRACTICE

The most common approach to risk assessment described in the literature is the use of an initial assessment, which is supplemented where necessary by more specific assessments of particular identified risks, and this approach will be followed here.

Suicide

Suicide is a relatively rare but serious event. Risk of suicide, like other risks, varies in immediacy and severity. All patients with serious mental health problems are at elevated risk of completed suicide. Fenton (2000) has identified that suicide is the primary cause of premature death in schizophrenia and Appleby (2000) has reported that 50% of completed suicides in the UK have had contact with psychiatric services at some time and 25% in the year before death, so that suicide is strongly associated with mental illness. Some cases of severe and immediate risk of suicide will be obvious from evidence such as failed suicide attempts or planning an imminent attempt and in these cases immediate hospitalisation may be life-saving. In most cases, the evidence will be less clear-cut and clinicians will need to blend their knowledge of the patient, the patient's current state and current circumstances with their knowledge of actuarial risk factors.

Table 10.1 presents a list of risk factors for suicide in the general population. These factors may have additive effects, although, within particular diagnostic groups, other additional factors may also apply. Most notably for people with mental health problems there is a hugely increased risk of completed suicide in the period immediately following discharge from hospital (Appleby et al 2001). Data from the Department of Health (1993) suggests a lifetime risk of suicide in schizophrenia of 10% and a 15% lifetime risk for the affective disorders, personality disorders and alcohol dependence, although Inskip (1998) has more recently recalculated the lifetime risks to be 6% for affective disorders, 7% for alcohol dependence and 4% for schizophrenia. A sophisticated assessment of suicide risk will balance identified risk factors against protective factors ('reasons for living'), such as concern for children, religious beliefs and fear of pain (Linehan et al 1983).

Communication of intent is normal in suicide (Shneidman 1993). When an initial assessment indicates a risk of serious self-harm or suicide, a more detailed assessment of the individual's intent and plans is required. Exploring these topics may be distressing for some, although equally other patients may find relief in discussing these matters. This assessment may follow a funnelling approach, beginning with open-ended and fairly general questions and leading on to more specific and direct questions. For example:

Table 10.1 Suicide risk factors

Variable	Risk
Age	Increases with age but young men and young Asian women may be at elevated risk
Gender	Men at greater risk than women
Physical health	Chronic pain Chronic life-threatening illness
Psychological health	Hopelessness (Feeling that things can never get better) Helplessness (Feeling that one is beyond help) High levels of psychological distress Experience of significant loss Depressed mood Agitation Low self-esteem Disturbing delusions and hallucinations
Personality factors	Impulsiveness (manifest in deliberate self harm and aggression)
Social situation	Social isolation and lack of friends and supports Interpersonal conflict with significant others Social upheaval: imprisonment, divorce, retirement, accommodation changes, recent discharge from hospital
History	Recent discharge from hospital Deliberate self-harm or suicide attempt in previous 12 months History of impulsive acts Family history of suicide
Diagnosis	Any major illness, personality disorder or substance misuse – risk rises if comorbid for any of these disorders
Intentions	Stated intention to kill self Formed suicide plans
Situational factors	Easy access to a lethal method of suicide

Q. Have you been thinking about death or dying recently?
A. Yes, just about all the time since I broke up with my boyfriend.

Q. That sounds awful; have you been thinking about harming yourself or killing yourself?
A. Yes, I have, I just can't bear it any longer, I just want it all to stop.

Q. Have you thought about what you would do, how you might kill yourself?
A. Yes, I have, I thought I would probably take an overdose.

Q. *OK, have you thought about what tablets you would take?*
A. *Yes, I thought I would take all my olanzapine and probably some aspirin as well.*

Q. *How many olanzapine and aspirin tablets have you got?*
A. *I've got my normal month's supply of olanzapine and I bought 150 aspirin last week.*

Q. *Have you thought about where and when you would do it?*
A. *Yes, I would do it here, when my mum goes up to my aunt's for the weekend.*

Q. *When will that be?*
A. *Next weekend.*

Q. *How likely is it that you will go through with this?*
A. *I will do it, I'm absolutely determined, I just can't bear this any more.*

Suicidal thinking has been associated with the experience of unendurable psychological distress resulting in a constriction of thinking that leaves the individual able to see only two ways forward – death or the continuance of unendurable and inescapable distress (Shneidman 1993). With this in mind, it is vital to explore the patient's hopes and plans for the future or their fears about the future, to find out whether they are able to see any way out of their current problems and to discover the level of distress they are experiencing. The answers to these questions will determine whether you need to probe further, using a more direct approach of the type illustrated above to determine the nature, seriousness and immediacy of the risk. This view also suggests therapeutic ways forward through tackling the distress and through helping the patient to see that they have options available to them other than suicide.

One should always bear in mind that patients who are hallucinated or delusional may plan to kill themselves for unpredictable or psychotic reasons ('to save the world') and others may go out of their way to conceal suicidal plans and intent from clinicians, so that an inquiring mind and a degree of healthy scepticism may help to keep your patients alive. The collection and synthesis of this information should provide an indication of the likelihood that the patient will act upon their feelings. Analysis of previous attempts at suicide may provide valuable information concerning current intent. These events can also be assessed by means of a functional analysis that retrospectively looks at the antecedents and behaviours involved, as well as the consequences. Table 10.2 presents areas for enquiry in a functional analysis following a suicide attempt.

Table 10.2 Assessment of intent following a suicide attempt

Antecedents	Was the act prepared for in advance?
	Were steps taken to deal with the aftermath, such as a will or suicide note?
Behaviour	Was the person alone when suicide was attempted?
	Were any steps taken to avoid the person's discovery by others?
	What is the person's perception of the lethality of the method they used?
Consequences	Was any assistance sought after the event?
	Did the person resist assistance from others?
	Does the person express any regret at the failure of the attempt?

Violence

Research over many years has identified a number of actuarial factors associated with violent behaviour (Table 10.3).

Violence is common in society and is fundamentally an interactive phenomenon (Whittington & Wykes 1996, Spokes et al 2002). The presence of the risk factors listed in Table 10.3 does not mean that violent incidents will inevitably occur but it does suggest that risks may be heightened, particularly when a predisposed individual meets particular situational triggers. The utility of these risk factors lies in the fact that they help to flag up the need for a careful assessment of a patient's presenting risks.

As with the assessment of suicide risk, the assessment of risk of violence should begin with initial general questions adopting a neutral but interested tone and a non-judgemental approach, employing prompts, paraphrasing and other active listening techniques as appropriate. If the initial assessment indicates areas of heightened risk, then the clinician should proceed to more specific and detailed questioning. The aim of this questioning will be to elicit and detail the following:

◆ how the patient experiences and copes with frustration and anger
◆ their involvement in fights and other forms of violence both as a juvenile and as an adult
◆ their involvement in any violent gangs or subcultures (e.g. street gangs, the Hell's Angels, organised football hooliganism)
◆ any history of emotional, verbal or physical abuse of partners, family members or children
◆ any history of sexual aggression or offending
◆ any arrests, criminal record or unconvicted involvement in violent offending

Table 10.3 Violence risk factors

Variable	Risk
Age	Risk declines with age
Gender	Traditionally thought that men are more likely to be violent than women but recent clinical evidence challenges this
Physical health	Head injury Pain Intoxication with drugs or alcohol Dementia Confusion/delirium
Psychological health	Excessive stimulation Disinhibition Hallucinations Delusions Anger Fears for personal safety
Personality factors	Low intelligence Impulsiveness (manifest in deliberate self harm and aggression) Antisocial personality traits Racism Pleasure, including sexual pleasure, from use of violence
Social factors	Lack of remorse for previous violent acts Unstable living arrangements Poor educational attainment Member of a violent gang or subculture
History	Exposure to violence in the social milieu Previous history of violent behaviour History of impulsive acts
Diagnosis	Any major mental illness, personality disorder or substance misuse – risk rises if comorbid for any of these disorders
Intentions	Stated intention to harm or kill others Formed plans for attacking others
Situational factors	Easy access to weapons/carries a knife, gun or other weapon

Table 10.4 Assessment of intent following violent behaviour

Antecedents	Circumstantial factors that motivated client
	Provocation
	Drug or alcohol intoxication
	Treatment status
Behaviour	Was behaviour planned or impulsive?
	Was behaviour directed at a specific individual?
	Were weapons used?
	How was the behaviour stopped, and by whom?
Consequences	Degree of resultant harm or damage
	Victim empathy
	Positive reinforcers for past behaviour
	Current perception of past behaviour

- any episodes of indiscriminate verbal or physical hostility
- any history of violence to health or social care staff
- any history of damage to property, or arson
- any history of violence driven by hallucinations or delusions.

If the patient gives a history of violence then it is also vital to establish the level of planning involved, any use of weapons and current access to or possession of weapons.

As with suicide risk, independent sources of information should be sought, careful attention should be paid to the circumstances of all documented incidents of violence and due weight should be given to threats and expressed violent intentions. In some circumstances it will be appropriate to obtain copies of an individual's criminal record from the police to inform the risk assessment and for the clinical team to refer the patient on to specialist forensic services for an opinion on the risks presented by that individual and for advice on their future management.

Also, as with suicide and self-harm, the analysis of incidents may provide useful information for the prevention of future incidents. A functional analysis, similar to that outlined for the assessment of acts of self harm, can be conducted to elicit this information (Table 10.4).

Assessment of intent to harm

In all cases where a patient expresses intent to seriously harm or kill a particular individual, group of people or class of person, it is vital to assess the level of risk. This will mean using good empathic communication skills to elicit from the patient feelings of hopelessness, frustration, anger or rage in relation to their current circumstances. It is also important to determine the focus of their anger and the detailed where, when and how of their thoughts or fantasies of revenge, including the frequency and intensity of these thoughts and the degree of control that the patient has over these thought processes, together with the strategies they employ to manage these feelings. As a general rule, the level of short-term risk rises with greater intensity of these thoughts, together with preoccupation and voluntary indulgence in violent fantasies, although practical obstacles such as not knowing the whereabouts of the intended victim may reduce these risks. In all cases where there is judged to be serious risk to others, a forensic opinion should be sought.

MANAGING RISK IN CLINICAL PRACTICE

As has been stressed throughout this chapter, clinicians do not just assess risk, rather risk assessment is the first stage in planning care and managing identified risks. A completed risk assessment will form the basis for development of treatment strategies and plans designed to manage identified risks by reducing or eliminating them or reducing their frequency and severity (Snowden 1997), and also by reducing the likely impact on all concerned should untoward events occur. Each individual patient's key worker, care coordinator or other main professional carer is responsible for formulating a risk management plan on the basis of a comprehensive analysis of risk and for securing agreement with the plan of all the individuals and agencies involved in that person's care.

Building from the comprehensive risk assessment, which quantifies and describes risk in all relevant areas (e.g. self-harm/suicide; risk to children; risk of violence; abuse/exploitation; relapse; non-engagement), for each identified area of concern, the risk management plan should describe:

◆ circumstances associated with risk behaviours
◆ early warning signs of risk
◆ a description of what must change to reduce risk
◆ strategies to enable change to occur
◆ an assessment of the client's likely collaboration with each strategy
◆ the roles and responsibilities of those involved in the client's care
◆ responsibilities for responding to emergency situations
◆ dates for routine review and circumstances that would necessitate an immediate review.

Given the dynamic nature of risk, all risk assessments and hence all risk management plans have a limited life and must be reviewed at regular intervals and whenever there is any significant change in the patient's circumstances or condition. Good communications between all parties underlie the successful management of clinical risk.

CONCLUSIONS

This chapter has presented a framework for understanding risk assessment and management, together with a description of the principles that underpin these processes. Risk is dynamic and constantly changing and the assessment of risk to the self and to others is a key element in care planning. This has been presented here in a staged way, although, in the fires of clinical practice, the sequence and inclusion of elements may vary considerably. The assessment of risk underpins all multidisciplinary decision-making regarding the relative merits of possible treatment options. Risk can only be managed and never entirely eliminated, so untoward events, including violent incidents, suicides and homicides, will occur from time to time. Good risk assessment, coupled with the appropriate communication of risk information and good multidisciplinary and interagency collaboration to manage identified risks, will reduce the frequency of these events and also help to protect individual practitioners and their employing organisations when tragedies occur.

Summary of practical strategies identified

◆ All patients should receive regular risk assessments, not simply to determine the possibility that they will harm themselves or others but also to identify factors that may compromise their health or the health of others they encounter.

◆ The validity of clinical risk assessments will depend on the application by staff of various principles that underpin the process (Box 10.1).

◆ Whether assessing risk to the self or to others, the process is similar and involves an initial assessment of risk of specific types, followed, when concerns are identified, by a more detailed assessment of the likelihood of the occurrence of a particular type of harm together with its probable impact if it does occur.

◆ Risk factors for self harm/suicide and violence are presented in Tables 10.1 and 10.3 and can be used to help inform initial assessments.

◆ Assessment of history is crucial to risk assessment, so details of previous risk behaviours should be sought and analysed in detail to help determine the likelihood of their recurrence (Tables 10.2, 10.4).

Summary of practical strategies identified (*cont"d*)

◆ When potential risks are identified a more detailed assessment of current intent should be undertaken; this should follow a funnelling process, beginning with open-ended, indirect enquiries and leading to more specific, direct questioning.

◆ Comprehensive risk assessment is the bedrock for good clinical risk management; this involves the development of a risk management plan, which identifies strategies to reduce both the severity and frequency of risk behaviours and to mitigate their impacts if they do occur.

◆ Risk is dynamic and will vary over time as people and circumstances change, so risk assessments must be subject to regular review.

References

Appleby L 2000. Prevention of suicide in psychiatric patients. In: Hawton K, van Heeringen K (eds) The international handbook of suicide and attempted suicide. Wiley, Chichester

Appleby L, Shaw J, Sherratt J et al 2001 Safety first: national confidential inquiry into suicide and homicide by people with mental illness. Department of Health, London

Beauford J E, McNiel D E, Binder R L 1997 Utility of the initial therapeutic alliance in evaluating psychiatric patients' risk of violence. American Journal of Psychiatry 159:1272–1276

Beck A T, Weissman A, Lester D, Trexler L 1974 The measurement of pessimism: the hopelessness scale. Journal of Consulting and Clinical Psychology 42:861–865

Beck A T, Steer R A, Kovacs M, Garrson G 1985 Hopelessness and eventual suicide. A 10 year prospective study of patients hospitalized with suicidal ideation. American Journal of Psychiatry 142:559–563

Carson D 1997 Good enough risk taking. International Review of Psychiatry 9:303–308

Department of Health 1990 The care programme approach for people with a mental illness referred to specialist psychiatric services. HC(90)23/LASSL(90)11. Joint Health and Social Services Circular, Department of Health, London

Department of Health 1993 The health of the nation: key area handbook, mental illness. Department of Health, London

Department of Health 1996 The protection and use of patient information. Department of Health, London

References (cont'd)

Department of Health 1999a Saving lives: our healthier nation. Department of Health, London

Department of Health 1999b A national service framework for mental health. Department of Health, London

Department of Health 2002. National suicide prevention strategy for England. Department of Health, London

Douglas K, Cox D, Webster C 1999 Violence risk assessment: science and practice. Legal and Criminological Psychology 4:184–194

Doyle M, Dolan M 2002 Violence risk assessment: combining actuarial and clinical information to structure clinical judgements for the formulation and management of risk. Journal of Psychiatric and Mental Health Nursing 9:649–657

Fenton W S 2000 Depression, suicide and suicide prevention in schizophrenia. Suicide and Life-Threatening Behavior 30:34–49

Grove W, Meehl P 1996 Comparative efficiency of informal (subjective and impressionistic) and formal (mechanical, algorithmic) prediction procedures: the clinical-statistical controversy. Psychology, Public Policy and Law 2:292–323

Hart S D 1998 The role of psychopathy in assessing risk for violence: conceptual and methodological issues. Legal and Criminological Psychology 3:121–137

Inskip H M, Harris E C, Barraclough B 1998 Lifetime risk of suicide for affective disorder, alcoholism and schizophrenia. British Journal of Psychiatry 172:35–37

Keirle P 1997 Psychiatric patient violence: assessment and management of risk. British Journal of Community Health Nursing 2:191–194

King E A, Baldwin D S, Sinclair J M A et al 2001 The Wessex recent in-patient suicide study, I: Case-control study of 234 recently discharged psychiatric patient suicides. British Journal of Psychiatry 178:531–536

Kraemer H, Kazdin A, Offord D et al 1997 The MacArthur risk assessment project: coming to terms with the terms of risk. Archives of General Psychiatry 54:337–343

Linehan M M, Goodstein J L, Nielsen S L, Chiles J A 1983 Reasons for staying alive when you're thinking of killing yourself: the reasons for living inventory. Journal of Consulting and Clinical Psychology 51:276–286

Monaghan J 1981 Predicting violent behaviour. Sage, Beverly Hills, CA

Monaghan J 1988 Risk assessment of violence among the mentally disordered: generalising useful knowledge. International Journal of Law and Psychiatry 11:249–257

Shneidman E 1993 Suicide as psychache. Jason Aranson, Northvale, NJ

Simpson P D F (in preparation) Formal and informal risk assessment.

Snowden P 1997 Practical aspects of clinical risk assessment and management. British Journal of Psychiatry 170(suppl 32):32–34

Spokes K, Bond K, Lowe P T et al 2002 HOVIS – the Hertfordshire/Oxfordshire Violent Incident Study. Journal of Psychiatric and Mental Health Nursing 9:199–209

Whittington R, Wykes T 1996 Aversive stimulation by staff and violence by psychiatric patients. British Journal of Criminology 35:11–20

Annotated further reading

Department of Health 2002 National suicide prevention strategy for England. Department of Health, London

Required reading for all mental health practitioners – the government's suicide prevention strategy

Duggan C (ed) 1997 Assessing risk. British Journal of Psychiatry 170(suppl)32

This comprehensive account of contemporary knowledge concerning risk assessment has been collated into a single British Journal of Psychiatry supplement by Conor Duggan. The contributors are eminent clinicians and academics who deal with a diverse range of issues from sexual offending to the rights of the person who is being assessed for levels of risk. Overall the text is rather more analytical than practical but nevertheless equips the reader with a sound grasp of relevant issues.

Hawton K, Van Heeringen K (eds) 2000 The international handbook of suicide and attempted suicide. Wiley, Chichester

This large and expensive edited volume will provide the reader with a comprehensive international 'state of the art' overview of all aspects of suicidal and suicide prevention

Royal College of Psychiatrists 1998 Management of imminent violence: clinical practice guidelines to support mental health services. RCP, London

These guidelines were developed to reflect the current levels of knowledge concerning the effective and appropriate treatment of potentially violent persons. They are based upon a rigorous and systematic review of research evidence as well as the views of practitioners, service users and their carers. They are fundamentally predicated upon the provision of an environment that reduces the likelihood of violence but also deal with the management of actual violence.

Gunn J, Taylor P 2001 Forensic psychiatry: clinical, legal and ethical issues, 2nd edn. Butterworth-Heinemann, Oxford

A revised and updated version of this comprehensive textbook, which integrates forensic treatment with its wider legal and moral ramifications. The book is written in an easily accessible format and provides practice-orientated recommendations for this field of care.

Shneidman E 1993 Suicide as psychache: a clinical approach to self-destructive behaviour. J Aronson, Northvale, NJ

A volume by Edwin Shneidman, the American founder of modern suicidology, which is very readable and will acquaint the reader with Shneidman's theory of suicide and practical approaches for understanding, managing and working with suicidal patients.

Section 3

Interventions

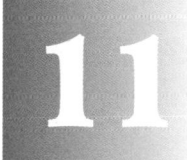

Dealing with voices and strange thoughts

Jem Mills

KEY ISSUES

- Voices and strange thoughts as part of the normal range of human experience
- Adjusting the helping process to suit individuals
- Encouraging service users and professionals to work alongside each other
- Using specific assessments to develop shared understanding of the problem, based on psychological models
- Developing ways of coping with voices and strange, worrying thoughts
- Exploring and testing out the specific beliefs about symptoms that are associated with a person's distress

INTRODUCTION

For half a century the most effective treatment for people with psychosis has been, and still is, to take powerful antipsychotic drugs. Despite the effectiveness of these substances, the majority of people taking them continue to experience some level of distressing symptoms. Other difficulties that people have with the chemical approach include the burden of unwanted effects and forgetting or deciding not to take the advised course. It is, then, a great advantage that this approach can now be complemented by other, more palatable interventions.

Psychological approaches to voices and strange thoughts have, in recent years, shown some remarkable developments. The application of cognitive–behavioural therapy to these problems is a predominantly British endeavour and one that is showing some success (NHS Centre for Reviews and Dissemination 2000). While we pride ourselves on these innovations we also need to take up the complex question of how to make the approaches more readily available to the people who need them.

This chapter deals with that challenge. I have attempted to identify important elements of the approach that might be useful to those mental health professionals seeking to help people with these problems. I have avoided producing a 'cook book' of techniques in the hope that the reader will realise the importance of the process of helping someone with voices or strange thoughts. In the spirit of collaborative working I have tried to present some ideas about dealing with these problems in a way that might be accessed by anyone. With this in mind I have also taken up the challenge of avoiding technical language, hence the use of the terms 'voices' and 'strange, worrying beliefs' rather than 'hallucinations' and 'delusions'. This use of language reflects another emergent principle of the work, namely that people with these problems experience something that is quite naturally human. Their tragic predicament is the disabling regularity of, and great distress over, intense psychotic experience, rather than the phenomenon itself.

Intervening too soon is often the cause of common problems encountered by mental health professionals learning to help people with psychosis. The

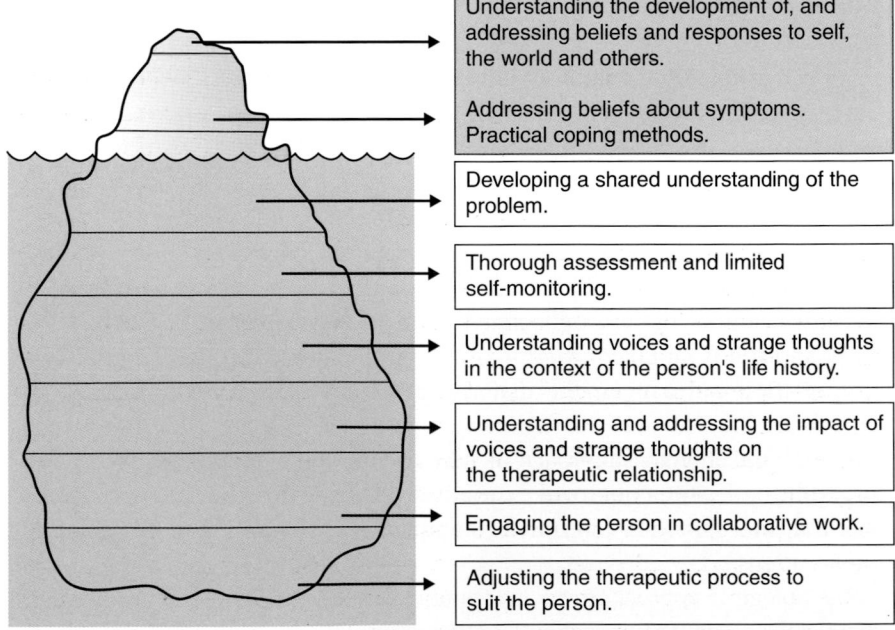

Figure 11.1   Iceberg model showing the importance of low visibility work in psychosis.

iceberg model (Fig. 11.1) shows that there are a number of things to consider before crossing the water line into practical interventions. Sometimes the steps below this line are overlooked because they have a low visibility and there is currency in being seen to be doing something. Sometimes the professional assumes that enough information has been gathered to suggest a solution to the problem. Whatever the reason, it is important to develop conceptual ways rather than intervention-led ways of understanding the person's experience. People want to tell their stories and in doing so seek to understand their experiences more fully. Mental health services can all too often trample on this need in the rush to explain people's experiences in professional terms (Johnstone 2000). Repeated experience of this can make people wary of opening up to others. It is therefore important to pay attention to the process of helping. The practical interventions shown in the shaded area of Figure 11.1 are often the icing on a cake that has taken a long time to cook. Essential to the recipe is attention to those processes that underpin the interventions.

ADJUSTING THE THERAPEUTIC APPROACH TO SUIT PEOPLE WHO EXPERIENCE PSYCHOSIS

Naïveté

It is very hard to understand what it must be like to have psychosis and this can often make empathising with the sufferer difficult. Adopting a naïve approach is helpful in a number of ways. It gives a clear message that you are interested in finding out about a person's problems and that you are not setting yourself up as an expert. It also allows you to explore people's thinking on their terms. The approach involves an open questioning style. You should try to put your own expectations out of mind and explore people's own understanding of their problems. Adopting the principle that you might think the same way given similar circumstances is helpful. If the story seems difficult to understand at first, do not assume that this is the storyteller's fault. Allow the confusion to wash over you and ask for clarification as you go. Many times, adopting this approach has led to new insights into problems that were already considered well understood.

It will probably be necessary to adjust your therapeutic approach when beginning to help people with voices and strange thoughts. Usual ways of working such as hour-long, weekly sessions, setting tasks to be completed between sessions and having an active and lively pace may well be appropriate for some people. However, it might be that some people have never been asked to participate actively in their care. It is also possible for people to be hampered by difficulties with concentration and motivation. Consideration should be given to how individuals' particular problems might affect the therapeutic process. This often means:

- being flexible about the timing and frequency of sessions
- negotiating regular breaks
- regularly checking out how the person is finding the experience
- agreeing to stop the session if necessary
- being creative about the setting for the session.

In practice this means having an open discussion about expectations for the work ahead. It is important to set out the options and to explore any likely obstacles at an early stage. When in doubt, start slowly and build the pace after reflecting on the process together. Another difficulty with this approach can be that people are not used to the increased sense of responsibility that often comes with collaboration. Again, adjusting the pace of work helps this. The guiding principle should be one of moulding the process to suit individuals, rather than the other way around. This was helpful in Nigel's case:

Case study – Nigel

Nigel had been referred by his occupational therapist for some specific help in coping with voices. He found discussing them very upsetting and was understandably wary. He also had problems at home with his heating breaking down and had to visit the local inpatient unit to use its bath. It was suggested that working upon his voices would be hard with so many practical problems taking up his time. He agreed that he was distracted by these difficulties and that he did not want to add to his stress. This approach acknowledged his difficult circumstances and made his well-being a clear priority. It also gave the message that learning to deal with his voices would involve some effort on his part, requiring him to devote time and motivation to the process. However, Nigel was keen to start something and so a suitable compromise was negotiated. After some discussion he decided that he would call in over the following month when attending appointments with his occupational therapist. He wanted us to get to know each other and as the visits progressed he started asking questions about the ways we would be working together. After a month his home life was more stable and Nigel felt able to begin. It was quickly established that even thinking about his voices was distressing, so to lessen this distress it was agreed that appointments should last no more than 20 minutes. As the work progressed Nigel felt confident about trying more frequent and longer sessions.

This tailoring of the approach began to sow the seeds of some important principles that would guide the process of helping Nigel to deal with his voices. These principles apply generally to helping people with these problems:

- Alleviating distress is the prime focus of the work.
- Staying engaged with the process is more important than pushing ahead for results.
- The way to tackle big problems is to break them down into manageable steps.
- Each step of the process is openly negotiated.

Engaging the person in collaborative work

Collaboration in this sense involves the person with voices or strange thoughts working alongside the professional. The term implies that both parties have a role to play in the development of new understandings and coping methods. The venture is characteristically open and honest within the confines of a professional relationship. The professional needs to be clear about the boundaries of the therapeutic relationship, including rules of confidentiality and duty of care. Because of this, collaboration can also be threatening to both parties. People with these difficulties have often had little active involvement in their own care. For some the idea of participation is a welcome and refreshing change. For others the increased responsibility can be quite daunting and unwelcome. Some can feel quite hopeless about the prospect of change while others might be weighed down with low motivation. An individual's ability to participate will guide the pace of the process. If the person is not able to take part in decision-making it will be very difficult to proceed. With this in mind it is often useful to discuss how the referral came about. Useful questions will include:

- Was the referral made collaboratively?
- What are the person's expectations?
- What has been said about the service on offer?
- How does it feel to consider new ways of dealing with psychotic symptoms?

As with the previous section the guiding principle here is that large obstacles are tackled in small steps. Any difficulties with collaboration should be identified and the problem solved. For instance, the person may have worries about medication being increased or reduced as a result of disclosing information about symptoms. A common worry is that full and open discussion of symptoms will lead to admissions or labelling of the person as mad.

Open discussion about the limitations of medication is often useful. Curson et al (1988) show that the majority of people taking neuroleptic medication continue to have residual symptoms. It is commonly thought that, when leaving hospital, rather than having experienced a complete recovery, people with voices and strange thoughts have improved to a degree where they are able to avoid talking about them. Acknowledging that residual problems are sometimes to be expected rather than seen as a sign of relapse can relieve fears about disclosure. Often the early practical stages of helping a person can be beneficial in demonstrating the value of collaborative work. It is important to foster this approach rather than pressing ahead with interventions that might be passively received by the unmotivated person.

UNDERSTANDING AND ADDRESSING THE IMPACT OF SYMPTOMS ON THE THERAPEUTIC RELATIONSHIP

The therapeutic relationship is vital to this kind of work. Voices and strange thoughts can have a profound effect on a person's ability to maintain a relationship of this nature. A popular training exercise for mental health professionals involves a role-played interview between two people while a third person whispers into the interviewee's ear. The result is meant to approximate what it might be like to hear voices and answer questions at the same time. People find themselves losing concentration, feeling wary of the interviewer and having seemingly inappropriate emotional responses. This simple exercise can be a useful and powerful learning tool.

Chadwick et al (1996) suggest that the professional should assume that a person's symptoms will be active in a new and potentially threatening situation such as an assessment interview. For instance, it is expected that voices will comment on the interview and that people prone to feeling paranoid will often have misgivings about the interviewer.

Predicting that voices and strange thoughts will occur in the session

It is useful to bring this subject up early on by asking whether the voices are speaking during the interview and whether they are commenting on the process. It can be useful to state that other people often find symptoms disruptive. Stating that it is common for people's voices to make comments, especially negative ones, about the interviewer is often useful. Once this is out in the open then difficulties arising from the predicament can be solved. Sometimes voices warn against disclosure of information to the interviewer. This can lead to the person feeling unsafe and can disrupt the development of trust. Interestingly, some people find that voices are not present during conversations with others. As will be mentioned later, talking aloud often forms part of the person's repertoire of coping skills. However, this was not the case with Lucy, who found her voices warning her that her problems would not be taken seriously.

Case study – Lucy

Lucy, while living in a local authority group home, was referred to the local mental health centre asking for help with voices. She had four voices that she recognised as deceased family members. She had a lot of difficulty concentrating during the assessment interviews owing to them saying that she was evil and worthless and than no one would believe her story. She believed that they had power over her and that they could harm her by urging her to take an overdose. We noted that it was very difficult for Lucy to discuss her voices during our sessions together. After a while, she was able to say that they were commentating on the interviewer. However, she felt very uncomfortable talking about the content of their comments. We discussed the reactions of people that I had seen before and I told her that one man had found his voices saying that I would not be interested in his story and that I would laugh at him if he told me. Lucy was able to say that, although she did not think that I would laugh at her, something similar worried her. I asked her if the voices had ever told her something that later turned out to be false and she replied that it happened all the time. She realised that there was a possibility that they were wrong on this occasion but said that the thought of being mocked was too much to bear. On further questioning it became clear that being mocked would mean having everyone she knew knowing about her voices and laughing at her because of them. Once this was clear we were able to discuss the boundaries of confidentiality. Lucy was surprised at how little information would have to be passed around the professionals at the mental health centre, and her fears that someone at her home might find out about her through their own community nurse were alleviated. Despite feeling nervous about trying, Lucy agreed to disclose a little of the voices' content and then see if the information got back to her friends. She returned the next week more confident that the process was safe despite what the voices told her. We acknowledged that it had been good to discuss this and Lucy agreed to bring up similar worries if they occurred again.

The process above includes:

◆ assuming that voices will comment on the interview
◆ being willing to address openly any warnings the voices are giving about the interviewer
◆ showing that voices commenting in this way is a usual occurrence
◆ acknowledging that disclosing details of the voice content can be very distressing
◆ moving the discussion away from the specific to more general aspects of the voices – such as whether they always tell the truth
◆ trying to identify information that might reassure the person hearing voices
◆ negotiating a small test of whether the voices will react in the predicted way
◆ discussing the results of the test and making plans for the future.

UNDERSTANDING VOICES AND STRANGE THOUGHTS IN THE CONTEXT OF THE PERSON'S LIFE HISTORY – WHY ME? WHY NOW?

The psychosocial model of voices and strange beliefs presented in this chapter highlights the role that attribution or meaning has to play in the experience of distress. Put simply, if people believe their voices or strange experiences are an asset, or at worst a minor inconvenience, then they will not be distressed by them. Indeed, as long as a person is able to get on with their daily life without causing concern to others they will be unlikely to come into contact with mental health services and there are many examples of people like this (Romme & Escher 2000). One way of understanding this is that these people have a story about themselves and the world around them that places a benign or advantageous meaning on the experience of voices or strange thoughts.

The cognitive psychology that underpins many psychosocial interventions is very interested in the relationship between emotional distress and the meaning ascribed to events (Grant et al 2004). A fundamental aspect of this perspective is that we create meaning on the basis of our previous experience. Voices and strange beliefs are understood to be expressions of personal meaning within a psychosocial framework. For instance, voices can be understood as types of thought that are heard audibly (Fowler et al 1995). It becomes apparent that previous life experience is then crucially wrapped up with voices and strange beliefs. People often intuitively know this and express a strong need to understand voices and strange beliefs in the context of their life history. Their experience of contact with mental health services can be demoralising and invalidating if this need is not met. This is often the case when voices or strange thoughts are seen as randomly generated symptoms of an underlying mental disease or syndrome.

With this in mind, it is understandable that people often learn to keep strange ideas or voices to themselves if reporting their presence is seen as a sign of being unwell. This can (often with good cause) lead to worries about increased medication, reduced leave and delayed discharge from hospital. Once people are convinced that talking about their distressing experiences will not automatically lead to these consequences, they can be relieved, interested and sometimes excited by the opportunity to discuss them in greater depth. Sometimes people want to directly address the question 'Why has this happened to me?' Sometimes they desperately want someone to understand and validate their experiences. Either way, the isolation associated with leaving them undiscussed can often become a source of stress in itself, adding to the vicious cycle by increasing preoccupation and conviction in worrying beliefs.

Voices, strange thoughts and traumatic life events

There is a significant body of literature pointing to the relationship between voices and traumatic life events (Romme & Escher 2000). It is probable, given the reports of people under extreme stress, that the ability to hear voices is actually a naturally occurring protective mechanism in humans (Kingdon & Turkington 1994). It could be that voices protect people from highly upsetting memories, even when the voices themselves are distressing. Some research has demonstrated a connection between intrusive, humiliating voices and events such as personal attack, sexual abuse and bullying (Hardy 2003). The exact link between voices, strange thoughts and trauma is not clearly understood. However, it can be relieving for a person to understand that this is a common reaction. A significant proportion of people with voices or strange thoughts may be experiencing post-traumatic stress disorder that has gone undetected. It may be that these people could benefit from specialist psychological help.

Reviewing life history

Reviewing the person's life history can reveal several key things:

◆ Thematic review of experiences and how they were interpreted can help to build a picture of the person's beliefs and general outlook
◆ Exploration of specific events preceding the onset of voices or strange beliefs can highlight connection, e.g. abuse and humiliating, derogatory voices
◆ An understanding of the people's beliefs about themselves, other people and the world in general can illuminate their attitudes towards voices and strange beliefs, as well as mental health services.

A succinct way of helping people with reduced concentration to undertake this work is to discuss life events in 5-year chunks. This can be done at a pace that suits the person and often requires at least one meeting for each 5-year period. When people have difficulty remembering, aids such as photographs, heirlooms or other family members can be helpful. Once the person's life experience is explored they can be assisted to explore connections between their resultant beliefs and attitudes and the problems they are experiencing in the here and now. This involves spotting broad themes such as whether they were extrovert or introvert as well as specific attributions such as 'when that happened it convinced me of this'. It can be helpful to keep questions in mind such as:

◆ If childhood experiences teach us about ourselves, other people and the world in general, what lessons did this person learn?

◆ What strategies did this person learn in response to their view of the world?
◆ How did schooling and mixing with peers affect these beliefs and strategies?
◆ What other significant relationships did the person have and what was learned from these?
◆ What was going on in the person's life just before voices or strange thoughts appeared?

Case study – Dan

Dan was experiencing great distress over his belief that certain people were able to steal his personality from him. He had been taking medication for nearly 3 years with some effect but still avoided social contact because of his fear. He was not at all convinced that he merely had an illness and was pleasantly surprised to find me interested in his version of events. I told him that other people often found it useful to go over things in some detail and that I was interested in helping him this way. We agreed that I could ask questions and that he could stop at any time if he found them too much. We also discussed how he sometimes became wary of people showing interest in him as he feared they might be attempting to steal his mind. I suggested that if he started to feel this way we could stop and address it directly and if reassurance was not helping we could try another day.

Dan described his life in 5-year periods over eight meetings. He found himself feeling as if his mind were being stolen during one session when he was describing a very upsetting relationship break-up. We dealt with this as planned, with good effect. After the eight sessions he requested that I write down the story for him as he found it helpful to read it at times when he felt anxious. The main points of Dan's story were:

◆ *His stepfather used to beat him violently when he was young*
◆ *His older brother left home when Dan was very young*
◆ *Dan's younger stepsister received much more favourable attention*
◆ *He was always told by his family that he was stupid*
◆ *He regularly experienced feelings of dissociation as a young child*
◆ *As a teenager, Dan used a lot of cannabis*
◆ *At 18 he had a relationship with a girl at college who left him and soon after got engaged to one of Dan's friends.*

We discussed in detail his experience of dissociation and I showed him some literature describing it. Dan agreed that he probably had experienced dissociation as a child and that there were a lot of similarities with the feelings he experienced when his girlfriend left him. We discussed how dissociative states can leave people feeling very vulnerable and that, combined with his heavy cannabis use, this could have left him open to the worries he developed about the friend who, as he put it, 'stole the mind, then the girlfriend'.

From that point on he had become concerned about a plot involving various people to wreck his prospects at college and in relationships by stealing his personality. We were able to see that his general view of people as untrustworthy had an effect on this. Later we drew on this understanding to develop specific tests of his belief that people were stealing his mind.

The work of collaboratively developing a shared understanding of the problem involves linking life history with understandings of stress and vulnerability and psychological; models of voices and strange beliefs.

THOROUGH ASSESSMENT AND LIMITED SELF-MONITORING

Assessment methods are discussed in detail in Chapter 8. The process of assessing voices and strange thoughts is vital for a number of reasons. First, a comprehensive understanding of the problem is essential in the search for new ways of dealing with the problem. Secondly, the process itself can be useful in helping the person experiencing symptoms to gain a better understanding of them. It can also be a time when principles that underlie the work ahead are first established.

Activities that promote this opportunity include:

◆ working collaboratively to collect information on the symptoms
◆ examining the way that stress precipitates the symptoms
◆ looking at the way vulnerability factors like poor social support affect the problem
◆ promoting the idea that symptoms are on a continuum with normal psychological processes.

The assessment process often blends with the relationship-forming process. The endeavour should be collaborative – i.e. done with, rather than to, the person experiencing symptoms. (Follow Ch. 8 for guidelines to the assessment interview.)

Specific questionnaires that are useful in assessing the nature of and fluctuations in a person's experience of voices or strange, worrying thoughts are given in Box 11.1.

Box 11.1 Questionnaires that assess experiences of voices or worrying thoughts

◆ The Topography of Voices Scale (Hustig & Hafner 1990)
◆ The Cognitive Assessment of Voices Schedule (Chadwick & Birchwood 1994)
◆ The Hallucinations Rating Scale (Haddock, unpublished scale, 1994)
◆ The Delusions Rating Scale (Haddock, unpublished scale, 1994)
◆ The Beliefs about Voices Scale (Chadwick & Birchwood 1995)

Specific information relevant to the assessment of voices will include:

◆ the characteristics of the voice (e.g. identity, age, loudness, how threatening it is)
◆ what the voice says exactly; this often relates to other problems that the person has, such as low self-esteem
◆ the person's explanation of how the voice is heard (e.g. telepathy, radio waves)
◆ what it means to the person to hear voices (e.g. madness, specially gifted)
◆ whether the voice makes commands and if so how easy it is to resist these at different times.

Specific information relevant to the assessment of strange, worrying thoughts includes:

◆ what the central belief is about (e.g. 'there is a plot against me' or 'I am being experimented on by aliens')
◆ what general rules and assumptions the person has developed in response to this belief (e.g. 'never trust new people', 'do not talk to the neighbours' or 'do not go out at night')
◆ what specific situations this leads to difficulties with (e.g. not being able to reply to the lady at the paper shop when she says good morning, or avoiding catching the bus)
◆ how much conviction the person has in these beliefs (e.g. 0–100%)
◆ how much distress the beliefs cause
◆ how much time is spent thinking about the beliefs.

Information that is useful to collect on both voices and strange, worrying thoughts includes:

◆ how easily ignored the problem is
◆ triggers that start the problem off
◆ things that make it better or worse
◆ ways of coping with the problem.

Experiences of failure should be avoided, particularly in the early stages of the process, as this can disrupt enthusiasm and hope. If there is any doubt over people's ability or motivation to monitor and record information, it is probably best to avoid it. These methods may be considered later if levels of concentration and motivation improve. Once it is collected, the assessment information will help with the development of a conceptualisation of the person's problems, i.e. a way of understanding how it all links together. This is one of the most important aspects of this type of work. Without a shared understanding of the problem, the process of learning to deal with symptoms can become overprescriptive, unstructured, disorganised or even demoralising.

DEVELOPING A SHARED UNDERSTANDING OF THE PROBLEM

There are a variety of psychological theories or models of voices and strange thoughts. These are helpful in piecing together the information gained during the assessment phase. The application of these ways of understanding symptoms to the actual experience of the person who has them forms the basis of a shared understanding of the problem. The professional's skill and experience in this part of the helping process will show in how involved the person feels with the development of the explanation. It takes practice to relate theoretical models to these problems. The result should be an individualised picture based on an understanding of the theory. In practice, the shared understanding is constantly developing as new information arises. It is also guided by the following principles:

◆ Voices and strange thoughts become largely understandable once enough information about the person's experience of them has been gathered
◆ Many of the characteristics of voices and strange thoughts fluctuate as if on a continuum so that, for instance, levels of conviction in strange, worrying thoughts vary and voices change in volume
◆ All psychotic experience is on a continuum with normal psychological functioning so that symptoms represent an extreme of normality rather than something that is categorically different
◆ Developing a shared understanding of psychosis is underpinned by a knowledge of theoretical models.

Only three models will be presented here for simplicity. The Further reading section at the end of this chapter lists a number of practice manuals, each of which contains a review of theoretical models.

Stress and vulnerability

There are a number of theories relating stress and vulnerability factors to voices and strange thoughts. A classic one is Zubin & Spring's (1977) stress vulnerability model. It proposes that the problem is episodic and precipitated by a variety of factors. Stressful life events are said to interact with vulnerability factors, determining whether someone is pushed over a threshold. Vulnerability factors include family history of psychosis, birth complications, poor social support, poor self-care, lack of sleep, etc. The model in Figure 11.2 shows that if several of these factors are present then just a small amount of stress may tip the balance.

The model allows for conversations about the nature of voices and strange thoughts such as:

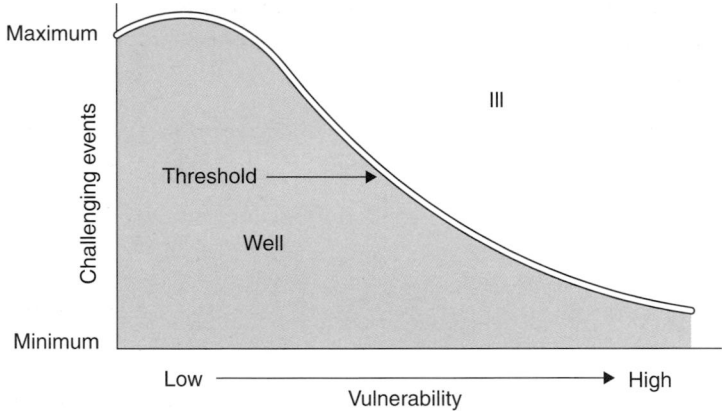

Figure 11.2   Zubin & Spring's model of the interplay between stress and vulnerability in episodes of schizophrenia. (With permission from Zubin & Spring 1977.)

- ◆ symptoms appear to be an extreme form of normal experiences
- ◆ all people have a degree of susceptibility to psychosis
- ◆ voices and strange thoughts are precipitated by stress
- ◆ looking after physical and social needs can protect against psychosis.

Kingdon & Turkington (1994) review the literature that supports these ideas. It is suggested that results from sleep deprivation and sensory deprivation experiments, along with studies of people's reactions to extreme stress, show that in these circumstances psychotic experience is the most common reaction. Indeed, when asking groups of mental health professionals whether they have ever had an auditory hallucination, I have found the majority report that they have, at least once. Feeling paranoid or thinking someone is watching you is, of course, commonly seen as being within usual human experience. This kind of information can be reassuring to people with voices and strange thoughts. Another useful discussion advocated by Kingdon & Turkington (1994) is one about the cultural differences in the way people who have these problems are received. In much of Western culture, people who hear voices, for instance, are feared, whereas in Native American culture hearers of voices are often revered as being in contact with spirits. This can be especially helpful to people whose self-esteem is badly affected by hearing voices.

A powerful message from the stress vulnerability model is that there are things the person with psychosis can do to help towards reducing vulnerability to voices and strange thoughts. These include:

- ◆ trying to maintain a regular sleep pattern
- ◆ reducing alcohol and drug intake
- ◆ maintaining self-care (e.g. in diet and hygiene)

- keeping in touch with supportive friends and family
- keeping active (e.g. keeping up exercise or some form of employment)
- taking regular medication.

A review of the person's previous experiences of relapse or recent history of voices or strange thoughts will often show changes in many of these areas. It can be encouraging to know that there is more to managing voices and strange thoughts than being a passive recipient of medication.

The ABC model – the relationship between voices and strange thoughts and a person's responses to them

The ways of dealing with voices and strange thoughts addressed in this chapter have an underlying assumption that a person's responses to a problem are central to how it is experienced. One of the central messages of cognitive therapy of psychosis, for instance, is that a person's beliefs about voices and strange thoughts are strongly associated with the way that person reacts, both emotionally and practically. How people actively respond to their voices and strange thoughts can play a large part in whether or not the problems escalate.

The ABC model shown in Box 11.2 is central to this way of working and helps to unravel the various facets of a problem. This is of course a grossly simplified description but it is where most conversations with people experiencing these problems will start. The important points are, first, to establish what factors precipitate the problem or, as is the case with voices and physical concerns, the exact nature of the voice or feeling. Secondly, it is important to ascertain what interpretation is being made of the event – i.e. exactly what the person thinks about the event, voice or feeling. Lastly, it is vital to note all the ways in which the person responds to the problem – i.e. what emotions, thoughts, actions or physical feelings occur.

Box 11.2 The ABC model

- **Activating events**: with strange, worrying thoughts these will be trigger situations, such as a stranger making eye contact in the case of paranoia; with voices the voice itself is classed as the activating event; in other cases such as physical symptoms of anxiety the symptom itself can be classed as the initial event
- **Beliefs** about the event or symptom
- **Consequences** of the problem, including emotional responses such as depression or anxiety or actions such as hiding in a bedroom or shouting at neighbours

Box 11.3 Some responses to problems

Emotions
◆ Becoming depressed and hopeless
◆ Feeling stressed and anxious
◆ Feeling angry towards people

Thoughts
◆ Spending time worrying about the problem
◆ Generally spending a lot of time thinking about the problem
◆ Thinking of the worst possible scenario

Actions
◆ Keeping a special lookout for the problem
◆ Spending time alone
◆ Complying with demands that voices make
◆ Being aggressive to others

Physical feelings
◆ Tense muscles
◆ Headaches
◆ Any physical sign of stress that could be mistaken for something else, such as thinking that dizziness has been caused by being poisoned

These responses are often helpful, such as removing oneself from a threatening situation, but they can also have unhelpful consequences, as in the case of Ken (mentioned later), who threatened his neighbours with a bat. Many of the responses that people have to symptoms are understandable but in the end feed back into the problem. These may include responses such as those given in Box 11.3.

It is important to use the thorough assessment methods mentioned earlier to ascertain as many of these responses as possible and to think about what effect they in turn might have on the problem.

Different levels of belief

When trying to understand strange, worrying thoughts it can be helpful to think in terms of three levels. At the centre of a person's problem with strange, worrying thoughts there will be a core belief. This is often related to self-esteem and contains meaning about relationships with other people and the world in general.

The next level corresponds to general rules or assumptions on which the person acts. Much of the time we are unaware that we are living by these rules, sometimes recognising only that we end up responding to events in similar ways.

The third level concerns specific situations – e.g. the specific judgements or predictions we make about particular events. If these three levels are pictured as a target with the core belief at the centre (Fig. 11.3) then what emerges is a model that is helpful in directing which beliefs to address at what times.

The first step in helping someone to cope with strange, worrying thoughts is to start with situation-specific beliefs – i.e. at the outer ring of the target. Moving inwards towards the assumptions and core beliefs requires a degree of specialist skill and good supervision. It is therefore inadvisable to tackle beliefs at this level without appropriate training or supervision. Core beliefs are by nature firmly held in place and premature intervention can strengthen them, leaving the person feeling worse (James 2001).

When summarising a person's problem using this model it is helpful to acknowledge emergent themes from the rules or assumptions level – i.e. the second level of the target. This is done to support the rationale for addressing the situation-specific beliefs that cause distress in the person's everyday life. This will often mean enquiring about general attitudes towards other people and will lead to a wider picture that includes the person's world view. Pointing out the link between assumptions and beliefs about specific events will begin to reveal the person's tendency towards jumping to conclusions. Developing a shared understanding of the person's expectations about others will open up discussions about events that the person has had mixed feelings about. People who operate on fixed generalisations often jump to conclusions

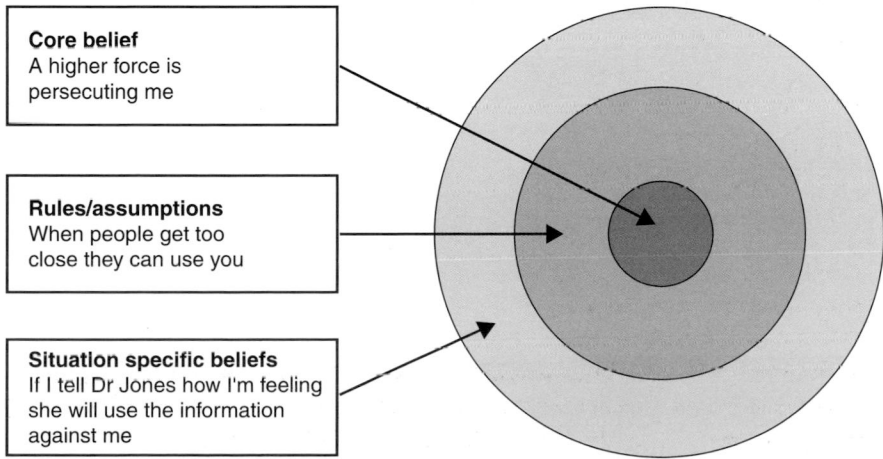

Core belief
A higher force is persecuting me

Rules/assumptions
When people get too close they can use you

Situation specific beliefs
If I tell Dr Jones how I'm feeling she will use the information against me

Figure 11.3   The target model of beliefs.

about others. Consequently they find themselves in situations that are expected to turn out badly only to find that the opposite is true. Acknowledging this jumping to conclusions style of summing up situations is often the first step towards acting differently in them and will be discussed later in relation to helping people respond differently to their beliefs.

The following case studies illustrate the usefulness of different models.

Box 11.4 shows the ABC model for David.

Box 11.5 shows the ABC model for Lorna.

Box 11.6 shows the ABC model for Carol.

Case study – ABC model, David

David had a single female voice that sounded like one of his primary school teachers, Miss Rochefort. The voice would tell him that he was useless and stupid. He found attempting anything new very distressing and would feel hopeless after making even the slightest mistake. He found that situations like these would start the voice off and would consequently avoid them as much as possible. Using the ABC model above we were able to discuss a specific recent example and identify what was particularly distressing for him. David had been advised by his key worker to try and get to know people at the local day hospital but was very worried about what to say. When he thought about approaching someone, his voice started.

Box 11.4 ABC model – David

Activating event: In this case, the voice of Miss Rochefort was saying 'You'll never be able to talk properly; they'll all find out you're stupid'.

Belief: David was convinced that he would be unable to start a conversation and that he would look foolish; he also predicted that this would lead to everyone at the day hospital thinking he was stupid and that, as a result of this, nobody would want to know him.

Consequence: He started to feel very tense and anxious. He found himself shaking and feeling quite flushed. This convinced him even more that he would mess up any attempt at a conversation. As a result he avoided talking to anyone that day and went home feeling dejected and worried that he had let his key worker down.

Case study – ABC model, Lorna

Lorna also found herself worrying that people would reject her, but for different reasons. Lorna heard the voice of a famous dead writer urging her to commit suicide and join him. She found talking about the voice very upsetting and had until recently denied hearing voices at all. She found that having a normal conversation with people helped to distract her from the voice. Unfortunately, the voice would often start taunting her when she woke up in the middle of the night. Although there was a member of staff awake during the night at her home she would not seek help and had on occasion overdosed on her medication. Weeks after the following event she was able to describe it in some detail.

Box 11.5 ABC model – Lorna

Activating event: Voice repeatedly saying 'Go on do it, come to me'.

Belief: 'If I tell the night staff about this they'll think that I'm mad, they'll tell everyone else in the house and no one will want to know me. If people find out I'm hearing voices I'll be put in hospital and be given electrical treatment like my mum. The voice will make me kill myself.'

Consequence: Lorna buried her head under her pillow and screamed for the voice to leave her alone. This woke up the person in the next room who complained the next morning. Lorna denied that anything was wrong and started spending more and more time alone in her room. She began to feel quite depressed as a result.

Stress and vulnerability model – Lorna

One thing that Lorna found helpful was discussing the relationship between stress, vulnerability and hearing voices. She was also particularly taken with the idea that, in some cultures, voice hearers are respected. She was able to identify aspects of her lifestyle that might make her vulnerable to hearing voices. These included:

◆ *spending too much time alone*
◆ *not sleeping very well*
◆ *acting on her low opinion of herself (e.g. never putting her own needs first)*
◆ *always turning down offers of support.*

   We talked about studies that showed that people's thinking changes when they are deprived of sleep (see Kingdon & Turkington 1994 for a review). Lorna could relate this to her own experiences over the previous month, which had seen her becoming increasingly worried about not sleeping. She found herself in a vicious cycle where sleep was prevented by worrying that the voice would start as a consequence of not sleeping. These night-time experiences had provided a hotbed for worry about what the other people in her house thought about her. One of the first steps towards reducing the distress caused by her voice was to make changes in these areas. She decided to visit her family more. As well as feeling more comfortable with talking about her voice with them, she also found that the long walk to her mother's house was good exercise and this helped her to sleep at night.

Case study – target model of beliefs, Carol

Carol was troubled by a belief that other people could hear her thoughts. Her mother had been a strong believer in psychic powers and had often talked of receiving telepathic messages. Carol's worries led her to trying very hard to avoid having critical thoughts about other people in case they heard them telepathically. At its worst Carol could not face people and worried that they would reject her if they knew she was having bad thoughts about them. After a number of assessment sessions we were able to start thinking about her beliefs using the target model. She had a core belief that she was guilty and evil and this seemed related to her worries about people finding out what she was really like. She was often anxious in the television room of her shared house.

Case study – target model of beliefs, Carol (*cont'd*)

The target model for Carol is shown in in Figure 11.4.

Using this model we were able to make a list of specific situations that caused Carol distress. She could not recall whether she had ever later discovered her first impressions of a situation to be wrong. She started to look out for these situations and talked with a few people that she trusted. She eventually decided that she did sometimes jump to the wrong conclusions, but not always. Carol was later able to find ways of entering situations that she had avoided for a long time. While she still had the belief that people could read her thoughts, she found that focusing on specific beliefs about here and now situations helped her to find ways of coping. We were also able to use the ABC model in trying to understand more about the specific situations that caused her distress. One that regularly upset her was meeting with her psychiatrist. Although she got on very well with him she found herself trying to control her thoughts so much that it interfered with her concentration.

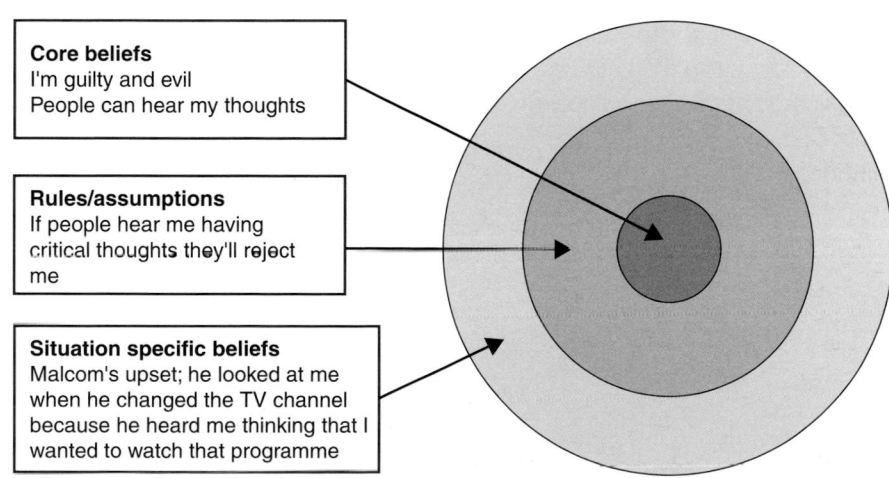

Core beliefs
I'm guilty and evil
People can hear my thoughts

Rules/assumptions
If people hear me having
critical thoughts they'll reject
me

Situation specific beliefs
Malcom's upset; he looked at me
when he changed the TV channel
because he heard me thinking that I
wanted to watch that programme

Figure 11.4　The target model of beliefs – Carol.

> ### Box 11.6 ABC model – Carol
>
> **Activating event**: Carol had a thought about not taking her new medication.
>
> **Belief**: 'He can hear me thinking this. He will think that I am going to stop taking my tablets and put me on a section because of it.'
>
> **Consequence**: Purposely repeating the thought: 'I will take my tablets'. Feeling afraid and not paying attention to the meeting.

Checking for shared understanding

The collaborative effort in developing shared understanding involves the mental health professional in presenting an appropriate model from the ones mentioned above. The skill in this lies in one's ability to describe the model in lay terms using individualised information. Wherever possible, use the person's own language to describe symptoms and difficult situations. The general principle is to develop the information in small steps. This can involve pausing after each idea or small set of ideas. Connections between concepts can be highlighted so that the whole picture builds up slowly. Each pause should be accented with a check for understanding and an invitation to elaborate further if the person feels that important points have been missed. Finally, it is useful to check for understanding by asking the person to repeat an impression of what has been discussed. In Carol's case above, a conversation similar to the one below was helpful in establishing a shared understanding.

JM:	Carol, I'd like to spend some time making sure that we understand this problem in the same way; how would that be?
Carol:	How?
JM:	Well, how about if I tell you what my understanding is and you can tell me if that's right?
Carol:	OK.
JM:	Well, from what you've said it seems that a lot of your distress comes from worrying about people hearing your thoughts. Is that right?
Carol:	Yes, people do hear my thoughts.
JM:	And you find that very upsetting.
Carol:	(Nods.)
JM:	And you were saying that, because of this, you spend a lot of time checking people's expressions to see if they have picked up on what you're thinking.
Carol:	Yes, I have to watch people all the time.

JM:	And this is because you worry that people won't want to know you if they find out you've had bad thoughts about them.
Carol:	That's why I have to stop myself thinking bad thoughts.
JM:	Yes, and you were telling me earlier that that's what was happening when the doctor said you looked distracted.
Carol:	I worried that he'd have me taken in.
JM:	Yes, because you worried that he could hear you thinking about your tablets.
Carol:	But he always says that he can't hear me thinking. Sometimes I worry for nothing.
JM:	How about if we try and pull all of this together?
Carol:	What do you mean?
JM:	Well it seems that all these things go together somehow. You have this worry about people hearing your thoughts because you think they won't like you if they hear them. This leads you to look out for it happening. Is that right?
Carol:	Yes.
JM:	And when you are looking out for signs of this you often find this makes life quite difficult around other people because you're watching them carefully and trying not to have bad thoughts. Have I got that right?
Carol:	Yes, I have to watch myself and everyone else.
JM:	But sometimes you get it wrong and find out that even though you really believed that someone could hear you thinking they couldn't all along. It's like if you really expect them to hear you hard enough you convince yourself that they can.
Carol:	It's so hard.
JM:	You must work very hard at keeping all this under control.
Carol:	(Nods.)
JM:	So let's see if we can sum this up. Stop me if I get this wrong. You really worry that people can hear your thoughts and that if they do they won't like you. (Pause.) This means that you try to control your thoughts and look out for signs that people can hear them. (Pause.) The problem makes life very upsetting sometimes. (Pause.) And we know that, at least sometimes, people can't really hear your thoughts even though you really believed they did. How was that Carol, does it sound like I've got it right?
Carol:	I think so.
JM:	Did I miss anything out?
Carol:	Well, only that my Mum always said that I was telepathic as a child.
JM:	OK, so that might explain where the worry came from. I need to see if I've explained myself properly, Carol. Can you say something about how you understand this problem?
Carol:	What like you just did?
JM:	Yes, but from your point of view.
Carol:	Well it's the same. I get upset because people can hear me thinking bad things about them.

JM:	And what do you do about that?
Carol:	I stop myself having bad thoughts and watch out for them getting upset. But sometimes people just get upset and it's nothing to do with my thoughts, but I can't tell the difference.
JM:	How about if we try and find some things that might help with this problem?
Carol:	Like what?
JM:	Well you said that when you told your friend that you have this worry you felt better about it and stopped watching her for a while. Maybe we could look at why that was helpful.
Carol:	All right.

Small summaries and reflective statements along with regular requests for feedback were helpful in breaking down the information. This helped Carol to piece it together with me and in the end we had some common ground to start from. This enabled us to move on to discussing ways of coping with the problem.

COPING WITH VOICES AND STRANGE, WORRYING THOUGHTS

The way people respond to symptoms of psychosis can be compared to the way people respond to headaches. Headaches are a common experience but everyone has different ways of dealing with them. Some people reach for tablets immediately while others try to get on with whatever they are doing. Others would never or only rarely take medication. A similar picture emerges from talking to people with voices or strange, worrying thoughts, especially if the person has been experiencing the problem for a long time.

Coping methods are not always helpful in the long term and some only partially reduce the distress associated with the problem. With this in mind it is useful to spend time developing three aspects of coping:

1. increasing the effectiveness of current coping methods
2. reducing the use of harmful ways of coping
3. introducing previously untried methods.

The first step is to examine current ways of coping. These might fall into one of the following categories (Table 11.1).

Building on coping methods

The person may have a variety of ways of coping with symptoms. It will be helpful to discuss how effective each one is. Some people use their coping

Table 11.1 Ways of coping	
Distraction	**Interacting**
Voices and strange, worrying thoughts: Listening to music Reading aloud Counting backwards from 100 Describing an object in detail Watching TV	**Voices:** Telling the voices to go away Talking to the voices while pretending to use a mobile phone Agreeing to listen to the voices at particular times **Strange, worrying thoughts:** Testing out beliefs (see next section)

Activity	**Social**	**Physical**
Voices and strange, worrying thoughts: Walking Tidying the house Having a relaxing bath Playing the guitar Singing Going to the gym	**Voices and strange, worrying thoughts:** Talking to a trusted friend or member of the family Phoning a helpline Avoiding people Going to a drop-In centre Visiting a favourite place	**Voices and strange, worrying thoughts:** Taking extra medication Using ear plugs (voices) Breathing exercises Relaxation methods

methods only when the symptoms are very bad, while others get through most days using them. As before, thinking about recent examples often helps, especially when detail is needed. When trying to develop the coping method's effectiveness consider the following:

◆ What type of coping method is it (distraction, activity, interacting, social or physical)?
◆ How could it be made more absorbing or intense?
◆ Are there any similar ones that might be more helpful?

Spending time thinking about what the essential qualities of a coping activity are (Table 11.2) can help in the process of making it even more effective.

The next step will be to practise the new or improved way of coping, repeatedly. This is started during a session and practised in between. When the person feels confident other methods can be added to the repertoire.

Coping methods with harmful effects

Methods of coping often emerge that are effective but costly in the long term. However, the person may feel reluctant to give them up if they are seen as

Table 11.2 Essential qualities of coping activities

Problem and coping method	Possible effective ingredients	Intensified version
Marie believes that the Masons are plotting to kidnap her sons. She finds that when she is anxious it can help to lie on the sofa and watch TV	Relaxation Distraction	Lying in a hot bath with aromatherapy oils Listening to soft music and reading magazine
Jonathan finds that having to talk to his friend on the phone sends his voices into the background	Speaking aloud Distraction Social contact	Visiting parents or friends and talking about things other than his voices

the only means of control. The use of these should also be explored in detail. These ways of coping can themselves become uncontrolled, causing problems of their own. This can be especially true for the use of alcohol and drugs. Serious problems of this nature will need to be dealt with separately (see Ch. 14).

A balanced view of the short- and long-term effects of coping methods will inform any discussion of this nature. The short-term usefulness should be acknowledged but offset against the damage likely to occur in the medium and long term. Harmful ways of coping include ones that:

◆ eventually cause more emotional distress
◆ are detrimental to physical health
◆ actually involve physical harm
◆ lower confidence and self-esteem
◆ cause other people to react badly.

Examples are included in Table 11.3.

Considering what the effective part of the coping method is can lead to more suitable alternatives. This often means undertaking a collaborative period of trial and error where the person agrees to try out new ideas that have been discussed and practised in session. Examples are included in Table 11.4.

If a less harmful version of the same coping method cannot be identified then the person may agree to using it less often if other alternatives are suggested. Again, every effort should be made to maximise the beneficial effects of the coping method. This will include thinking of ways to make distraction methods more absorbing or social methods more engaging.

Table 11.3 Harmful ways of coping

Problem	Coping method	Short-term effect	Medium/long-term effect
Ken hears voices that sound like his neighbours planning to break into his flat	Threaten them with a bat	Voices stop, leaving Ken feeling safer	The police are called and they take the neighbours' side. People in the area avoid Ken. He begins to feel that everyone is against him
Carrie hears voices saying that she is a prostitute	Shouts at the voices during meal times	Feels that she has made her point and that the voices will stop for a while	Staff ask her to leave and eat in her room. Carrie begins to feel depressed about having no one to talk to
Mark believes that he has defrauded the benefits agency and that he will be prosecuted	Visits the benefits office daily to confess	Feels reassured when he is told that there is no problem	Has little time in the day to do things he enjoys. Later thinks that it is too serious for the desk clerk to know about and feels even worse

Table 11.4 Alternative coping methods

Problem and coping method	Possible effective ingredients	Alternative coping method
Ken threatens his neighbours with a bat because of the voices he hears	Activity Exercise Adrenaline	Kicking a football very hard and chasing it in the field behind his house
Barbara feels embarrassed when she is compelled to shout at her voices while walking down the street	Answering the voices Talking aloud	Pretending to use a replica mobile phone and answering the voices in a normal voice
Cyril feels upset when his neighbours get angry about him playing his music very loud to drown out the voices	Distraction	Listening to the same music on a personal stereo

DEALING WITH STRANGE, WORRYING BELIEFS

Any attempt to deal with this problem should take into account the effects of:

- ◆ the distress associated with the belief
- ◆ the preoccupation with the belief
- ◆ the strength of belief (conviction)
- ◆ the person's responses:
  - ● acting as if it were true
  - ● looking out for things associated with the belief
- ◆ the increased tendency to jump to conclusions.

As seen earlier, people respond to problems in ways that are designed to keep themselves safe. However, these responses can in fact make the problem worse and this process is just as evident with strange, worrying beliefs (Fig. 11.5). To emphasise that this way of responding to beliefs is part of human nature, rather than being unique to those experiencing psychosis, we can use the example of superstitious beliefs.

It is part of being human that people often have strong beliefs despite having little or no real evidence to support them. Superstitious beliefs are like this. For instance, there is no conclusive evidence of unfortunate events being precipitated by ignoring magpies, walking under ladders or putting new shoes on a table. It is, however, common for people to believe these things. These

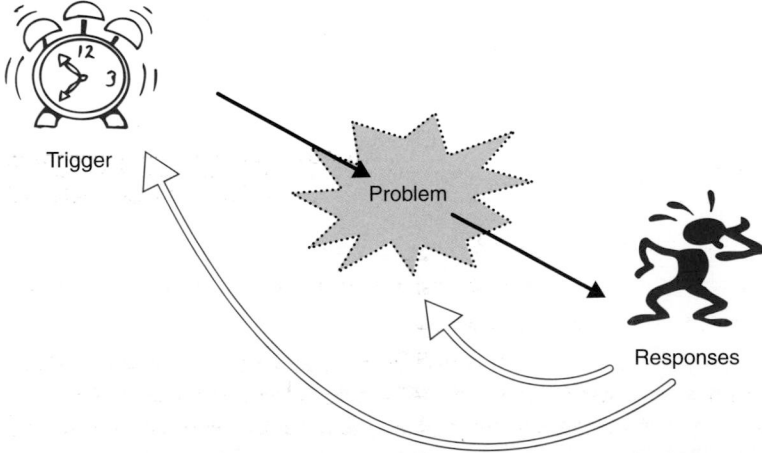

Figure 11.5   A generic view of how responses can feed back into a problem.

examples can serve to highlight two of the processes that affect people when they have strange, worrying beliefs:

◆ looking out for signs that support the belief as well as ignoring evidence against it (consciously and unconsciously).
◆ acting as if the belief were true.

Keeping a lookout

Consider people who worry about not saying hello to every magpie that they come across. When confronted with a situation that makes this inevitable, such as seeing seven all together while driving along a fast road, such a person would naturally feel quite distressed. Once the worrying belief is activated, in this case 'that unfortunate events come after ignoring magpies', the person will be on the lookout for bad luck. This happens purposefully as well as automatically. The automatic process is the same one that causes us to notice more Volkswagen camper vans if we are thinking about buying one. Of course, if something is being looked out for more then it is much more likely to be noticed. In this way, people concerned with magpies increase the number of unfortunate events that they notice. Strong beliefs also cause us to ignore evidence against them. Strong prejudicial beliefs, for instance, survive this way. Hence the person who worries about having ignored a magpie is also more likely to discount automatically any good events that happen that day.

The same process applies to all strange and worrying beliefs. The more time a person spends dwelling on a belief the stronger it gets, as more supportive evidence is collected and refuting evidence is ignored. Therefore one of the first steps in coping with strange and worrying beliefs is to find ways of being less preoccupied by them (Box 11.7).

Box 11.7 Tips for dealing with strange, worrying beliefs

◆ Preoccupation leads to greater conviction
◆ Greater conviction leads to more distress
◆ Distress is what we work with
◆ Helping someone to be less preoccupied with their distressing beliefs will help to prevent increasing conviction; commonly helpful coping strategies include absorbing and distracting activities such as structured time with trusted friends (e.g. playing a game or going shopping)

Acting as if the belief were true

A second process that leads to the maintenance of strange, worrying beliefs is that of responding to them as if they were true. This is understandable given that we all have a powerful need to protect ourselves from harm. Unfortunately, the avoidance of predicted harm strengthens the notion that it would have happened if action had not been taken. Take, for example, somebody who avoids putting new shoes on the table, believing it will lead to tragedy. If no such tragedy occurs the person will explain this in terms of the safe handling of shoes rather than attributing it to sensible precautions. Following this pattern can intrude more and more on a person's quality of life. People with distressing beliefs often find themselves so convinced of them that they adapt their lives around the belief to a disabling extent.

Jumping to conclusions

When we are tired or experiencing distress we tend to leap to conclusions that are not always accurate. A classic analogy used to illustrate this is that of waking up in the middle of the night to the sound of breaking glass. Imagine that this happened to you and that you were alone in the house. Would you feel anxious? What would be the first conclusion to enter your mind? Most people answer that they would feel distressed, thinking that an intruder had entered the house. The story continues that on bravely venturing downstairs you discover that your cat has woken up and broken a vase while exploring the mantelpiece. The jumping to conclusions style of thinking in this case would have been helpful in preparing to deal with an intruder. However, the resolution of the story points to the frequent false alarms set off by this quick but often inaccurate automatic thinking process.

Jumping to conclusions is something that people with voices and strange beliefs are particularly prone to. Garety & Hemsley (1994) describe some research that involved asking people to guess the proportions of coloured beads in a hidden jar as they were taken out one at a time. It was discovered that people with psychosis were more likely to come to a firm conclusion after fewer beads had been drawn. So, although it is naturally human to jump to conclusions on the basis of small amounts of information, it seems that this is more pronounced for people experiencing strange, worrying beliefs. Jumping to conclusions too quickly can lead to regular misunderstanding of events. Thus people can often find themselves making mistaken assumptions about people and situations. Unfortunately, if this is followed by the types of response mentioned above, the mistaken assumption can become increasingly believable as it is bolstered with more supportive evidence and the seemingly protective effects of evasive action.

Exploring the effects of jumping to conclusions – testing beliefs

As mentioned earlier, this phase is impossible to engage in successfully without the thorough groundwork described in the first part of the chapter. A shared rationale for exploring the effects that jumping to conclusions has on a person's lifestyle will emerge from assessment and the development of coping techniques. As the work continues, opportunities should arise to discuss recent examples of how the tendency to view the world in a certain way leads to mistaken assumptions. This happened in Neil's case.

Case study – Neil

Neil had been seen on six occasions for help with his voices and paranoia. He found it particularly difficult to trust people and this was exacerbated by the voices, which would tell him that people were collecting information about him so that he could be banned from the ward. At the beginning of the session Neil was asked how the previous few days had been and he described an upsetting event that had taken place the day before. It transpired that he had gone to attend a discussion group facilitated by his primary nurse Sue (whom he was just beginning to trust). When he entered the group room Sue was sitting with her back towards the door. The voices told him that she did not want him there and for a while he was convinced that she would turn around and ask him to leave. Neil bravely stayed and was eventually greeted by Sue as she turned around. Neil was quite shaken by the experience but remained in the group despite not contributing a great deal. This became an ideal opportunity to discuss Neil's tendency towards jumping to conclusions that did not always turn out right. The discussion ended with the following summary:

JM: *Neil, this event seems quite important, I think it tells us a lot about the kinds of situation that you find difficult.*
Neil: *How do you mean?*
JM: *Well, it seems to me that this tendency you have to think of the worst in certain situations causes you a lot of grief. Let's imagine that you had left the group room when you felt sure that Sue was against you. How would you have felt?*
Neil: *Well I probably would have gone back to my room and wound myself up about it.*
JM: *Right, but you didn't, you took the plunge and stayed.*
Neil: *Yeah, sometimes it's easier than others.*
JM: *OK, I wonder if there might have been other occasions when you jumped to a conclusion that someone was against you and later found out that they were OK?*
Neil: *It does happen sometimes but, most of the time, I avoid people that I'm not sure about.*

Case study – Neil *(cont'd)*

JM: I wonder if sometimes you avoid people who are actually OK but you don't get to find out?

Neil: I suppose that could happen, but it's better to be safe than sorry!

JM: That's true, it is good to be safe, but I wonder if there's such a thing as being too safe. I mean, what kind of effect does this strategy have on your life?

Neil: Well, you know that it makes me very edgy around people and that I sometimes upset them because I have a go. But I'm not about to start running up to people with open arms just because I sometimes make mistakes.

JM: I don't think that's what I'm going to suggest.

Neil: What then?

JM: Well, how about looking at the people that you think might be OK? Is there any way we could check out to see if you're jumping to conclusions with them?

Neil: You mean like Sally? I suppose I could stop and say hello to her rather than keep walking by.

JM: That sounds like the kind of thing. Let's see if we can work this out as something for you to try in the week.

A specific test was then negotiated with Neil. He was encouraged to work out the details following the guidelines given in Box 11.8.

A test is, generally, more effective the simpler it is. In the case above, for instance, Neil decided that he would spend 5 minutes talking to Sally to see if she would (as he predicted) turn nasty towards him. The specific signs of nastiness that he expected to see were written down, as well as his own evidence for and against the prediction. One strong piece of evidence was his 'gut feeling' about the situation. After he discovered that Sally was in fact very pleasant towards him, we discussed the results and Neil decided that it might be worth exploring other areas where his strong intuitive sense might lead him to jump to incorrect conclusions.

Pitfalls to avoid include:

◆ imposing your own ideas for a test
◆ any approach that involves you trying to prove something to the client
◆ lack of preparation and preliminary discussion.

ADDRESSING BELIEFS ABOUT VOICES – EXPLORING CONTROL OVER VOICES

Most people, when asked about how much control they have over their voices, will report having very little or none at all. Voices can make people feel weak, hopeless and powerless. With this is mind, a significant step towards

Box 11.8 Guiding principles for tests of strange, worrying beliefs

- Start with beliefs about specific events so that the knowledge that beliefs are sometimes wrong can be used as a method of coping with future events.
- Ask whether the person has ever jumped to a conclusion that was later found to be wrong.
- Explain common effects of factors such as stress and lack of sleep on thinking (e.g. selective attention and jumping to conclusions) – ask if anything like this could be happening.
- Clarify a particular belief about a particular situation that the person feels able to tackle.
- Discuss the evidence for and against the belief using a naïve approach that allows a development of the person's own perspective with as few suggestions from you as possible.
- Discuss the quality of the evidence for the worrying belief. People often base important predictions and conclusions on intuition or insufficient information.
- Work together to devise a way of safely testing the belief.
- Take time to prepare the test, including recording predictions about what might happen and what this might mean.
- After carrying out the test, spend time discussing the meaning of what happened; ask how the client might use the information gained.

dealing with voices can be discovering just how much control can be gained over them.

Previous discussions about the nature of voices will be essential to this work. If a person is to give up an idea that voices are uncontrollable because they come from an outside source then consideration must be given to the alternative explanations. Without the underpinning work described earlier, people can be faced with frightening misconceptions about voices and what it means to have them. As discussed previously, accounts of voices that emphasise the role of stress and vulnerability will be crucial to this foundational work.

Helping a person to develop a greater sense of control over a voice involves identifying, clarifying and testing out the specific beliefs that are held about the power of the voice. In essence the method is similar to the guidelines for testing out beliefs set out in Box 11.9. It is worth reviewing how this process relates specifically to beliefs about the power of voices.

The case study of Anne-Marie is an example of exploring control over voices.

Box 11.9 Guiding principles for testing beliefs about voices

◆ Discuss the person's current beliefs about how controllable the voice is.

◆ Discuss the link between lack of power over the voice and the distress it causes.

◆ Review the person's evidence for having no control over the voice. This usually amounts to 'not being able to switch it off'.

◆ Discuss how having more control over the voice would affect the person's level of distress.

◆ Discuss actions that demonstrate a person's control over things such as a radio, car or heater. This discussion explores the idea that turning things up and down is as good a demonstration of control as switching them on and off.

◆ Propose that being able to make the voice louder then quieter, at will, would demonstrate a high degree of control over it.

◆ Collaboratively plan a test of whether the person can develop this kind of control. This involves:
   ● picking a useful coping method developed during previous work
   ● making the voice louder by listening to it intently (this may have to involve bringing the voice on by thinking about it)
   ● using the coping method to reduce the volume of the voice
   ● repeating this process until the person can call up the voice, make it louder and then reduce the volume at will.

◆ Review the person's previous ideas about control over the voice in relation to this process and develop ideas for further coping.

Case study – Anne-Marie, turning the voices up and down

Anne-Marie was very distressed by a voice that sounded like her late grandfather's. The voice would comment on her actions and say very upsetting things about her. At its worst the voice shouted that she was evil and demanded that she hurt herself. Earlier work with Anne-Marie had concentrated on understanding the experience of hearing voices. She developed ideas around stress and vulnerability and was able to identify a number of factors that would make her particularly vulnerable to hearing voices. For instance, she had a poor view of herself, having been regularly beaten by her grandfather when she was a child. She had experienced bouts of depression on and off for most of her life. Two family members on her mother's side experienced emotional problems requiring long-term medication. Her sleep was regularly disturbed and she frequently forgot to take her

Case study – Anne-Marie, turning the voices up and down (cont'd)

tablets, owing to waking up late. Anne-Marie was very worried about upsetting people and consequently found spending time in new social situations very difficult. She had recently been introduced to a new keyworker and two new residents at the group house where she lived. This stress, coupled with her particular vulnerability, had, she thought, led to her problem with the voice becoming worse.

Practical ideas developed from this understanding included working to improve sleep, asking a friend who called by her room every morning to remind her to take medication and talking to her new keyworker about her shyness with a trusted person present. Anne-Marie later found that talking aloud was helpful in reducing the volume of her voice. She would sing along to her stereo in her room, talk to her friend or read the newspaper to a fellow resident whose sight was bad. She found all these things to be helpful to a greater or lesser degree. Anne-Marie's voice had reduced in intensity and frequency but it was still very distressing to her, especially as she believed that it might make her harm herself and that she had no power over it whatsoever. She looked to the times that she had very nearly followed its instructions to hurt herself and thought that without the reassurance and help of either her best friend or her sister she would not have been able to resist. She saw these near misses as proof that she could succumb if the voice pushed too hard when she was alone.

Exploring control

Anne-Marie agreed that worrying about the power of the voice was one of the worst aspects of the problem. She was also intrigued by my suggestion that her seeking help from her sister and friend was a successful coping method rather than a failure to cope. We used her demonstrating control over her stereo as an analogy. She identified that she could show that she was in control of her stereo by turning it on and off, changing the tape in it or turning the volume up and down. I suggested that the last method might be useful for our purposes and began:

JM: *So, Anne-Marie, are you saying that if you were able to change the volume on the stereo, turning it up and down when you decided, you would be showing you were in control of it?*

AM: *Of course I can control the volume, I have to in case the others complain about the noise.*

JM: *Yes. How about thinking about the voice in the same way?*

AM: *What, turning it up and down?*

JM: *Yes. If you could turn the volume of the voice up and down just like that, how would that be?*

AM: *That would be great but I can't see it happening.*

We discussed the arrangements for trying this out, including the art of bringing the voice on. Anne-Marie was very unsure of this and wanted to try it out with her friend first rather than with me. We set this up and agreed that she should have something to do shortly afterwards in case the voice became very distressing; she

Case study – Anne-Marie, turning the voices up and down (cont'd)

also informed her keyworker what she was going to do. We spent the next session discussing her success in bringing the voice on and planning the test. Anne-Marie brought a newspaper to the session and spent 15 minutes thinking about and listening to the voice for 1 minute followed by reading aloud for 2 or 3 minutes. After 15 minutes she was happy that she could bring the voice on, make it louder and then reduce the volume at will. We discussed what this meant to her. She was excited about the finding but remained a little cautious.

Over the coming weeks she tried the technique regularly and eventually decided that she did indeed have more power than the voice. This helped to decrease her fear of hurting herself and we discussed the implications that this might have for her. Anne-Marie began to be a little more adventurous socially, chancing that the voice would increase with stress. It did worsen on a few occasions but she was happy to just ignore it or to continue a conversation rather than leave, which is how she would have responded previously.

Useful ideas from Anne-Marie's experience of exploring control include:

◆ Use an effective coping method that is already well practised
◆ Use analogies relevant to the person's lifestyle (e.g. in Anne-Marie's case the stereo volume)
◆ Move forward at the person's own pace
◆ Practise turning the volume of the voice up and down until it becomes easy.

CONCLUSIONS

I am always humbled by people's ability to bear the adversity associated with voices and strange thoughts. Often people have adapted their lifestyle so much that the small sense of well-being they do have feels precariously balanced. It is enthusing to be able to offer some degree of help to a group of people who have historically had limited access to anything other than drug treatments. However, learning to deal with these problems can in itself be worrying and so I have tried to emphasise the sensitive nature of this approach. There is a fine balance in the therapeutic stance between caution and confidence. For instance, offering suggestions tentatively, and carefully negotiating the pace of the process, while maintaining a quiet confidence that small things can helpfully change, is a useful position to adopt.

There are many ways that the ideas presented in this chapter can be taken forward practically. Putting the ideas into practice and discussing them with people who experience symptoms is by far the most effective method. However, launching into radically new ways of working without having someone to help you reflect is unwise. Meeting with an experienced professional for regular supervision sessions is vital in the development of any new skills and for many professionals it is necessary for continued registration. Further reading from the list at the end of the chapter will be essential for the person looking to develop skills beyond those covered here. Workshops and conferences around the subject are frequent in the UK and can provide a useful as well as cost-effective further introduction. There are a number of courses that prepare professionals to work in this way; a few of which are listed at the end of the chapter. In my experience, courses that can demonstrate a high level of skills-focused training are most useful. This can be verified if the course includes high levels of practice scrutiny through the mediums of role play, feedback on taped clinical work, and supervision.

Dealing with voices and strange thoughts is a challenge to those who experience it as well as to those from whom help is sought. With the right support, however, the process can be both fruitful and rewarding.

Summary of practical strategies identified

◆ Sharing worrying experiences with a trusted person and understanding it in the context of life history.
◆ Having that person, or someone else, to help work out practical strategies.
◆ Trying to maintain a regular sleep pattern.
◆ Reducing alcohol and drug intake.
◆ Maintaining self-care (e.g. diet and hygiene).
◆ Keeping in touch with supportive friends and family.
◆ Keeping active (e.g. exercise, some form of daily activity or employment).
◆ Taking regular medication.
◆ Reducing potentially harmful ways of coping.
◆ Building up useful coping methods and learning new ways of coping from other people. These might include:
  ● telling the voices to go away
  ● agreeing to listen to the voices at a particular time
  ● using ear plugs
  ● learning relaxation methods
  ● having a relaxing bath
  ● talking to friends
  ● playing a sport or exercising
  ● reading or watching television.
◆ Working with a trusted person to explore levels of control over voices.
◆ Working with a trusted person to test out beliefs about events or voices.

References

Chadwick P, Birchwood M 1994 The Cognitive Assessment of Voices Schedule. In: Chadwick P, Birchwood M, Trower P (eds) 1996 Cognitive therapy for hallucinations, delusions and paranoia. Wiley, Chichester, pp 195–200

Chadwick P, Birchwood M 1995 The Beliefs about Voices Questionnaire. In: Chadwick P, Birchwood M, Trower P (eds) 1996 Cognitive therapy for hallucinations, delusions and paranoia. Wiley, Chichester, pp 201–202

Chadwick P, Birchwood M, Trower P (eds) 1996 Cognitive therapy for hallucinations, delusions and paranoia. Wiley, Chichester

Curson D, Patel M, Liddle P, Barnes T 1988 Psychiatric morbidity of a long stay hospital population with chronic schizophrenia and implications for future community care. British Medical Journal 297:819–822

Fowler P, Garety P, Kuipers L 1995 Cognitive behaviour therapy for psychosis, a clinical handbook. Wiley, Chichester

Garety P, Hemsley D 1994 Delusions: investigations into the psychology of delusional reasoning. Psychology Press, Hove, Sussex

Grant A, Mills J, Mulhern R, Short N 2004 Cognitive behavioural therapy in mental health care: a contextual guide to practice. Sage, London

Hardy A 2003 Investigating hallucinations in psychosis in relation to trauma history and post traumatic stress disorder. Paper presented to BABCP annual conference, University of York, 18 July

Hustig H, Hafner R 1990 Persistent auditory hallucinations and their relationship to delusions of mood. Journal of Nervous and Mental Diseases 178:264–267

James I 2001 Schema therapy: the next generation, but should it carry a health warning? Behavioural and Cognitive Psychotherapy 29:401–407

Johnstone L 2000 Users and abusers of psychiatry: a critical look at psychiatric practice. Routledge, London

Kingdon D, Turkington D 1994 Cognitive behavioural therapy of schizophrenia. Lawrence Erlbaum, Hove, Sussex

NHS Centre for Reviews and Dissemination 2000 Psychosocial interventions for schizophrenia. Bulletin on the effectiveness of health service interventions for decision makers 6:3. Available on line at: http://www.york.ac.uk/inst/crd/ehc63.htm

Romme M, Escher S 2000 Making sense of voices: a guide for health professionals working with voice hearers. Mind Publications, London

Zubin J, Spring B 1977 Vulnerability: a new view of schizophrenia. Journal of Abnormal Psychology 86:260–266

Annotated further reading

Bentall R (ed) 1989 Reconstructing schizophrenia. Routledge, London

This text examines the historical development and debate over the current relevance of the disease concept of schizophrenia. It provides part of the theoretical backdrop to the approaches described in this chapter.

Chadwick P, Birchwood M, Trower P 1996 Cognitive therapy for hallucinations, delusions and paranoia. Wiley, Chichester

Fowler P, Garety P, Kuipers L 1995 Cognitive behaviour therapy for psychosis, a clinical handbook. Wiley, Chichester

These two books are essentially treatment manuals. Either will be of use to the professional with training in cognitive–behavioural therapy (CBT) seeking to cross over to working with people experiencing psychosis. Alongside good supervision, either will provide a valuable guide to this process.

Grant A, Mills J, Mulhern R, Short N 2004 Cognitive behavioural therapy in mental health care: a contextual guide to practice. Sage, London

This text describes the techniques of CBT and goes on to show how they can be applied to a wide variety of problems in a range of healthcare settings, including specialist community teams and residential units. This will useful to people who are new to CBT as well as specialists seeking to use their skills in new settings.

Haddock G, Slade P (eds) 1996 Cognitive behavioural interventions with psychotic disorders. Routledge, London

A broad range of approaches under the umbrella of CBT is introduced in this book. It will be of use to the person seeking an introduction to the field.

Kingdon D, Turkington D 1994 Cognitive behavioural therapy of schizophrenia. Lawrence Erlbaum Associates, Hove

Another treatment manual. One of the strengths of this book is the clear and practical description of the normalising approach. The whole text is clearly presented, providing an ideal first stop for the person developing a practical interest in this type of work.

Kingdon D, Turkington D 2002 The case study guide to cognitive behaviour therapy of psychosis. Wiley, Chichester

An in-depth description of helping people with voices and strange beliefs. Each chapter is given over to one person's therapy. The authors each describe their own professional background and approach prior to describing the work undertaken.

Annotated further reading (_cont'd_)

Nelson H 1997 Cognitive behavioural therapy with schizophrenia: a practice manual. Stanley Thornes, Cheltenham

This very practical manual covers a wide range of strategies used within CBT. Again useful for a person with some experience or at least good CBT supervision. The text covers strategies for overcoming a range of common obstacles.

Romme M, Escher S 2000 Making sense of voices: a guide for health professionals working with voice hearers. Mind Publications, London

Romme & Escher's work is invaluable to this way of working. Many of the ideas developed in the psychosocial interventions movement originated with them.

Wykes T (ed) 1998 Outcome and innovation in psychological treatment of schizophrenia. Wiley, Chichester

A more recent review of the state of the art in psychological approaches to serious mental health problems. The text describes emerging applications of CBT, including problems arising from cognitive deficits and dissatisfaction with medication. The book will be of use to those interested in recent developments in the field as well as to people involved in the development of services or training programmes.

12

Dealing with blankness and deadness

Jem Mills, Sue Kerr and Sally Goldspink

I developed a feeling of blankness and deadness which has stayed with me. To this day I have felt I have died inside and have lost all my inner energy. Because of this I thought I was going to die, which is very frightening.

(Ch. 1)

KEY ISSUES

◆ Understanding the context of reduced energy, motivation and connectedness

◆ Developing a shared understanding of the problem

◆ Working to achievable goals at a realistic pace

◆ Getting back into the social world

◆ Gradually increasing mastery and pleasure activities

◆ Mindfulness meditation as a concentration aid

INTRODUCTION

The above quote highlights an area that is often ignored or undervalued in conceptualising serious mental illness. To be 'mad' is to be 'raving', 'crazed', a 'lunatic' – all of which conjure images of dynamic movement, erratic, inexplicable and often violent behaviour, as if the person is removed from humanity through the grip of some terrifying alien force. These stereotypical images do not include people who 'look, act and feel numb', or people who have 'lost all their inner energy'. They do not include the person sitting on a sofa smoking endless cigarettes and getting up only to make a cup of tea (and leaving milk, sugar and the used tea bag in a mess afterwards). Neither does it include the individual who spends 2 hours getting out of bed, puts on the same clothes as worn for the last week and then falls asleep in the chair half an hour after getting up. Nor does it explain people whose families think they no longer have any feelings for them because they hardly talk and only reply 'yeah, I'm OK' in a flat and uninterested voice when asked how they are.

Bleuler (1983) describes these 'hidden' symptoms as 'the loss of feeling felt, the numbness perceived, the lifelessness experienced'. These hidden symptoms are the concern of this discussion. They are the so-called 'negative symptoms'. Although mostly associated with a diagnosis of schizophrenia, negative symptoms cover a range of health and social factors. In this chapter we critically examine the illness concept of negative symptoms presenting a variety of perspectives, which will hopefully inspire more comprehensive assessment and creative approaches to negative symptoms. We underline the value of reaching beyond traditional views of negative symptoms and emphasise the importance of taking an individualised perspective. With this in mind we have drawn on the eloquent first-person account in Chapter 1 to describe ways of dealing with blankness and deadness.

AN ILLNESS PERSPECTIVE

A diagnosis of schizophrenia is generally made when individuals experience positive symptoms (hallucinations and/or delusions) at the onset and during the acute phase of their illness. Often these persist as residual symptoms. However, the severe positive symptoms are often transient, although a percentage remain despite treatment with neuroleptic medication. The positive symptoms are so called because they are 'outside the normal range of experience', although more recent debate on the symptoms of mental illness has quite rightly pointed out that some positive symptoms are experienced by a wider population than those diagnosed as mentally ill (see Chs 4, 11). Even so, hallucinations and delusion still remain a foreign experience to most people.

Negative symptoms, conversely, are defined as a 'failure' of everyday functions. They have the capacity to affect all aspects of functioning. Speech, behaviour, level of enjoyment, motivation and concentration can all be adversely affected (Table 12.1). Unfortunately, as the features of negative symptoms are essentially an absence rather than an addition, they are harder to recognise as abnormal and can be misidentified as an aspect of a sufferer's personality or as wilful behaviour on their part. It follows that they could therefore be seen to be within an individual's control. It is this mistaken view of control that can lead to judgemental attitudes that adversely affect treatment philosophies

Table 12.1 Main negative symptom groups	
Negative symptom	**Observed behaviour/consequence**
Blunted affect: 'Decreased range and intensity of emotional responsiveness'	Diminished or absent facial expressiveness during interactions with others Unchanging, monotonous or inexpressive voice tone when conversing Lack of gestures when conversing
Alogia: 'Poverty of thought'	Little or no spontaneous speech Little said during interactions Speech conveys little actual information Stopping in the middle of a conversation and forgetting what was said
Avolition: 'Loss of motivation or drive'	Difficulty in following through on activities Lack of interest in doing things Sitting around doing little or engaged in activities requiring little effort (such as watching TV)
Anhedonia: 'Diminished capacity to experience pleasure'	Lack of enjoyment from recreational activities Inability to feel close to others, such as friends and relatives Difficulty in experiencing pleasure from anything
Inattention:	Becoming easily distracted during conversations Difficulty in focusing attention on a task such as reading a magazine article or getting dressed Stopping midway through something, such as a task or conversation

Adapted from Watkins 1996.

and outcome. An example of this is someone who finds it difficult to get up in the morning being thought of or described as 'lazy', as the observer believes the person is wilfully staying in bed rather than battling with symptoms. This mistaken view, that the sufferers are more in control and just need to 'pull themselves together', has been exhibited by professional carers as well as by family and other informal carers (Oliver & Kuipers 1996).

In thinking about positive and negative symptoms in this way, we should be aware that the two can and do coexist within the individual's experience of illness. The manner in which they are related and coexist has been the subject of debate for some time. Although positive and negative symptoms are distinguishable in a number of ways (including possible biological processes and response to medication), our understanding of the interrelations between the two is mediocre (Smith et al 1998). As mentioned earlier, serious mental illness is often associated with the presence of the positive symptoms and yet for some the first evidence of onset comprises behavioural changes, such as withdrawal or a decrease in interest or hygiene. We therefore need to be careful that we do not give primacy to the positive symptoms in our treatment strategies. Negative symptoms have the capacity to cause long-term distress to clients, professionals, family members or lay carers.

PROBLEMS WITH THE ILLNESS PRESPECTIVE

Put simply, Bentall (2003) makes a strong case that the idea of schizophrenia as a diagnosable illness is misleading and unhelpful. He argues that it is scientifically invalid and confusing since a century of research has revealed the following firm discoveries. Schizophrenia is an illness with no exact set of signs and symptoms, there is little agreement among researchers about what causes it and the course and outcome of the illness vary dramatically amongst sufferers. This is not to say that people do not experience serious and debilitating emotional and psychological problems, merely that the concept of schizophrenia may not be a useful way of describing those problems.

The further subdivision of symptoms of schizophrenia into positive and negative symptoms is also widely debated (Liddle 1987). More research has been devoted to establishing the nature of the negative symptom syndrome than to finding ways of helping the people who experience it and yet there is still much to know (Hogg 1996). Despite evidence that positive and negative symptoms of schizophrenia vary independently throughout the course of treatment (Strauss et al 1974), the notion that these problems are a subgroup of symptoms remains intact. It may be true that feelings of blankness and deadness have a biological basis; however, an arguable effect of exclusively retaining this view is that alternative explanations are marginalised and consequently left unexplored in clinical practice.

WITHDRAWING FROM A DANGEROUS OR HOPELESS WORLD

Imagine the worst moment of your life. Extend it to an hour, a day, a year, years on end, moments stacked up and lost forever. This is the stultifying process of madness. This is why mental patients look, act and feel numb. To be in perpetual suspended animation is better than never ending pain.

(Unzicker 1989)

Low levels of functioning may be a deliberate strategy to cope with frightening beliefs and voices (Strauss et al 1989). Close reading of Unzicker's comments above highlight this possible protective function for negative symptoms in that they are 'better than being in never-ending pain'. Venables & Wing (1962) reinforced this idea that withdrawal is associated with decreased ability to cope with sensory input and is, therefore, a possible defensive strategy. Strauss et al (1974) also pointed to the interaction between services and people experiencing low motivation and energy. They described how professionals have a tendency to withdraw from people showing little or no response to therapy. This sends a message of hopelessness to the person on the receiving end that ultimately increases withdrawal from life.

The possibility that sufferers are in some way cocooning themselves for a period of recuperation highlights the need for caution in all aspects of intervention. The individual with negative symptoms can often seem to be passive and compliant, which may induce a practitioner to become prescriptive and authoritarian. ('All he needs is a good shove! If you go soft on him, he won't do anything, believe me!', as was once said to one of us.) It is of great importance when planning interventions not to fall into this trap. The impact of blankness and deadness is so great that overzealous plans can exacerbate unhelpful beliefs or voices, drive the individual further into withdrawal and/or cause the individual to resort to other protective strategies such as avoidance of therapy or, in extreme cases, even physical violence. This perspective has implications for adjusting the approach to people with this kind of problem. This includes taking small steps at a slow pace and tackling small, achievable goals that benefit the person's life. Also, this view has important implications for assessment and planning interventions:

◆ Consider how the person's behaviour might be protective
◆ Consider alternative ways of coping that the person has or can learn
◆ Find out what negative experiences the person has had with mental health services.
◆ Expect mistrust at the outset and accept this as understandable
◆ Consider how the person's environment might be interacting with their problems, e.g. would coming out of their shell bring increased criticism or stress that might trigger past problems?
◆ Professionals need to recognise and manage their own feelings of hopelessness if improvements come slowly by:
  ● expecting a slow pace and encouraging small manageable steps forward
  ● seeking effective supervision regularly
  ● regularly monitoring their own reactions to the work.

DEALING WITH LOSS AND ASSOCIATED DEPRESSION

There is a strong link between depression and schizophrenia, with as many as 25% of people diagnosed with schizophrenia thought also to experience clinical depression.

Beck et al (1979) associate depression with thoughts about loss and a feeling of hopelessness about the future. Given the stigma around mental health problems and the downward social slide of many people experiencing them, depression seems a highly likely reaction. Teasdale et al (2002) describes how people with long-term depression become depressed about depression. It is easy to see how the same could happen with other mental health problems. Some of the symptoms in Table 12.1, such as lack of interest and pleasure, could be caused by depression, which may require special exploration and different treatment, either pharmacological or psychosocial.

It is advocated that special attention be given to mood, anxiety and suicidality in any assessment strategy. The Manchester Symptom Severity Scale (KGV; Ch. 8) includes these items and can be used to identify depression, or a specific tool such as the Beck Depression Inventory could be used. Even with the presence of depression we still need to ask if this is a natural result of the debilitating effect of the symptoms. Gilbert (1992) presents a view of depression as a natural reaction to battling an immovable problem. It literally makes us stop and wait for help. Battling with voices and strange thoughts on a daily basis could easily be viewed in such terms.

Implications of this perspective include assessing and dealing with depression by:

◆ adapting Beck's (1995) mastery and pleasure work
◆ helping the person to come to terms with loss events
◆ helping to build a more hopeful view of the future.

MEDICATION EFFECTS

'Some side effects of neuroleptic drugs can mimic or compound problems with negative symptoms' (Watkins 1996, p. 41). For instance, Healy & Farquhar (1998) explored the effects on a group of junior doctors of taking one dose of droperidol. They found a wide range of effects but all noted a strong feeling of being cut off from the world that lasted anywhere between a few hours and a week. All the participants reported a deadening of their emotions and some even felt quite depressed. It is very common for people taking neuroleptic drugs to experience reduced imagination, creativity and sense of engagement with the world. Most see this as a necessary trade for the period of stability that medication brings. It would seem that the new atypical neuroleptics do not cause as many problems in this regard. However, it should be acknowledged that medication may cause behaviours that appear to be negative symptoms. Implications for dealing with blankness and deadness include:

◆ discussing people's experience of taking medication and working collaboratively towards a helpful balance between helpful and unhelpful effects
◆ using side-effect inventories such as the Liverpool University Side-Effect Rating Scale (LUNSERS, see Ch. 8)
◆ considering newer drugs with fewer side effects
◆ consulting a pharmacist.

VICIOUS CYCLES OF SOCIAL ISOLATION AND INSTITUTIONALISATION

It has long been recognised that spending periods of time in a psychiatric institution can lead to many of the experiences listed in Table 12.1 (Watkins 1996). Indeed, Wing (1978) identified that levels of withdrawal from life, blunted emotions and lack of motivation are strongly associated with how much time a person spends doing nothing. Since mental health services in the UK have become more community-based and incidences of these experiences continue, it has been argued that something else must be occurring (Hogg 1996). However, this assumes that people with mental health problems who move to community-based accommodation leave behind the restrictions of institutional life. Priebe & Turner (2003) argue that this is not the case and that a process of re-institutionalisation is occurring. They point to the increasing structure of community-based services such as assertive outreach and the proliferation of supported accommodation, as well as the increase in forensic beds and use of the Mental Health Act.

Regardless of whether the process of institutionalisation still ensnares people with mental health problems, if one follows Wing (1978) then it is doing nothing that leads to increased feelings of blankness and deadness. This relates well to theories of social skills deficits that work from a skills atrophy perspective. Put simply, if you don't use it you lose it (Bellack et al 1997). The experience of trying to deal with serious mental health problems as well as living independently, or even with assistance, must be an enormous task. It is well documented that when faced with this task people find themselves socially cut off through either exclusion or self-isolation (Halford & Hayes 1995). It then follows that over time a person's social confidence might well decrease and a vicious cycle of increasing withdrawal and social apathy might emerge. Implications for dealing with feelings of blankness and deadness include:

- understanding the social context of the person's difficulties
- structured assessment of the person's social opportunities
- identifying any circumstances in which the person is more socially active and drawing on strengths
- exploring the person's past levels of social interaction
- discussing specific areas of social confidence that might be lacking.

DEVELOPING A SHARED UNDERSTANDING

Research indicates that the characteristics of therapists are indicative of positive outcomes in therapy and are as important as, if not more so than, the model of therapy itself (Luborsky et al 1985). We have outlined a number of different perspectives from which to view feelings of blankness and deadness. Our view is that consideration of all of these alongside an adjusted therapeutic stance is essential to helping people with these difficulties. The various perspectives can be summarised using the diagram in Figure 12.1. This diagram could be used as an aid to assessment as well as to generate an ongoing formulation of the problem.

Increased motivation and improved confidence are goals that many individuals share. A helpful aspect of focus in this work will be to 'normalise' individuals' experiences and build on their desire to change, no matter how small that change may be.

Often, professionals view individuals with mental health problems as collections of symptoms to be cured or deficits to be rectified. With regard to blankness and deadness, it can be helpful to become interested in people's strengths and interests. A person's environment can be seen as a source of resources to be tapped. It is interesting how often an individual with feelings of blankness and deadness will be described negatively in a professional's presentations of problems. Consider the statements below:

Mr Jones suffers from negative symptoms. The only time he ever leaves his home is to collect his benefit as he says he 'can't be bothered' with any other daytime activity arranged by his care worker.

This statement sends an implicit message about Mr Jones. The basic message is that he is a difficult case, has little if no motivation and has rejected all the efforts of his care worker to improve his lot.

Suppose, however, that the statement is changed to:

Mr Jones has a strong feeling of deadness. He feels numb most of the time. Despite this he retains the skills necessary to collect his benefit from the post

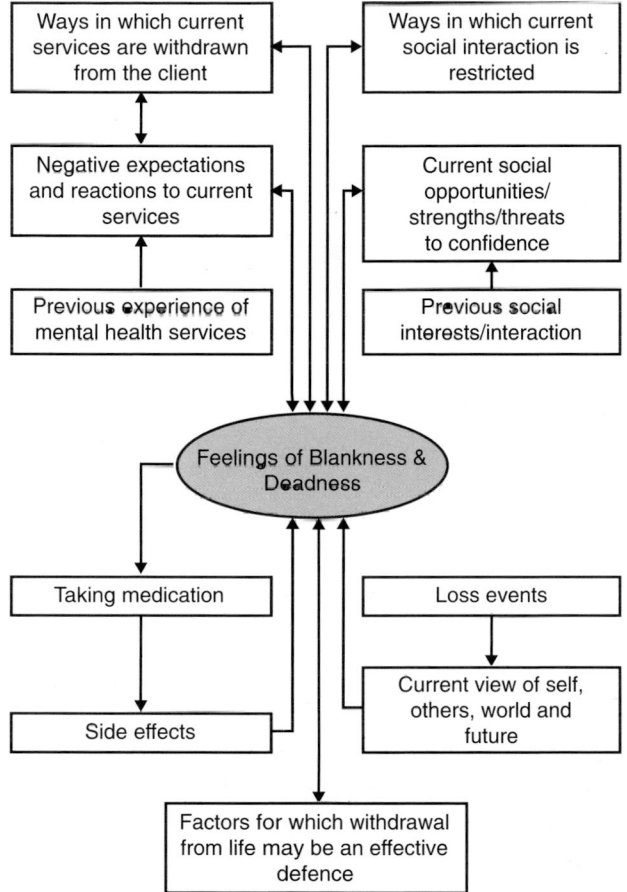

Figure 12.1 Interaction between potential processes associated with feelings of blankness and deadness.

office on the correct day. At the present time Mr Jones and the care team have not been able to expand on this skill base.

From this perspective the future becomes one of possibilities rather than predicted and expected failures. 'The only time' previously mentioned becomes a valuable exception and indicator of health to be explored. From here it becomes possible to identify skills, strengths and motivators. To address any beliefs or behaviours that compound the effects of problems and to be able to work therapeutically with individuals, we must first explore our own attitudes. Box 12.1 invites you to do this through a reflective exercise.

Box 12.1 How would you feel?

You are in hospital recovering from an acute relapse. Your hallucinations were very vivid and disturbing, yet despite these symptoms you realistically assessed your needs and entered hospital voluntarily. You have accepted medication, even though you doubt its effectiveness. As you have got 'better' the voices have lessened in volume and abuse, but you are constantly tired. The simplest thing exhausts you. It feels as if you have some sort of virus. You have had these feelings before, during and after your last admission. You don't want this illness to get the better of you – you have a lot to gain from being well. You are determined to fight it!

Every morning the ward staff run a group from 9 am to 10 am. You have decided to attend this as it provides a focus for the start of the day and may help you recover quicker. The first morning after you have made this decision you wake at 8.30 am but can't seem to get up. You are tired and yet you've only just woken up. Finally, you manage to get out of bed. It's now 9.05 am. You drag yourself to have a wash. This makes you feel a bit better. It's now 9.20 am.

You postpone having a cup of tea and go straight to the group. You sit down. The group goes quiet. Everyone is looking at you. The staff member who's running the group waits a minute before addressing you. 'Good morning X. While I would like to welcome you to this group can I remind you that it starts at 9 am and not 9.20 am. I mention this as it's not fair on other members and disruptive to the group if people come and go whenever they feel like it'.

How would you feel?

GETTING BACK INTO THE SOCIAL WORLD

When positive life changes occur and people develop valued social roles their mental health difficulties improve (Romme & Escher 2000). Certainly this is apparent from the first person account in Chapter 1 and, given the role of social factors discussed so far and further expanded in Chapter 18, working towards increased social confidence would seem essential to dealing with feelings of blankness and deadness. Planning this work would usefully emerge from an individualised understanding of the person's social situation and personal resources. It might usefully include many of the following:

◆ Volunteering to take more responsibility for things at home
◆ Family work focused on communication between the client and family members or supported housing workers
◆ Joining a group, either therapeutic or social
◆ Spending more time with one trusted person

◆ Looking at work opportunities or training
◆ Practising particular social interaction skills in real life.

INCREASING MASTERY AND PLEASURE ACTIVITIES

Beck's (1979) seminal therapy manual for helping people with depression introduced the notion of planning certain types of activity that have been dropped from a depressed person's life. The theory in depression is that a numbing of emotional response and reduction in energy lead a person to get less out of their activities and so they are avoided. The net result is that the person begins to feel more negative about life and themselves, which compounds the feelings of depression. Kingdon & Turkington (1994) suggest that this approach if modified can be helpful with feelings of blankness and deadness. It involves:

◆ a comprehensive assessment of the person's current activity (Box 12.2)
◆ identification of activities the person used to be involved with that gave a feeling of achievement (mastery activities) or pleasure
◆ looking at possibilities for developing similar activities
◆ making it clear that these changes in themselves will not bring back previous feelings of energy but that avoiding them is likely to compound feelings of blankness and deadness
◆ grading each activity as far as it needs to be in order for the person to find it manageable; this can mean steps as small as:
  ● open eyes
  ● sit up in bed
  ● swing legs to side of bed and wait 2 minutes
  ● stand up

Box 12.2 Assessment tools to be used

◆ KGV
◆ Social Functioning Scale
◆ Side-effects of medication (LUNSERS)
◆ Functional analysis
◆ Activity schedule
◆ Mastery and Pleasure Inventory
◆ Motivational interview
◆ Negative Symptom Checklist

- ◆ giving positive feedback to any efforts made
- ◆ expecting and rolling with set backs
- ◆ supporting the person through what can be a long process.

Activity-based interventions for feelings of blankness and deadness can take time to develop. The steps mentioned earlier to avoid feelings of hopelessness in clients and professionals are particularly relevant here.

MINDFULNESS MEDITATION AS AN AID TO CONCENTRATION

Prior to writing this section I sat in a chair next to the window in my office. I rested the backs of my hands on my legs and looked out, over some rooftops to the sea beyond. I noticed nearby trees swaying in the breeze and the sounds of children playing at the school next door. I then became aware of some tension in my shoulders and relaxed it a little by raising them and letting go. I began by listening to my breathing. At first I noticed myself *trying* to breathe *normally* then I let go and just listened to and experienced my natural breaths. As I breathed, my mind wandered to the sounds of footsteps outside my door; I had images of who I thought these people might be and then remembered that I was supposed to be focusing on my breathing. I gave a mental shrug and gently returned my attention back to my breathing only to find myself distracted again and again until I felt tired. Gradually, the rate at which my distracting thoughts came slowed and I was able to focus on my breathing for slightly longer periods. The whole process took about 10 minutes but seemed much longer.

This type of breathing technique is commonly used in mindfulness meditation and many people experience it in similar ways to the description above (Thich Nhat Hanh 1991). The concept of mindfulness derives from a Buddhist tradition (Batchelor 1997) and has been incorporated into cognitive therapy approaches to depression (Zindel et al 2002). Used regularly, techniques such as these can help people to be more aware of their emotional and psychological experiences (Teasdale et al 2002). It can also help to reduce stress and develop levels of concentration (Thich Nhat Hanh 1991).

When introducing this with people experiencing mental health difficulties it is useful to emphasise the gentle nature of the technique. People generally find it difficult, so highlighting the fact that there is no such thing as getting it right, only watching what happens when you try, is a helpful approach. Starting breathing meditation together for a few minutes at a time and then discussing what happened can be a good way of demonstrating the unique but similar nature of people's responses. Discussing effects and the pace of expanding practice is important, especially as some people find it frightening to let go of their thoughts and feelings in this way.

Case study – Mark

Mark is a 32-year-old man with a 3-year diagnosis of paranoid schizophrenia. He came to the attention of the psychiatric services following an incident in which he is believed to have jumped from a bridge while actively psychotic. At the time of the incident Mark believed he was being hunted. Subsequently, Mark sustained a number of fractures.

The diagnosis of schizophrenia was made following the incident described above. At this time, Mark disclosed a 10-year history of social withdrawal, and a family history of schizophrenia (father, brother and sister).

Mark was prescribed 30 mg of haloperidol and continued to take that dose for the following 2 years. He was seen on a monthly basis by a social worker. The social worker reported that, other than a lack of any social interests, Mark appeared to have recovered. A subsequent restructuring of services meant that he was reallocated and consequently reassessed by the rehabilitation services.

Observed behaviour
Mark slept for 16 hours each day. His waking time was spent 'staring at a newspaper or the TV'. He ate or drank what was put in front of him. His domestic chores were done by his mother. He appeared unable to initiate any conversation and his responses were monosyllabic. Mark denied any positive symptomatology, although he rated high on the Negative Symptoms Checklist.

One important exception to the observed behaviour was Mark's consistency and punctuality when asked to attend appointments with the psychiatric services. This may be partly explained by Hatfield & Lefley (1987), who suggest that routine and order can be of particular benefit to people living with schizophrenia. In other words, by knowing where they are going and what to expect, people can prepare themselves and thus exert a degree of control over events. It was felt to be important that professionals mirrored Mark's behaviour and were also consistent and punctual.

It was recognised that Mark was at risk of self-neglect and potential self-harm. This was felt to be due to the decline in his interest, confidence and overwhelming sense of hopelessness, along with an inability to express his thoughts and feelings. The aim of engaging Mark and monitoring any changes should be the focus of interventions.

One caution in Mark's presentation was that his medication might have been contributing to the behaviours diagnosed as negative symptoms. A LUNSERS was carried out and Mark did score highly. These results highlighted the need for a formal review of neuroleptic medication. A case was presented for changing to an atypical antipsychotic. The multidisciplinary team were understandably cautious, owing to Mark's history of self-harm and his difficulty in expressing the content of his inner world.

Specific areas of difficulty identified through the ongoing process of assessment were:

◆ *difficulty with concentration*
◆ *lethargy*
◆ *excessive sleeping.*

Case study – Mark (cont'd)

At this point it was not possible to carry out a functional analysis as described in Chapter 9. This was because of the disabling nature of Mark's illness and his inability to verbalise his problems. To attempt to carry out such an assessment at this stage might well have resulted in alienating him. It was therefore decided to proceed with the engagement process and try to develop an observed problem statement, as detailed in Box 12.3.

To reinforce and expand upon the positive, consistent, punctual behaviour already noted, a plan was drawn up to provide daily contact with the rehabilitation services. The idea to maintain social contact was discussed with Mark. He consented to the intervention as he said he liked the notion of having 'something to get up in the morning for'. He also liked the idea of seeing the staff as they were his only contact with the world and thus helped him stay in touch with reality.

This acceptance was the first indication that Mark had some insight into his situation. He later confided that he was, in fact, terrified of his psychotic experiences and had found that they had previously become worse when he attempted any social contact. As a consequence he had lost the ability to communicate even on the most basic of levels. Mark also believed that his slowness and difficulty in making decisions irritated people.

Mark's difficulties were discussed with him in the context of his illness. Within this, his social isolation was reframed as coping strategies he had developed in order to maintain a safe and manageable environment. To improve the quality of his daily life he was encouraged to utilise and reframe other strategies.

As an addition to the assessments discussed earlier, the Allen Cognitive Disability Assessment (Velligan et al 1995) was carried out by an occupational therapist. This assessment identified the difficulties Mark was experiencing in planning activities and problem-solving, along with a severe lack of social skills. Mark's care package was deemed to require input from a number of professionals. This was not only to ensure that Mark had the benefit of a pool of skills but also to expand his number of contacts. By providing a consistent approach they were able to address a number of problems and defined goals listed in Table 12.2.

One year on from the start of this process, Mark trusted the staff enough to tell his side of the story.

Mark's story *My life changed completely when I was 11 years old and my family moved into the town. My dad left us because he was ill. We had to be quiet when he was around. Then my brother became ill and he was just the same, then my sister became ill and I was just waiting for my turn. I was terrified all the time; everything was weird. I couldn't understand what was happening and everyone seemed to be out to get me. I felt like a time bomb, I don't remember jumping off the bridge, but I remember waking up in hospital feeling like a 'numbskull'. My mind was empty. I thought that this was what the illness was all about. I didn't think of questioning anything, in fact I just didn't seem to think, because I wasn't as scared of feeling numb.*

Case study – Mark (cont'd)

Mark identified this time of feeling numb as a healing process, which resonates with the observation that some negative symptoms are protective and defensive. Mark is now engaged in an active rehabilitation programme and has set himself a number of short-term and long-term goals.

Box 12.3 Interventions

Observed problem statement:
Mark exhibits low levels of motivation, and social withdrawal, leading to a lack of purpose or enjoyment in all activities.

Long-term goal:
To engage Mark. Increase motivation, interest, enjoyment and improve social networks.

Action:

1. To offer a consistent, supportive, non-threatening environment for Mark.

2. To formulate a shared understanding of Mark's internal world and the threats proposed by the external world.

Table 12.2 Problems and goals – Mark

Problems	Goals
I have minimal conversation with people	To have conversation with support worker for 15 minutes every day
I am socially isolated	To attend day-centre communication classes for 1 hour a week To visit my mother for 2 hours each week
I have minimal knowledge of what 'normal' behaviour is	To attend mental health awareness sessions on Wednesdays for 1 hour
I find it difficult to plan things to do during the day	To make an activity schedule on a daily basis with occupational therapist

CONCLUSIONS

Individuals with mental problems often tread a fine line between overstimulation, which is likely to precipitate voices or strange beliefs, and understimulation, which precipitates feelings of blankness and deadness. Unfortunately, people who feel dead to the world cause little fuss and are often suffering in less dramatic ways; therefore they are easy to forget. This is wrong. The people suffering in this way are often criticised as being lazy, selfish and generally beyond help because they seem to have no inclination to help themselves. It is fundamental to the therapeutic relationship that clinicians explore their own beliefs and assumptions before attempting to work with clients; only then can the focus of the relationship be based on the expectations, beliefs and experiences of the individual. A client-centred interpersonal relationship, which focuses on the conditions of accurate empathy, non-possessive warmth and genuineness, is a prerequisite to working collaboratively with individuals to enable them to identify personal strategies for improving their motivation and confidence and providing an informed vantage point to manage and live according to their own needs and wishes. A truly longitudinal and flexible approach to dealing with feelings of blankness and deadness is needed if clinicians are to collaborate with individuals and their carers in managing the impact their problems have on their daily life.

Summary of practical strategies identified

- ◆ It is essential to take a long term approach.
- ◆ Understanding what messages services are sending a person can shed light on withdrawal.
- ◆ Goals must be achievable and realistic for the client.
- ◆ Take steps towards finding valued social roles.
- ◆ Develop social confidence by practising specific skills in real life situations.
- ◆ Activity scheduling can help to lift energy and mood levels.
- ◆ Mindfulness meditation can aid concentration.
- ◆ It is essential to work at the client's pace.

References

Batchelor S 1997 Buddhism without beliefs: a contemporary guide to awakening. Bloomsbury, London

Beck J 1995 Cognitive therapy: basics and beyond. Guilford Press, New York

Beck A T, Rush J A, Brian F, Emery G 1979 Cognitive therapy of depression. Guilford Press, New York

Bellack A, Meuser K, Gingerich S, Agresta J 1997 Social skills training for schizophrenia: a step by step guide. Guilford Press, New York

Bentall R 2003 Madness explained: psychosis and human nature. Penguin, London

Bleuler M 1983 Schizophrenia determination. British Journal of Psychiatry 143:78–79

Gilbert P 1992 Depression: the evolution of powerlessness. Lawrence Erlbaum, Hove, Sussex

Halford W, Hayes R 1995 Social skills in schizophrenia: assessing the relationship between social skills, pathology and community functioning. Social Psychiatry and Psychiatric Epidemiology 30:14–19

Hatfield A B, Lefley H 1987 Families of the mentally ill: coping and adaptation. Cassell, London

Healy D, Farquar G 1998 Immediate effects of droperidol. Human Psychopharmacology 13:113–120

Hogg L 1996 Treatment for negative symptoms. In: Haddock G, Slade P (eds) Cognitive–behavioural interventions with psychotic disorders. Routledge, London

Kingdon D, Turkington D 1994 Cognitive behavioural therapy of schizophrenia. Lawrence Erlbaum, Hove, Sussex

Liddle P 1987 The symptoms of chronic schizophrenia: a re-examination of the positive-negative dichotomy, British Journal of Psychiatry 151:145–151

Luborsky L, McLellan A T, Woody G E et al 1985 Therapist success and its determinants. Archives of General Psychiatry 42:602–611

Oliver N, Kuipers E 1996 Stress and its relationship to expressed emotion in community mental health workers. International Journal of Social Psychiatry 42:150–159

Priebe S, Turner T 2003 Reinstitutionalisation in mental health care. British Medical Journal 326:175–176

Romme M, Escher S 2000 Making sense of voices: a guide for health professionals working with voice hearers. Mind Publications, London

Smith D A, Mar C M, Turoff B K 1998 The structure of schizophrenic symptoms: a meta-analytic confirmatory factor analysis. Schizophrenia Research 31:57–70

Strauss J, Carpenter W, Bartko J 1974 The diagnosis and understanding of schizophrenia. Part III: Speculations on the processes that underlie schizophrenic signs and symptoms. Schizophrenia Bulletin 11:61–69

Strauss J S, Rakfeldt T J, Harding C M, Lieberman D 1989 Mediating processes in schizophrenia: towards a new dynamic psychiatry. British Journal of Psychiatry 155(suppl 5):24

Teasdale J D, Moore R G, Hayhurst H et al 2002 Metacognitive awareness and prevention of relapse in depression: empirical evidence. Journal of Consulting and Clinical Psychology 70:275–287

Thich Nhat Hanh 1991 The miracle of mindfulness: a manual on meditation. Rider, London

Unzicker R 1989 On my own: a personal journey through madness and re-emergence. Psychosocial Rehabilitation Journal 13:16

References (cont'd)

Velligan D I, True J E, Lefton R S et al 1995 Validity of the Allen Cognitive Levels Assessment: a tri-ethnic comparison. Psychiatric Research 56:101–109

Venables P H, Wing J K 1962 Level of arousal and the subclassification of schizophrenia. Archives of General Psychiatry 7:114–119

Watkins J 1996 Living with schizophrenia: an holistic approach to understanding, preventing and recovering from negative symptoms. Hill of Content, Melbourne

Wing J 1978 Social influences on the course of schizophrenia. In: Wynne L, Cromwell R, Matthysse S (eds) The nature of schizophrenia: new approaches to research and treatment. Wiley, New York

Zindel V, Segal J, Williams M, Teasdale J 2002 Mindfulness-based cognitive therapy for depression: a new approach to preventing relapse. Guilford Press, London

Annotated further reading

Bellack A, Mueser K, Gingerich S, Agresta J 1997 Social skills training for schizophrenia: a step by step guide. Guilford Press, New York

This book provides a comprehensive guide on how to incorporate social skills training into everyday clinical practice.

Watkins J 1996 Living with schizophrenia: an holistic approach to understanding, preventing and recovering from negative symptoms. Hill of Content, Melbourne

This small, easy-to-read, thought-provoking book provides the reader with an insight into the problems caused by negative symptoms. The author has wide experience in dealing with the subject matter. There are many logical and practical strategies given to aid any practitioner who wishes to work in collaboration with clients who experience negative symptoms.

13

Working with families and informal carers

Catherine Gamble and Geoff Brennan

I have never received any services and none have been offered. I've not been given any information on what might be available. I feel totally ignored by all.

(Missed Opportunities 2003)

Carers are hugely appreciative of those practitioners who understand the reasons behind any emotion-focused coping and work constructively with it.

(Lyn Shore, Ch. 2)

KEY ISSUES

- ◆ Exploration of evidence-based family interventions
- ◆ Reducing stress and burden in the family environment
- ◆ Identifying who to work with and why
- ◆ Relating how to use family intervention in clinical practice

INTRODUCTION

With the introduction of Standard 6 of the national service framework and the National Carers Strategy we could be forgiven for thinking that things have changed for carers. Indeed, if we look at a national survey conducted by Rethink Mental Illness (2003), there is some evidence that this is the case. In a survey of over 1000 carers, 47% felt that standards of mental health care had improved for carers in the previous 3 years. Despite this, there is still a long way to go, as the quote at the head of the chapter indicates.

Historically, families have been as much burdened by the mental health system as by the illness. This may seem like a contentious statement but, as illustrated all too often, they have been (and often are still) perceived as part of the problem, if not the cause of serious mental illness. The reality is that the treatment of serious mental illness would not be possible without them. Community care would be exclusive, expensive and unfeasible (Nolan 1996). In the main, it is dependent on the participation of families and informal carers as they represent the major resource and support network.

WHAT CONSTITUTES A FAMILY?

This question is often raised when practitioners begin to explore the structures and systems within which their clients live. It is no longer applicable to see the 'family' as the traditional nuclear, two-up two-down, 2.2 children, mum and dad family. Yet some practitioners continue to see this as the only system possible – hence the routine response, 'there are no families where I work, all my clients live alone'. We have personally used the interventions with gay couples of both sexes, stepfamilies, single lone carers, flatmates and significant others. We also believe that hostel workers who have long-term relationships with clients could and should be considered to constitute 'family'. In addition, we have noticed that 'family' is sometimes used as shorthand for 'mother'. Mothers are often left with the emotional and practical responsibilities of care. However, if we unquestioningly accept this assumption, we are ignoring the influence and needs of siblings, fathers, grandparents and other extended family members. Serious mental illness reaches out into these people's lives and this should never be trivialised. As a general rule, if the question 'Who should I work with?' is raised, the simple answer should be 'Whoever the client wants you to'.

So what about the case where a client says 'I don't want my family to know anything'? In this situation we need to ascertain whether the family will be taking an active caring role after our involvement. If so, how should we prepare and support them? Indeed, consider whether, if the above statement were reframed to: 'I don't want my GP to know anything', would this be accepted, if the client was to return to primary care and the community? If we are honest, the request would probably be questioned and even ignored. We would rationalise our actions by reinforcing the importance of a GP's role in aftercare – so they must have the information they need. Yet, clients never spend as much time with their GP as they do with their informal carers. In our experience, as someone becomes more in control they often re-evaluate this position. If the family is involved in care, professionals must assist and respond to this re-evaluation. (For further discussion, surrounding issues of confidentiality and family inclusion see Ch. 6)

Even in the event of the person maintaining their position, the carer could access agencies external to the mental health system who would be in a position to assist them. Examples of such agencies are Rethink, the Manic Depressive Fellowship, Saneline and numerous local carer organisations. Nevertheless, just referring on is no longer acceptable as it is often asking the family to face something that they are not prepared for. We have to recognise that you do not throw a pebble in a pond without a ripple effect. Mental illness does not affect the individual in isolation. We have, in reality, a duty of care to carers, which becomes evident at times of direct threat to them; for example if a client is saying they will harm them.

The issue then becomes: at what point do we need to inform the carer of issues that will directly affect them? It is obvious that an argument can be made for an all-inclusive attitude as, by definition, carers are directly affected because of their role. The National Service Framework (Department of Health 1999) supports this view as it determined the right of any 'individual who provides regular and substantial care for a person on (the) Care Programme Approach' to 'have an assessment of their caring, physical and mental health needs, repeated on at least an annual basis'. Also, to 'have their own written care plan which is given to them and implemented in discussion with them'.

This does not mean that families should be perceived as needing 'treatment from professionals who know best', but does acknowledge the strain caused by everyday caring. (For essential elements of a carer's plan, see Box 13.1.)

Box 13.1 The carer's plan (Department of Health 1999)

The carer's plan should include:

◆ Information about the mental health needs of the person for whom they are caring, including information about medication and any side effects that can be predicted, and services available to support them

◆ Action to meet defined contingencies

◆ Information on what to do and who to contact in a crisis

◆ What will be provided to meet their own mental and physical health needs and how it will be provided

◆ Action needed to secure advice on income, housing, educational and employment matters

◆ Arrangements for short-term breaks

◆ Arrangements for social support, including access to carers' support groups

◆ Information about appeals or complaints procedures

Indeed, most families would rather be plain 'family' and not a carer in need of support.

ENGAGEMENT ISSUES

After being confronted by the array of negative assumptions and historical beliefs that some professionals and systems hold, it is not surprising that many families are initially suspicious when family work is suggested. Indeed, contrary to popular myths, this work does not involve interpreting family dynamics or parent–child relationships. As mentioned, providing families with support is essential if community care is to be effective. It is therefore imperative that professionals introduce the idea of family work when practical help and information is asked for – i.e. at a time of crisis. If the offer is taken up when it has been previously rejected this is not the time to think or say 'we told you so'. Instead, it is a time to listen and reflect on the families' experiences of service provision and ascertain what can be learnt and subsequently offered to address actual or perceived shortfalls. At this stage, some families may continue to refuse; however, this should not be perceived as rejection. The invitation must be left open, a lifeline given and contact maintained. In other words, families should be tentatively followed up. One advocated method is to write a letter or send an informal greetings card (as this is more likely to be opened than an official, Trust-franked, brown envelope) that seeks to ascertain how the family has been since you last met. Its content should contain a summary of what their situation was at the time of appraisal and an enquiry as to whether they need anything more. For example:

> *We are currently in the process of reviewing the families on our books. We were therefore writing to ascertain how you are getting on and how things are progressing. When we last met you described your situation to be … if you no longer feel able to cope with these circumstances or if any additional issues have arisen we would be happy to meet up at the earliest possible convenience.*

To enhance the engagement process it is essential that the following guidelines are adhered to and provided:

◆ Be flexible as to the time and venue – always be punctual and keep the appointment – if the family is late, wait for them – they may have been held up. If you rush off to do something else this will give the impression that they are not important and you are too busy to give them priority!
◆ Give a clear and non-judgemental rationale for family intervention.
◆ Use the problem-solving strategy outlined in the case study of Shirley to create solutions to overcome potential engagement barriers.

Case study – Shirley

Shirley is an elderly mother who has been supporting her son, who has schizophrenia, for over 20 years. He relapses frequently, despite taking regular medication. Shirley has coped in the past; however, the burden of living with her son is becoming too difficult and stressful, and she is very worried about how he will survive alone in the future. The 'young' community psychiatric nurse has suggested supporting Shirley with family work, but she is very sceptical because so many professionals in the past have come up with new ideas – but they have never amounted to much and they haven't stopped her son going in and out of hospital like a yo-yo.

Issue/engagement problem
Team members are concerned that Shirley's past experiences and her verbalised scepticism will reduce the likelihood of her engaging in family work. All the possible solutions to the question of how best to approach Shirley were formulated. They are listed in Table 13.1.

Choosing the 'best' solution
In this case, while solution 5 was acknowledged, it was clear that a combination of solutions 1, 2, 3, 4 and 6 could be productively used. From this exercise, team members could now devise a plan for how contact and initial meetings would be made and run, as they had considered potential engagement hitches and thought how to pre-empt them. They could now arrange to meet Shirley and review the effectiveness of their devised engagement solutions afterwards. Moreover, if they proved effective, the problem-solving strategy could be replicated with other families who express concerns about participating.

ASSESSMENT AND THE RATIONALE FOR IT

Considering that 'assessment' usually connotes a problem to be found or defined, we need to clarify what the process of assessment for family intervention means. To identify which family systems to work with, it could be argued that all you need to do is to use the rule of thumb shown in Box 13.2. However, although this is a useful indicator of stress within the family system, it does not tell us much more about what practitioners may face after initial contact. In order to gain the fullest picture of the system and roots of stress, we should employ a more rigorous process. This does not mean to say that we are advocating a long-drawn-out interrogation and questioning. Families are searching for recognition, support and help and we need to provide this at the earliest opportunity. It is important, however, that we have an identified framework within which to operate. There is nothing more insulting for families than to be given information they have found out for themselves. In order to know how to link our knowledge with their experience and expertise, we need to assess what their experience and expertise is. Otherwise some of the areas identified in Table 13.2 will be missed.

From this exercise it is possible to deduce that we are not looking for 'problems to solve' but 'strengths to build on'. Formalised assessment strategies to help with this process are as follows.

Table 13.1 Advantages and disadvantages of possible solutions

Solution	Advantages	Disadvantages
1. Contact Shirley and acknowledge frustrations	Giving mother permission to verbalise these will help to defuse potential anger	Could be perceived as patronising
2. Arrange to visit and acknowledge limitations of previous interventions and recognise the difficulties Shirley has had – 'That's why we are here, and we will provide greater support than you have previously experienced'	Sets boundaries, stops unrealistic expectations/plans being made, will reduce frustrations and increase confidence in the approach and the team members. Highlights the commitment and sustainability of new approach	May be too much to take in and thus may reduce confidence
3. During meeting, view family work as an experiment that will be reviewed regularly	Shirley may feel less pressurised by this idea, as her expertise and experience of past service/s is being listened to and she doesn't have to commit herself immediately	May not be embraced or taken on as real – 'Am I a guinea pig, then?'
4. During meeting, get agreement on a common goal	Shared goal will be seen as beneficial, and reduce the likelihood that family work will be perceived as undermining the mothering role	
5. Be aware of defensive responses	Letting it ride and meeting the prickly situation head on will check realities and prevent you from making wrong assumptions	Could all go horribly wrong and Shirley will be left feeling that her actions or behaviours are being criticised or pathologised
6. Look at possible provision for practical help and provide this	Taken seriously, Shirley will receive more support and appreciate the effort put in	

Box 13.2 A 'rule of thumb' for families to work with

◆ Carers living with clients who relapse more than twice a year despite taking regular medication

◆ Those who frequently contact staff for reassurance or help

◆ Home environments where there are repeated arguments, violence and/or the police are called

◆ Any carer who is looking after a client unaided

Source: Kuipers et al 2002

Table 13.2 Family areas of expertise

Participant	Expertise in
Client	Symptoms Treatment effects from service and individual level Strengths in functioning Knowledge and understanding of own family, culture, values and philosophy History of illness
Informal carer	History of prodrome and illness Early warning signs Assessment of stress Knowledge and understanding of own family, culture, values and philosophy Resource for client in family and wider systems
Professional	Knowledge of illness and treatment strategies Advocating within professional systems Illness effects on wider population Interventions to reduce stress and burden

Relative assessment interview

The Relative Assessment Interview (RAI) aims to obtain information about the relatives' behaviours, beliefs and subjective feelings towards the client, their illness and its consequences. It helps to elicit clients' and carers' positive and successful coping strategies and resources as well as their difficulties. The RAI covers seven main areas (Barrowclough & Tarrier 1995):

◆ background to the patient and family
◆ background information and contact time

- chronological history of the illness
- current problems/symptoms
- irritability or quarrels in the household
- relatives' relationship with patient
- effect of the illness on relatives.

Assessment procedure

In clinical practice, an issue that often prevails is how, when and where to conduct the above interviews. This is a difficult question to be definitive about, as it always relies on the time, place and person. Ideally they should be conducted on a one-to-one basis in a quiet, informal setting. It is also useful to gain consent to tape the interviews as it can be off-putting for the recipient if notes are constantly being made. An additional advantage of audio-taping is that it is sometimes hard to remember everything that is said.

Interviews can be time-consuming and it is not always possible to interview all family members. However, in our experience and that of others, when attempts have been made to incorporate more than one family member at a time, the sessions become confusing and the ability to take notes is reduced. Some family members may also not feel able to disclose or discuss some of the points raised in Table 13.2. Ultimately, the whole process is a negotiated engagement trade-off between what ensures comfort and safety for the individual and the professionals' need for information. When it comes to assessing client need, the same principles apply as those described in other chapters of this book.

Feeding back what has been learned to the family

In most cases, the assessment process will have facilitated family members to disclose a lot of information about their past experiences and current coping strategies. This may have provided an important engagement forum; however, to maintain this collaborative stance the information obtained must be handled proficiently. Indeed, if this is not the case, it could potentially alienate the family; there could be nothing worse than telling your story and then for professionals to disappear with the information, providing a vague and/or incomplete explanation as to what use will be made of it. It is therefore only respectful at this juncture to consider how knowledge gained should be assimilated and fed back. After completing initial assessment sessions, it is possible to sum up what has been learned into a strengths and needs format, as illustrated in Table 13.3.

This formulation can then be circulated and shared with the family for discussion. In the aforementioned case, the family was delighted that their

Table 13.3 Strengths and needs matrix

Strengths	Needs
All family members know the name of diagnosis, clearly recognise this as a serious mental illness. Perceive this as a biological illness that affects how the brain works and affects many aspects of their daughter's life Know the names of the tablets, recognise that they should be taken as prescribed Perceive illness to be a life long issue, recognise that hospital admissions cause huge problems for everyone Everyone signed up to wanting to find different ways of coping Have supported daughter for many years, even when there has been inconsistent treatment/support from services	More information about the illness and what causes it – an overview of how stressors and life events can exacerbate symptoms may be helpful To review everyone's perspective on how some behaviours, such as losing temper, irritability and isolation, can be attributed to some symptoms experienced To review and inform about medication dosage and other side effects Additional one-to-one work to deal with some pertinent concerns not related to family Outside support to reduce overall worries and responsibility for caring, e.g. currently helping with shopping, keeping house clean, washing up, being on the end of the phone – average 20 calls a day To exchange ideas and information on additional management re coping strategies and how to stay well

strengths had been acknowledged but were initially disconcerted about the level of need they had. Indeed, it formally highlighted how unsupported they all felt and, additionally, the daughter, i.e. the person with the mental health problem, had not realised how many times a day she communicated with her parents by telephone, and perceived this to be a critical revelation – 'You never told me you don't like me calling you!' To ensure that the engagement process continued smoothly, both had to be handled sensitively. This was done by redirecting and changing the perceptual experience of the situation by placing it into another context, using a technique called *positive reframing*. The positive aspect of this technique is that alternative explanations are proposed so that the meaning of the situation, and therefore its consequences, are changed. In doing so the presenting issue is viewed in a more positive light (San Blise 1995). For example, the following explanation was given to the family:

> *The number of calls may not be the prevailing issue. What was perceived*
> *from this feedback was that although you [talking directly to daughter]*

Box 13.3 Levels of intervention

Level 1: Engagement and communication support plus introduction to service provision and personnel
Care coordinator and/or team member liaises with all key stakeholders, sets up ongoing two-way communication with carer and provides generic information re service provision and personnel and practical help. Thus a collaborative treatment plan can be developed. Care coordinator and/or team member monitors carer response and client outcomes and if necessary recommends that the family graduate to Level 2.

Level 2: Communication support plus tailor-made information to maintain current coping strategies and develop relapse prevention plans
One or more team members with family-work training meet with carers and elaborate on previous assessments undertaken by providing tailor-made information. Thus collaborative relapse prevention and crisis plans are developed. Carer response and client outcomes are monitored. On completion, family workers liaise with care coordinator and key stakeholders and family reverts back to Level 1 or graduates to Level 3 as necessary.

Level 3: Full family intervention to enhance communication and coping styles
Trained family workers formally implement family intervention as described in this chapter. Carer response and client outcomes are monitored and, on completion, family graduates back to Level 1 intervention for ongoing support.

> *appreciate being able to call your parents frequently and you [talking directly to parents] don't mind being available to provide support, there are a number of things that you all [looking at everyone in the room] wished to change, so shall we now go on to consider how these may be resolved?*

This intervention defused potential disagreements and by doing so it was possible to prioritise the level of need and negotiate a formal plan of action. In this case the family was referred for Level 3 intervention (Box 13.3). In other cases it is possible, based on the assessment of need, to intervene with Level 1 or 2 interventions:

GETTING STARTED

Dealing with the family as a group

When thinking about working with family groups, professionals often fear that they will be confronted with situations that they cannot manage (Leavey et al 1998). They may feel overwhelmed or fear that they are going to be expected to sort everything out. This can be daunting and may be one of the reasons why families do not get seen regularly. Nevertheless, there are strategies to overcome some of these anxieties. First, no issue or problem can be formally addressed if everyone expects an overnight miracle, talks over each other and/or argues. Therefore, practitioners should not worry about lowering expectations and taking control. Many families express relief when they meet confident, knowledgeable, realistic practitioners who kindly but assertively deal with the prevailing issues. To achieve this, it is important to set simple, mutually negotiated ground rules within which all sessions can be conducted. These, as suggested by Kuipers et al (2002), could follow the guidelines outlined below, but you may wish to make them more idiosyncratic.

◆ Talk to people, not about them, and encourage the use of names, rather then using he/she
◆ Speaking time should be shared out equally, so that each person's view can be heard, listened to and respected
◆ Only one person may speak at a time, avoid interrupting each other and no one's opinion – including the family worker's – is any more important than the next person's.

Single practitioner or co-working pair?

One of the identifiable differences in models of family intervention is whether families are seen by single or co-working practitioners. While there are obvious resource benefits for single practitioners to see families, it should not be underestimated how stressful this can be on a long-term basis. The advantages of co-working tend to outweigh the disadvantages (see summary in Table 13.4). Furthermore, Leff & Gamble (1995) advocate that co-working should be considered for the following reasons:

◆ **Balancing alliances**: It is important for each family member to feel supported. This is difficult for a single person to achieve, especially if there are numerous family members present. A pair of family workers provide greater opportunity to form alliances with different members of the family. These alliances are not fixed but can shift between sessions or even within a session, according to the need.
◆ **Rescue operations**: Families are often in a state of emotional turmoil. It is easy for one family worker to get stuck in a maelstrom of emotions, or to be sidetracked and to lose the focus of the session. A second worker can help to maintain objectivity, rescue and intervene as necessary to bring the discussion back to the agreed topic.

Table 13.4 Advantages and disadvantages of co-working

Advantages of co-working	Disadvantages of co-working
Share the work and burden	Complicated to organise meeting times
Help when stuck	Rely on each other
Two views on the family	Too powerful for the family
Offer alliances to the family	
Advocate for the client	
Less overwhelming in pairs	
Role models	

◆ **Modelling the negotiation of differences**: (Families in which conflict erupts and it is difficult to resolve their differences through calm discussion.) Family work pairs can openly discuss differences between themselves, thus modelling a rational approach to disagreements. (This strategy is recognised to be only successful if the family workers have developed a trusting, open working relationship with each other.)

◆ **Sharing the emotional burden**: Work with families should not be taken lightly, as it involves a considerable emotional burden. Raw emotions are close to the surface and are readily communicated to the family worker. It is a relief to be able to share these feelings with a co-worker.

◆ **Two heads are better than one**: Some of the problems generated are difficult to solve. Two workers increase the chances of finding solutions to the large array of problems experienced by families and/or other members of the multidisciplinary team. Indeed, two family workers can help to *reduce the likelihood of satellite situations arising*, i.e. if family work is not perceived to be an integral part of everyday clinical work, it can occur in isolation and/or orbit around other work being undertaken with the client. Therefore, by liaising with the multidisciplinary team, one or both co-workers can share the responsibility of advocating for the family, in order to ensure that communication channels remain open and responsive to their prevailing needs. Likewise, such actions can help to promote the positive outcomes of family intervention, so they are valued by all, thereby increasing the likelihood of the intervention being offered to all those who are using the service.

Providing education

All the practical handbooks in family work advocate that education should be provided first and foremost. This is because providing information about serious mental illness helps to defuse some of the myths and misunder-standings that may be around for carers and clients (Fadden 1998). This is important as practical advice and information sharing is something that carers

> **Box 13.4** The Knowledge About Schizophrenia Interview
>
> ◆ Diagnosis
> ◆ Symptomatology
> ◆ Aetiology
> ◆ Medication
> ◆ Prognosis
> ◆ Management

have repeatedly asked for (Leavey et al 1998). In addition, it is recognised to be a positive way of improving optimism and may help the carer appreciate clients' viewpoints and increase their insight into why some respond as they do (Kuipers et al 2002).

As mentioned previously, it is often insulting for families to be told something they already know. Indeed, this is particularly the case for clients themselves – they rarely get the opportunity or permission to talk about what it is like to experience psychosis and yet, as we have seen, they are the experts. It is therefore strongly advised that a thorough assessment of knowledge is undertaken before embarking on an education session. The Knowledge About Schizophrenia Interview (KASI, see Box 13.4) was designed to be conducted informally (see Barrowclough & Tarrier 1995). It assesses knowledge, beliefs and attitudes about six areas of schizophrenia. Nevertheless, it is possible to adapt as necessary. Pre and post measures give an indication about how effective the sessions have been in achieving change to the areas in Box 13.4. Additional common problems when providing information can be summarised as in Table 13.5.

Problem solving

The core principle of family intervention is the ability to implement effective problem-solving strategies. Whilst all families have individualised coping strategies and must always be assumed to have strengths in this area, there are an array of challenges thrown up by the illness for which they may need assistance. Some families are stronger in this area than others. The majority really appreciate being given the opportunity to examine their current coping strategies and refine them to meet present and/or future situations. Indeed some families wish to revise some aspects of their management styles completely because they have found them to be ineffective and counter-productive. For example, a parent who constantly shouted at their child to get out of bed ended up becoming so exasperated they pulled the person down the stairs on the mattress.

Table 13.5 Problems and strategies in information provision

Common problems	Suggested strategies
Client is perceived as the poor sufferer, rather than the potential expert.	Model a positive attitude to client's knowledge. If necessary, make space and time for client to describe their experience and interpretation of symptoms. Treat this input with respect – encourage other members to listen and ask direct but non-confrontational questions
Professionals expect those present to assimilate knowledge and literature as they do and therefore avoid a formal session	Plan to go through the literature in a formalised, structured manner but do not over load – break frequently for questions to clarify what has been covered
Carers and clients assimilate knowledge differently	Base the sessions upon their own experiences and subjective reasons for the occurrence of the illness. Provide information on an ongoing basis. Use clear non-jargonistic literature. Talk in lay rather than professional language
KASI reveals high level of knowledge in one member	Use this knowledge by directly referring to this expertise in session
Client does not agree with diagnosis	Use information on psychosis, relate to general experience and externalise rather than personalise while asking client and carers to draw comparisons about the impact their experiences have on their lives. Avoid confrontation – and agree to disagree
Family produce practical issues that take priority over the session	Assess this need – is it likely that it will impede further progress if not immediately addressed? Act upon the practicalities if they are achievable and realistic in this time frame. Avoid brushing these issues aside – but make it clear that you will and can address them further on in the process
Not all members present	Continue with session. Leave leaflets for absent members. Ask who can relay the information from within the family. Check in subsequent sessions that this has been achieved
Carers and client feel awkward about saying things in front of each other	Conduct the sessions separately if necessary. Procure the consent of all to participate. Bring everyone together at a later date

Problem solving is an art. It is inherent for some – but not for others. Before starting to think about helping families with their problems, it is worth considering our own attitudes to problems and the skills we have to deal with them (Mills, unpublished data, 1995). Sometimes we can sort problems out reasonably quickly. On other occasions we put decision-making off. This usually occurs when we: (1) have already tried and the plan backfired horribly, (2) perceive the problem to be too large or (3) think it will upset others. Thus, it would appear that the ability to solve problems depends on motivation, personal disposition, culture, past experiences, emotional involvement and overcoming the fear of confronting difficult issues, others' expectations, losing control and change. Families' experiences are no different and it is important to realise that problems occur as a normal part of life and that finding ways to solve them is a skill that can be learnt and practised like any other. Indeed, learning to solve problems is a collaborative, constructive process that involves having a clear idea of how to negotiate, set an agenda and priorities, agree on goals and practise tasks (Kuipers et al 2002).

The format given in Box 13.5 provides a useful structure to guide families through a six-step problem-solving strategy.

Box 13.5 A six-step problem-solving strategy

Step 1: What exactly is the problem or the goal?
Talk about the problem until you can write down exactly what it is.
Ask questions to clarify the issue. Break down into smaller parts.

Step 2: List all possible solutions
List all ideas. Try to get everyone to suggest something. Do not discuss merits of ideas at this stage.

Step 3: Highlight the main advantages and disadvantages
Briefly highlight the main advantages and disadvantages of each suggestion.

Step 4: Choose the 'best' solution
Choose a realistic, achievable one that can be most readily carried out with the resources available (time, money, skills).

Step 5: Plan exactly how to carry out the solution
Consider resources needed. Plan each step, Try to consider hitches and pre-empt them. Reduce expectations if necessary.
Date and time of review: _____

Step 6: Review progress in carrying out homework
Praise effort, not achievement. Review progress on each step. Revise the plan as necessary. Continue to problem solve until stress resolved or goal achieved.

Source: Falloon & Graham-Hole 1994.

WORKING WITH A FAMILY: EVALUATING THE PROCESS

The following case study encapsulates what can be achieved and learnt from family intervention work.

What was known about the family

The genogram in Figure 13.1 identifies the constitution of this family and who was living in the household at the time. Mum and dad were born in Africa, but all the children were born in England. The genogram indicates that mum and dad are divorced and have been amicably so for 7 years. They have two sons and two daughters. Steve, the eldest, lives independently. Although interested in his family's welfare, he had work commitments so he envisaged being unable to attend meetings. David, the second son, has learning difficulties. Jayne, the elder sister, also worked but was keen to attend meetings if they were held in the evenings. Elizabeth, the youngest, was the index client.

Family history of illness

◆ Elizabeth first described hearing voices shortly after her 18th birthday.
◆ Her first admission was at age 19 following the loss of job and partner.
◆ Her mother visited the ward for several hours every day to bring food and assist Elizabeth to wash; Elizabeth hit her mother during this admission and ward staff asked her not to visit as often.

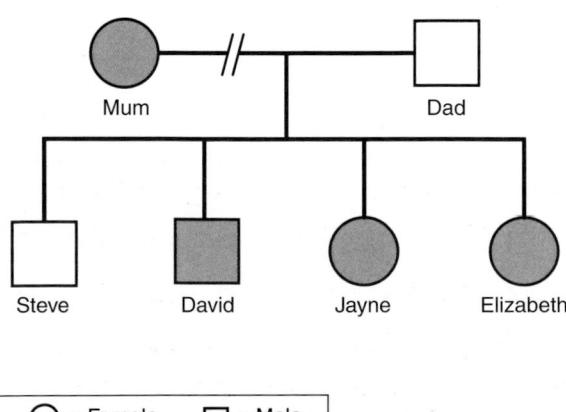

Figure 13.1 Genogram – case study of family intervention work.

◆ Flizabeth was discharged on depot medication; her mother was very concerned and took over the caring role, accompanied her everywhere and began to assist her in all aspects of daily living.
◆ Elizabeth became psychotic again and hit her mother on numerous occasions. Consequently was readmitted to hospital 2 weeks later.

Getting started

On this second admission, the family were recognised as needing more support than originally envisaged. Their needs fitted with a number of areas identified in the 'rule of thumb' (see Box 13.2) – i.e. mum was a lone carer whose responsibilities also included looking after someone with learning disabilities, and there had been violent episodes. The family accepted the offer of family work as part of the discharge plan. This work was advocated for by all members of the multidisciplinary team. This team ownership proved to be particularly important, especially in the light of the fact that the work would be conducted in the family home and that both family workers were full-time members of the acute ward team.

The following outline is intended to explain the sequence of events and acquisition of skills.

Providing information

Formal, interactive, information-sharing sessions were carried out in the home with all members of the household. Information leaflets, such as the ones issued by Rethink Mental Illness, were provided. Everyone was encouraged to read them and discuss the salient issues. During these sessions it was noticeable that no one felt awkward about interrupting each other. At this stage, ground rules were negotiated, which took some time for everyone to own and respect. In particular, everyone had a tendency to talk over others, or for Elizabeth. In this instance the suggested strategy (no. 1) outlined in Table 13.1 was utilised. Furthermore, the family had a reasonable level of knowledge. This had been gained from a visit to the local library and the Internet. Interestingly, they felt that this was generally negative with regard to prognosis.

Additional specific issues unearthed during the education session

Grandmother had been mentally ill: This information had not been elicited during admissions. It was highlighted that the mother was concerned that Elizabeth's life would follow the same path. However, the disclosure provided an opportunity to discuss the genetic and hereditary aspects of schizophrenia.

Mother thought that the illness had been caused by divorce: This belief was probed and challenged, by asking questions such as: 'Why has only one sibling become ill as a consequence?' and 'Why did it take 7 years to manifest itself?' After this style of questioning it was clear that other family members did not share their mum's belief. However, mum continued to feel guilty.

The family was unaware of negative symptoms: The issues that caused the family most concern were caused by the negative symptoms Elizabeth experienced. It was therefore clarified that an inability to be bothered about things, lack of motivation, and loss of interest, enjoyment and concentration were all recognised symptoms of the illness. As with other families, this aspect of the illness proved to be the hardest thing for them to comprehend. Therefore, it was deemed important to revisit this part of the education process when issues such as 'laziness' and 'can't be bothered' were raised in subsequent sessions.

The family viewed schizophrenia outcome as the same as learning difficulties: Because of the information they had gathered, the family believed that Elizabeth was facing a process of deterioration that would require her to have similar treatment to her brother David. This had a major impact on their caring strategies and was directly related to mum's beliefs and behaviours.

The workers were aware and curious about the culture of the family as neither was from a similar background: During these early engagement sessions, it was realised that there was a need to learn from the family about this important issue. Strategies used to aid this process were as follows:

– Outside agencies and colleagues from the same culture were contacted for advice.

– Family workers reiterated how important it was for them to learn from the family about this issue; everyone was encouraged to share and inform them when any cultural issues came up. Interestingly, all the children described themselves as English and saw England as their home. One of the family workers, although white, was not born in England and felt an alliance with the mother as a consequence. One area that the family did believe was culturally significant was the perceived power of the older sister, who, in the absence of the parents, was often seen as the adult in charge. This did have an impact on how the family dealt with issues as Elizabeth, being the younger daughter, was expected to respect her sister as she would her mother.

Enhancing communication

Specific issues

Using Elizabeth's 'expertise' and giving her room to speak: As mentioned earlier, during education sessions it was apparent that Elizabeth found it hard to communicate how her symptoms made her feel. Room was made for Elizabeth to relate her experiences and how she perceived them. This proved to be very cathartic for the family; they began to shift from the perception of 'Elizabeth's problem' to 'the problems caused by schizophrenia'. One particular comment made highlighted this:

> *It was a good idea, us all meeting in the comfort of our own home to discuss my sister's illness. We were all able to say how it felt and for the first time I realised that I knew very little about what she was suffering from or how much – the word schizophrenia meant nothing to me before but it's much clearer now. I used to think she was just being lazy until she told me in the meeting what it was really like.*

Reframing of mother's involvement: as sessions progressed the family reassessed the mother's involvement. In one session the comment was made that she 'interfered too much', which seemed to be reinforced by the family's experience when mum was asked not to visit the ward. Family workers focused on this statement and reframed it to the mother 'working very hard and needing a break'. This was felt to be important, as family members often criticise their previous care strategies without acknowledging their commitment to the individual. In this case, mum had indeed been working very hard and this was due to her obvious concern for her children.

Keeping Dad and Steve informed of the sessions as they were not able to attend: As dad and Steve were integral members of the informal care team, it was established that family members who could attend would take it in turns to relay what happened in the meetings to their brother and father.

Problem solving

Dealing with specific issues and problems generated by the illness is at the core of family work. As mentioned, one of the main areas of concern was the effects of negative symptoms on Elizabeth's functioning. Elizabeth's ultimate goal was to achieve some meaningful daily activity – i.e. she wanted a positive social identity and a job. However, she was having difficulty in socialising and in getting out of bed. Nevertheless, this ultimate goal proved to be an important key to gaining Elizabeth's and her family's cooperation. Family workers reiterated that in the long term this overall aim might be achievable. However, in these initial stages it was important to focus down on to a specific issue, identify objectives and plan small, achievable tasks that could be practised by the family. The six-step problem-solving framework was used to help frame their ideas. These are summarised in Box 13.6.

Box 13.6 Application of the six-step problem-solving strategy

Step one: What exactly is the problem or the goal?
Problem: 'Elizabeth is unable to get out of bed until after noon on most days.'
Goal: 'For Elizabeth to get up every morning from Monday to Friday by 10 am.'

Step 2: List all possible solutions
The family were encouraged to generate solutions. An exploration of each solution was not formally listed, as the family wished to discuss them and solve problems informally.

At this point it became obvious that mum was volunteering to do everything. The family workers challenged this and, subsequently, the family began exploring supportive roles that other members could undertake.

Step 3: Highlight the main advantages and disadvantages
As these were discussed, the family began to incorporate different aspects of different solutions. This often happens in problem-solving and workers need to be flexible enough to allow the ultimate solution to evolve. In this case, for example, it was clear that Elizabeth did not have an alarm clock. It was decided that she should have one but that this should not be perceived as the ultimate solution.

Step 4: Choose the 'best' solution
Through the above process the family identified the following as a solution they were willing to implement:

◆ Jayne to wake Elizabeth at 9 am when she gets up for her shower
◆ Family to leave Elizabeth and not scold her if she does not get up
◆ Mum to praise Elizabeth if she does get up.

Step 5: Plan exactly how to carry out the solution
It is clear from the above that the solution clearly outlines the role each person has to play in the solution. The solution also indicates what the family should do if Elizabeth is not able to get up.

Date and time of review
The solution, which was termed 'an experiment', was left with the family to practise for the following 2 weeks between sessions.

Step 6: Review progress in carrying out homework
Elizabeth did get up at 10 am twice in the 10 days.

While initially the family felt that the experiment had been of limited success, on examination it was felt by all that valuable lessons had been learnt. It became clear that Jayne had found consistency difficult and that the solution had asked for too much from her as well as from Elizabeth.

> **Box 13.6** Application of the six step problem-solving strategy (*cont'd*)
>
> What was also clear, however, was the family's satisfaction with the two successes. Mum in particular described a feeling of joy on these two occasions and related this feeling to an increased sense of hope and relief.
>
> Interestingly, when evaluating the session in which the solution had been formulated, the workers felt that they had contributed to the target being too high (i.e. for Elizabeth and family to be expected to achieve the goal on all ten occasions). This was fed back to the family and the workers focused more on the successful outcomes as valuable insights into effective problem-solving.
>
> From this it was identified that on the days on which the solution had been unsuccessful Elizabeth did not have anything meaningful to get up for. Therefore the strategy should be focused on those days when she needed to be up to attend work training.
>
> The family agreed to the change in goal to:
>
> **Goal:** For Elizabeth to get up on Tuesday and Thursday by 10 am in order to attend work training.

Subsequent problem-solving areas identified

Appropriate socialisation: Elizabeth asked for this to be considered and the problem was subsequently solved. The family openly discussed mum's anxiety when Elizabeth was alone or outside the family home. Eventually a solution was generated that involved Elizabeth going out with her sister and some friends. On these occasions they would take it in turns to ring home to say they were OK.

Combined with this solution was mum's awareness that Elizabeth was becoming less dependent on her. Such insights can exacerbate the feeling of losing control of the caring role; it is therefore important to generate ideas as to what this role could be replaced with. In this instance, however, mum was excited about returning to interests she had abandoned when Elizabeth became ill. Had this not occurred spontaneously, the family workers had planned to discuss mum finding replacement activities, such as visiting friends and relatives.

Elizabeth becoming independent: As the family work sessions progressed this issue became increasingly important to Elizabeth. She wanted an antidote to the 'patient role' and a more positive social identity within the household. It was important at this stage to focus on helping Elizabeth with social-functioning deficits. A programme was devised for her to do her own laundry and cooking. Interestingly, mum, who had previously carried out these tasks for the entire household, now asked if Jayne could also be included!

Coming off medication: As the family became more confident and Elizabeth regained control of her health, the issue of stopping medication arose. The workers discussed the need for maintenance medication and discussed the issue with the multidisciplinary team. Medication was eventually reduced to a small dose of oral medication.

Disengaging from family: As Elizabeth and her family progressed, the time between sessions was gradually extended. After 18 months the sessions were being held 2-monthly. It became clear that Elizabeth, who was now actively looking for a realistic work placement with her day service, viewed the family work as unnecessary as it reminded her of the period of illness. On one occasion the family workers went to the family home to find everyone out apart from mum. This was seen as a major change from initial visits, when she talked of her anxiety of letting Elizabeth go out alone. One more session was held to discuss family management in the case of relapse. To provide them with a clear framework within which to voice any future concerns, an early warning signs record was completed, as described in Chapter 18. Prior to formally discontinuing, the family were given a lifeline and informed that they could contact the team at any time in the future if they needed to.

Summary of practical strategies identified

◆ Education should be an ongoing, empowering process and should encompass the following topics: aetiology, symptomatology, diagnosis, medication course, prognosis and management.

◆ Cultural awareness and understanding must be acknowledged and incorporated.

◆ The intervention should be offered over a substantial period and tasks should be achievable, realistic and meaningful to the client's and family's long-term goals.

◆ Family workers should be flexible, knowledgeable and reliable and be able to access services and provide a range of options and opportunities.

◆ The philosophy of family work should be embraced and owned by the whole multidisciplinary team and be integrated into every treatment package (for ideas and further examples see Furlong & Leggart 1996, Smith & Velleman 2002, Sin et al 2003).

◆ Family work should be offered as and when it is required. Families who refuse should not be discriminated against (Budd & Hughes 1997).

References

Barrowclough C, Tarrier N 1995 Families of schizophrenic patients: cognitive behaviour intervention, 2nd edn. Chapman & Hall, London

Budd R J, Hughes I C T 1997 What do carers of people with schizophrenia find helpful and unhelpful about psychoeducation? Schizophrenia Bulletin 23:341–347

Department of Health 1999 A national service framework for mental health: modern standards and service models. The Stationery Office, London

Fadden G 1998 Family intervention. In: Brooker C, Repper J (eds) Serious mental health problems in the community: policy, practice and research. Baillière Tindall, London, pp 159–183

Falloon I R H, Graham-Hole V 1994 Comprehensive management of mental disorders. Buckingham Mental Health Service, Buckingham

Furlong M, Leggart M 1996 Reconciling the patients right to confidentiality and the families need to know. Australian and New Zealand Journal of Psychiatry 30:614–622

Kuipers E, Leff J, Lam D 2002 Family work for schizophrenia: a practical guide, 2nd edn. Gaskell Press, London

Leavey G, Healy H, Brennan G 1998 Providing information to carers of people admitted to psychiatric hospital. Mental Health Care 1:260–262

Leff J, Gamble C 1995 Training of community psychiatric nurses in family work for schizophrenia. International Journal of Mental Health 24:76–88

Missed Opportunities 2003 Carers UK. Available online at: http://www.carersuk.org

Nolan M 1996 Supporting family carers – the key to successful long term care? British Journal of Nursing 5:836

Rethink Mental Illness 2003 Who cares? The experiences of mental health carers accessing services and information. Available online at: www.rethink.org

San Blise M 1995 Everything I learned, I learned from patients: radical positive reframing. Journal of Psychosocial Nursing 33:18–25

Smith G, Velleman R 2002 Maintaining a family work for psychosis service by recognising barriers to implementation. Journal of Mental Health 11: 471–479

Sin J, Moone N, Wellman N 2003 Incorporating psycho-educational family and carers work into routine clinical practice. Journal of Psychiatric and Mental Health Nursing 10: 730–734

Annotated further reading

Atkinson J M, Coia D A 1995 Families coping with schizophrenia: a practitioner's guide to family groups. Wiley, London

Outlines the importance of providing adequate services and resources to families. The appendices provide an excellent comprehensive guide to setting up relatives' education groups.

Barrowclough C, Tarrier N 1995 Families of schizophrenic patients: cognitive behaviour intervention, 2nd edn. Chapman & Hall, London

Describes the history of EE and family intervention research. Its most relevant chapters include those that describe how to work proactively with families. The assessments that are referred to in this chapter, such as the RAI and the KASI, are included in the appendices.

Fadden G 1998 Family intervention. In: Brooker C, Repper J (eds) Serious mental health problems in the community: policy, practice and research. Baillière Tindall, London, pp 159–163

This chapter provides a concise overview of the effectiveness of family intervention and discusses the current issues surrounding its effective implementation into routine clinical practice.

Kuipers E, Leff J, Lam D 2002 Family work for schizophrenia: a practical guide, 2nd edn. Gaskell Press, London

This concise book outlines the Leff model of family intervention and includes brief clinical vignettes on how to provide information via education sessions, improve communication skills through goal setting and cope with negative emotions

14

Coexistent substance use and psychiatric disorders

Jood Gibbins and Cheryl Kipping

KEY ISSUES

◆ Prevalence of comorbidity
◆ Aetiological theories and reasons for use
◆ Clinical implications of comorbidity
◆ Policy guidance
◆ Assessment procedures
◆ Staged treatment approaches

INTRODUCTION

The coexistence of severe mental illness (SMI) and substance use disorder (SUD) – dual diagnosis – is an important challenge for psychiatry (e.g. Gournay et al 1997, Department of Health 2002a, Noordsy et al 2003). Although there is a growing research literature, evidence for the most effective service models and interventions is limited (Ley et al 1999). Much of the available research is derived from the USA, where the health-care context, configuration of services and treatment goals for substance use are different from those in the UK.

This chapter is divided into three sections. The first provides some background context, the second deals with assessment and the third with treatment approaches. A case study is included to illustrate the key points that have been made.

BACKGROUND CONTEXT

Prevalence

Despite concerns about substance use in people with SMI, it is difficult to establish prevalence rates because researchers have selected different samples and used different criteria for measuring both mental illness and substance use. It is recognised, however, that rates of substance use are higher among people with SMI than in the general population and some authors have suggested that substance use should be considered usual rather than exceptional in this group (Mueser et al 1995, Department of Health 2002a). Prevalence studies have reported incidences from 20% to 75% (Menezes et al 1996) but it is generally accepted that 30–50% of people with SMI also have problems with substance use. Working with people with a dual diagnosis is therefore part of routine work in any field of mental health and social care (Banerjee et al 2002). Overviews of prevalence studies can be found in Banerjee et al (2002) and Maslin (2003).

Aetiological theories and reasons for use

Many explanations have been provided for the high rate of SUD in people with SMI. Mueser et al (1998) identify four types of model:

Common factor: These models attribute coexistent substance use and mental illness to a common vulnerability factor. Possible common factors include: genetic, biological (e.g. poor cognitive functioning), psychosocial (e.g. history of childhood sexual abuse), environmental (e.g. homelessness) and personality (e.g. antisocial personality disorder).

Secondary substance use disorder: A primary mental illness is seen as a vulnerability factor for SUD in these models. There are two types: psychosocial risk factor models and the supersensitivity model.

The self-medication model is one example of a psychosocial risk factor model. It assumes that substances are used to alleviate particular symptoms of mental illness. For example, stimulants may be used to counter the negative symptoms of schizophrenia. A more general model is the alleviation of dysphoria model. This suggests that people with SMI are prone to dysphoria, which in turn makes them susceptible to using substances.

A multiple risk factor model is also proposed. This suggests that experiences such as social isolation, poverty and lack of structured activities, common in people with SMI, may contribute to dysphoria. This is additional to dysphoria associated with their mental illness; hence the person has been exposed to multiple risks.

The psychosocial consequences of mental illness can present other risk factors for substance use. For example, substance use may be a way of gaining acceptance into a social group to counter social marginalisation (Lamb 1982) or people may be introduced to substances through their contact with other mental health service users (Banerjee et al 2002).

The 'supersensitivity' model suggests that some people with a mental illness have a significant response to relatively small amounts of a substance. For example, a person with schizophrenia may relapse having taken only a small amount of cannabis.

Secondary psychiatric illness: This model posits that substance use is the primary problem and mental illness symptoms are experienced as a consequence. A variety of substances can trigger psychiatric symptoms. Examples include amphetamine use triggering a psychotic episode and alcohol use inducing depressive symptoms. Uncertainty remains about the role of substance use as a causative factor for mental illness but there is a growing evidence to indicate that cannabis use is a risk factor for schizophrenia, particularly in people with a pre-existing vulnerability (Arseneault 2002, van Os 2002, Zammit 2002).

Bidirectional: These models propose that the person is experiencing two unrelated disorders (a psychiatric disorder and SUD) that, over time, are likely to interact and exacerbate each other.

While these models provide a helpful conceptual framework for understanding comorbidity, evidence to support them is equivocal (Mueser et al 1998, Phillips & Johnson 2001). Noordsy et al (2003) argue that, given the difficulty of disentangling the primary/secondary distinction, it is best to assume that both are primary and treat them simultaneously.

Some reasons for severely mentally ill people using substances have been suggested but, as in people who do not have a mental illness, reasons for use are varied. These include dealing with negative feelings or situations (e.g. tension, anxiety, boredom, interpersonal conflict, lack of sleep), engendering positive feelings (e.g. enjoying the 'buzz', use to enhance celebrations) and responding to social pressures (use is the norm within a person's social circle).

It is unlikely that people use one drug or another simply because of their psychiatric diagnosis or symptoms; multiple determinants, including availability and cost, are likely to be influential. Evidence suggests that the substances used most frequently by people with a mental illness are alcohol and cannabis (Menezes et al 1996, Department of Health 2002a, Graham et al 2003).

Clinical implications

Regardless of the reasons for use, it is now well established that, in comparison to people with a mental illness alone, people who also use substances have significantly poorer outcomes. These include:

◆ increased rates of suicidal behaviour
◆ increased rates of violence

◆ higher rates of homelessness
◆ poorer medication adherence
◆ worsening of psychiatric symptoms
◆ increased rates of human immunodeficiency virus (HIV) infection
◆ increased use of institutional services
◆ greater contact with the criminal justice system (Banerjee et al 2002, Department of Health 2002a, Maslin 2003).

These outcomes clearly have important implications for the people themselves, their carers, the communities in which they live and services working with them.

Policy guidance for services working with people with a dual diagnosis

Despite growing concerns about dual diagnosis, it is only recently that guidance to inform service development has been produced. The key document is the *Dual Diagnosis Good Practice Guide* (Department of Health 2002a) which constitutes part of the *Mental Health Policy Implementation Guide*. As such, service providers in England must comply with it. The Guide argues that an integrated treatment model is required. This is one in which mental health and substance use interventions are provided at the same time, in one setting, by one team. It contrasts with the serial model, where mental health and SUDs are treated consecutively by different services, and the parallel model, where mental health and substance use interventions are provided at the same time but by different services. For people with a SMI the expectation is that the integrated approach will be provided within 'mainstream' mental health services.

Other documents impacting upon service development are the Health Advisory Service *Substance Misuse and Mental Health Co-Morbidity Standards* (Abdulrahim 2001) and *Models of Care for Treatment of Adult Drug Misusers* (Department of Health 2002b).

The Health Advisory Service document identifies standards for commissioning, interagency working, care organisation and service delivery. The standards are intended to be a tool for service development rather than targets against which services are monitored.

Models of Care (Department of Health 2002b) has been likened to a National Service Framework for drug services. The document is wide-ranging but includes a section on 'psychiatric co-morbidity' that draws heavily on the *Dual Diagnosis Good Practice Guide* and the Health Advisory Service Standards.

ASSESSMENT

Assessment of substance use should be integral to all mental health assessments. Sound assessment is essential for accurate diagnosis and safe and effective treatment. Up to 50% of substance use may be undetected in people with SMI (Osher & Drake 1996) and the most common reason for this is failure to ask (Noordsy et al 2003). Complex interrelationships exist between mental illness and substance use. If such relationships are not disentangled, misdiagnosis and inappropriate treatment can result (Carey & Correia 1998). Crome (1999) summarises these relationships:

- ◆ Substance use or withdrawal can produce psychiatric symptoms or illness
- ◆ Dependence, intoxication or withdrawal can produce psychological symptoms
- ◆ Psychiatric disorder can lead to SUD
- ◆ Substance use may exacerbate a pre-existing psychiatric disorder.

As well as its role in diagnosis and treatment planning, the assessment process is important for developing an empathic client–therapist relationship. The nature and strength of this relationship is a key influence on the outcome of interventions (Miller & Rollnick 2002, Repper 2002). Assessment should be conducted in collaboration with clients and, where appropriate, their carers, and should be sensitive, non-judgemental and confidential (Carey & Correia 1998). Judgemental attitudes, being confrontational, or overly directive, e.g. pushing someone towards abstinence before they are ready, can damage the client–therapist relationship and inhibit effective work. Lack of clarity regarding confidentiality may also be an inhibiting factor. Services should be transparent about their confidentiality policy and the circumstances in which it may be broken.

Assessment should not be thought of as distinct from treatment. It is important for engaging and educating the client, and enhancing motivation. From the outset, then, the worker's contact with the client constitutes an intervention.

Assessment of substance use is an ongoing process. It can take a considerable period of time to gain a detailed picture of a person's use, the way it developed over time and the impact it has on various aspects of their life, particularly when symptoms (of mental illness and/or substance use) impede this process. Patterns of substance use are also likely to change over time so it is important to regularly review the person's situation.

The Dual Diagnosis Good Practice Guide (Department of Health 2002a) identifies three components to assessment: detection and screening; specialised assessment, and risk assessment.

Detection and screening: specialised assessment

Substance use can be detected by self-report, laboratory tests and collateral information; however, the most common way of obtaining information is to ask people. Standardised instruments are available and, although few have been specifically designed for this client group, several have been evaluated in the SMI population (Carey & Correia 1998). The purpose of the various tools differs, e.g. some assess recent use, some lifetime use and some are designed to assess the severity of problems. Examples include:

◆ CAGE (King 1986)
◆ MAST – Michigan Alcoholism Screening Test (Selzer 1971)
◆ AUDIT – Alcohol Use Disorders Identification Test (Babor et al 1989)
◆ DALI – Dartmouth Assessment of Lifestyle Instrument (Rosenberg et al 1998)
◆ The Timeline Followback (Sobell & Sobell 1996)

Clinicians should be aware that screening techniques may not be sufficiently sensitive to detect problematic use in people with SMI. As their levels of use may be low, they may not meet the threshold criteria of a standardised instrument; however, even low levels of use can have serious consequences in the context of SMI.

Laboratory and other objective tests are important sources of assessment information. Urinalysis can be conducted 'on the spot' by using 'dip sticks' but more accurate results can be obtained by laboratory analysis. Approximate detection periods for drugs in urine screens vary; details are available in Banerjee et al (2002) and Department of Health (1999). Breathalyser tests assess alcohol use in the immediate past (a few hours) but blood tests, e.g. for liver enzymes, give a picture of the longer-term consequences of alcohol use. Low levels of substance use may go undetected by biological markers.

Finally, collateral sources, such as professionals and other agencies involved in a client's care, medical records, family and friends, can provide important information. This may detect hidden substance use and can also validate clients' self-reports.

Many components of a specialised substance use assessment are common to those of a comprehensive mental health assessment. In the remainder of this section the emphasis is on those components directly relating to substance use. Attention should be given to information that points to factors contributing to continuation of use; for example, using substances may be a way of dealing with bereavement. Substance use must be considered within the wider biopsychosocial context, not in isolation.

Components of a specialised substance use assessment include:

◆ current and recent use
◆ past use

- physical health (including consequences of use, e.g. liver damage, respiratory problems, blood borne viruses – Hepatitis B, C and HIV – accidental overdoses)
- mental health
- social situation (e.g. accommodation, support network, financial situation, education/employment, children)
- legal situation (users may be involved in illegal activity to support, or as a consequence of, their use)
- personal and family history
- clients' perceptions of their situation, reasons for using and motivation for change.

Risk assessment cuts across these areas. Information obtained within the context of each will contribute to the building of a sound risk assessment.

Current and recent use

Information is required to determine the nature and severity of use. Questioning should ascertain which substances the person is using, the amount being used, frequency of use, route of administration and an indication of how long the person has been using at the current level. To ensure that information is gained about the full range of substances being used (including prescribed and over-the-counter medications) prompting may be required. Additional questions may also be necessary to gain more detailed information, e.g. what strength of alcohol is being consumed, what time of day use commences, into which sites a person is injecting and which, if any, injecting equipment they are sharing. Figure 14.1 shows a table that could facilitate collection of such information.

To determine whether a person's use is reasonably stable from day to day, or whether there is a more chaotic picture, and to provide pointers as to whether physical dependence exists, a detailed account of the past five days use should be obtained. Some people will be able to provide accurate information over a longer period but poor recall will preclude this in others. Figure 14.2 shows a table that could be used to collect a 5-day substance use history. Factors that influence patterns of use over time should be explored; for example, the person may use one substance to counteract the effects of another or they may use heavily for a few days, perhaps after receipt of benefits, but not between times. Information about withdrawal symptoms is important for assessment of physical dependence and risk. Withdrawal seizures (from alcohol, barbiturates or benzodiazepines) and delirium tremens (alcohol) are life-threatening.

Observation is integral to the assessment process. The clinician should look for signs of intoxication or withdrawal, evidence of injuries and indicators of substance-misuse-related physical health problems.

Substance use information chart

Substance	Amount	Frequency	Route(s)	Prescribed or not	Duration at this level

Figure 14.1 Substance use information chart.

In conjunction with information about current and recent use, a substance misuse history is required. This should determine when the person began taking each substance they have used, factors that prompted use, how use has developed over time and the impact it has had on other aspects of the person's life (e.g. education, employment, relationships, finances, physical and mental health). Details of any periods of abstinence should be noted, along with information about how these were attained. Episodes of substance use treatment should be explored and aspects experienced as helpful should be identified. Obtaining a chronological account of a person's substance use and comparing this with their mental health history can be useful in gaining an understanding of the relationship between the two.

Client's perception of their situation, reasons for use and motivation to change

If realistic treatment goals are to be identified – goals set by the client and not imposed by the clinician – it is essential to understand the client's perceptions

Chart for completing five day substance use history

Day	Substances	Amount
Today		
Yesterday		
.......day		
.......day		
.......day		

Figure 14.2   Chart for completing 5-day substance use history.

of their situation, reasons for use and motivation for change. Clients often reveal their reasons for using during the assessment process, but a structured way of gaining this information is the completion of a decisional balance sheet. The client identifies the advantages and disadvantages (costs/benefits) of changing and not doing so. The perceived advantages may reveal strong motivators for continuing use, such as blocking out memories of childhood sexual abuse, reducing the intensity of hallucinations and giving the confidence to engage in social situations. The perceived benefits of change, however, often reveal strong motivators for the client to work towards reducing use, such as preventing a child being taken into local authority care, or a desire to go to college. If change is to be achieved it is likely that treatment interventions will need to address all such issues.

The importance of change and the confidence a person has in their ability to achieve it underpins their readiness to change (Rollnick et al 1999). Readiness can be assessed simply by asking people how ready they feel to change a particular aspect of their use, but a more quantitative assessment might be desirable. Clients could be asked to assign themselves a score on a numerical scale, where zero is not ready to change at all and ten is ready now. Alternatively, they could be given a pictorial representation of a 'readiness ruler', where one end is 'not ready' and the other end is 'ready'. The client identifies where on the continuum they see themselves (Rollnick et al 1999).

Risk assessment

Substance use can be a factor that increases the risks associated with mental illness, e.g. suicide and violence (Department of Health 2001), but there are risks more specifically associated with substance use that should be considered. Examples include accidents and overdose due to the sedating effects of some substances, contraction of blood-borne viruses from sharing injecting equipment, neglect of self and children, and involvement in the sex industry. With sensitive questioning, information about these risks can be obtained as part of the wider assessment. For more detailed information about risk assessment in the context of dual diagnosis see Alcohol Concern & Drugscope (2002) and Kipping (in press).

TREATMENT

Treatment of coexisting SMI and SUD requires integration of interventions from mental health and substance misuse (Department of Health 2002a). This section focuses on community interventions, since SUDs are environmentally sensitive conditions and the literature suggests that care provided in the context of the community is more effective in the long term (Drake & Mueser 2000). Inpatient care is addressed briefly.

Three main approaches underpin work with dually disordered clients: Prochaska & DiClemente's (1986) transtheoretical model of change, Osher & Kofoed's (1989) staged treatment model, and Miller & Rollnick's (1991) motivational interviewing skills approach.

Prochaska & DiClemente's model focuses on the client's level of motivation, i.e. their state of readiness to change. The stages are:

◆ **precontemplation**: no recognition of the problem and therefore sees no reason to change
◆ **contemplation**: recognition of, and thinking about the problem, exploring possibility of change
◆ **determination and action**: preparing to and making changes
◆ **maintenance**: maintaining changes and preventing relapse.

Relapse is integral to the model and individuals may move back and forth between the stages several times before achieving long-term change. Although this model is commonly used to understand SUD, it has applications to other aspects of treatment such as medication management (Rollnick et al 1999).

Osher & Kofoed's treatment model comprises four stages: engagement, persuasion, active treatment and relapse prevention. These stages closely relate to those in Prochaska & DiClemente's model and are more fully described below.

Throughout assessment and treatment, the main counselling approach employed is motivational interviewing, an effective evidence-based approach that assists people in making desired changes in their lives by overcoming ambivalence (Miller & Rollnick 2002). This section does not provide a detailed account of motivational interviewing; however, central to its purpose is developing discrepancy in clients between their current behaviour and any goals or hopes they have for the future. Traditionally, motivational interviewing has been linked to the persuasion stage of treatment; however, recent evidence suggests that motivational interviewing is particularly useful at the engagement stage (Zuckoff & Daley 2001, Handmaker et al 2002).

Motivational interviewing draws on the concept of ambivalence (being in 'two minds') to understand the dilemma substance users face between indulgence and restraint. The expression, clarification and resolution of ambivalence through eliciting 'commitment' talk are essential for creating readiness to change. Clients are encouraged to reflect on the antecedents and consequences of their substance-using behaviour and the relationship of substance use with other areas of their lives. The skills are applicable to group or individual interventions.

Table 14.1 shows how the stages of change and the staged treatment model link, and identifies treatment interventions, including motivational interviewing techniques, that can be utilised at each stage.

Although a sound evidence base exists to inform effective psychological treatment of people with SMI (Barrowclough et al 2000, Drake et al 2001), and SUDs (Department of Health 1999), the evidence base is less robust for effective treatment of co-occurring disorders (Jeffery et al 2000). Research, however, suggests that it is important to integrate interventions from both fields. Key components include engagement, persuasion and, in the active treatment stage, assertive monitoring, adopting a longitudinal view of treatment, using modified psychosocial and cognitive behavioural interventions, skills training, sophisticated prescribing and carer intervention (Drake et al 2001, Holland 2002).

Engagement

Engagement is the first essential stage of treatment, as this client group demonstrates a tendency to not engage with or disengage from services

Table 14.1 The stages of treatment–intervention matrix

Stage of change	Stage of treatment	Intervention
Precontemplation: No recognition of problem	Engagement	Relationship building Information gathering Screening and assessment Eliciting change talk Practical assistance Appropriate response to resistance Stabilising symptoms (SMI and SUD) Carers' needs evaluation
Contemplation: Recognition and exploration of the problem areas	Persuasion	Cost benefit analyses of change Specialised assessment Relationship building Information exchange Healthy social sampling Reframing events Negotiating appropriate goals
Action: Planning, rehearsing and refining strategies for change to reduce and stabilise symptoms and substance use	Active treatment	Detoxification or reduction strategies Review medication Coping skills training Lifestyle modification Psychoeducational work Group work for SUD and/or SMI Engagement into self-help groups Relapse prevention exploration and planning
Maintenance: Ongoing review and practice of strategies to maintain changes in the long term	Relapse prevention	Relapse prevention planning Healthy social sampling Therapeutic occupational roles Lapse analysis Consolidation of skills learned

(Mercer-McFadden et al 1997, Zuckoff & Daley 2001). Engagement is primarily concerned with the development of a therapeutic alliance. The strength of this depends, in part, on the value a client attributes to the service and, more strongly, on the approach the therapist takes (Miller & Rollnick 2002, Repper 2002).

Providing practical support, such as help with housing, physical health care, benefits or legal issues, can be an important engagement strategy. Such support often precedes interventions to reduce substance use and there is more emphasis on reducing harm and increasing stability of lifestyle and symptoms (Carey 1996, Oscher & Drake 1996, Banerjee et al 2002). Compliance with further treatment can be enhanced by eliciting the client's perspective and using an empathic, motivational approach to gain a clear idea of their needs and values (Daley & Zuckoff 1998).

Persuasion

The persuasion stage endeavours to help clients to explore and understand why they need to consider change and to strengthen their motivation and commitment to change. Developing discrepancy is crucial and represents the directive element of motivational interviewing. One method of achieving this is providing feedback and information (e.g. blood test results). This is not done with the intention of frightening or coercing clients; they are invited to consider the results and offer their own interpretation. The therapist uses active listening, accurately reflecting back to the client those aspects of use that appear problematic, thus nudging the decisional balance in favour of change. Examples of techniques for deploying discrepancy are included in Table 14.1.

Traditionally, substance use treatment has tended toward confrontation to break down the user's denial or resistance. The expression of client resistance has been shown to predict a lack of change in behaviour (Miller & Rollnick 2002). It is therefore essential to resolving ambivalence to respond appropriately to resistance. Motivational interviewing posits that denial is actually a misinterpretation of resistance, arising when a clinician offers an intervention that is not congruent with the client's stage of change. For example, someone who is precontemplative and needs engaging is unlikely to respond well to being offered a detoxification programme, which is an active treatment intervention.

Modifications to motivational interviewing for clients with deficits in cognitive functioning, such as SMI, are recommended. Modifications include presenting educational information in written form that is easy to remember, presenting information slowly and repeating it often, using memory prompts (e.g. diaries), rehearsing strategies and working in smaller groups than usual (Blume et al 1999).

Active treatment

It may take many months before clients are ready to participate in active treatment interventions for their substance use. Ideally, the aim should be abstinence, although this can be difficult to achieve and may require many attempts. The Department of Health (2002a) suggest that alternative short-term goals that are acceptable to the client and based on harm reduction principles are necessary to build confidence and skills, e.g. reduced substance use without impairment of functioning or adverse consequences. It is important for clinicians to acknowledge the achievement of any intermediate goals and to maintain an optimistic outlook (Gibbins 1998).

Specific treatment interventions can be delivered in groups or individually. These will vary for each client; however, the literature recommends two broad areas: coping skills training and lifestyle modification (Carey 1995). Carey emphasises the role substances play as social facilitators for people with mental illness. Social skills enhancement is therefore necessary if individuals are to derive sufficient social support without using substances. Craving, symptom and medication management, conversational, assertiveness and drug refusal skills are recommended. As noted, many people use substances to combat uncomfortable symptoms. Thorough, ongoing and educational collaborative reviews of medication, accurate monitoring of side effects and discussion about the interactions of medication and other psychoactive substances are necessary to reduce reliance on non-prescribed substances.

Research also suggests that peer influence, written participation, homework, family involvement and contingency management are useful interventions (Bellack & Gearon 1998). These authors also advocate highly structured skills training designed to 'reduce the load on memory and attention, and minimise demands on higher level cognitive processes' (p 758). They emphasise the role of rehearsing behaviours, over-learning key skills and the use of learning aides. Clients need to learn basic strategies, responses and thinking patterns through constant exposure and consistent therapeutic approaches to combat the array of symptoms and stressors in daily life. Bellack & Gearon also suggest that urinalysis contingency plans with modest financial reward and social reinforcement within the group can significantly enhance skills training.

Lifestyle modification

Substance use cessation will necessarily involve lifestyle changes at every treatment stage. This can be difficult for clients, particularly when substance use is central to their daily activities and social identity. Early avoidance of people and places associated with substance use, accompanied by structuring vocational and drug-free leisure time, is essential. Research increasingly emphasises the use of transitional or supported employment projects (Drake & Noordsy 1994, Carey 1996, Kavanagh et al 1998) as well as self-help groups (Ho et al 1999, Drake & Mueser 2000). These can provide invaluable structure, promotion of self-esteem and a context in which to establish non-using friends (Hodgson & Lloyd 2002).

Pharmacological considerations

A further treatment option is that of prescribing medication. Concerns often focus on achieving a therapeutic dose of psychiatric medication while safely managing potentially harmful interactions with alcohol or illicit substances. Unless clients are known to be using a substance that has a negative interaction with neuroleptic medication, the benefits of controlling psychiatric symptoms suggest that the prescribed regime should be continued (Carey 1995, Denison 2003). Overviews of these considerations are presented in Siris 1990 and Denison 2003.

Alcohol, barbiturates, benzodiazepines and opiates can lead to physical dependence if taken regularly over extended periods. Consequently, detoxification can be a complicated and uncomfortable process that carries certain risks, e.g. withdrawal seizures. Detoxification involves the substitution of these drugs with prescribed alternatives, which are reduced incrementally over time (Department of Health 1999). Inpatient care for this type of treatment is recommended, particularly since the cessation of substance use may reveal or initiate the re-emergence of psychiatric symptoms. Denison (2003) covers these topics comprehensively and specific guidelines on the management of dependence and detoxification are available in *Drug Misuse and Dependence – Guidelines on Clinical Management* (Department of Health 1999). Sophisticated prescribing for both SMI and SUD is needed, with regular evaluation of effects and interactions, including over-the-counter preparations, homeopathic remedies and common legal substances such as nicotine and caffeine.

In-patient care

Inpatient admission is primarily reserved for further assessment, accurate diagnosis, stabilisation, detoxification or specific medical intervention for both SMI and SUD (Bachman et al 1997, Drake & Mueser 2000). During admission, inreach from community services can help to establish links with outpatient resources, offering the client an opportunity to re-engage and renegotiate treatment goals. A long period of inpatient care solely to reduce access to substances is not recommended (Drake & Mueser 2000).

Relapse prevention

Both SUD and SMI are chronic relapsing conditions (Carey 1995, Birchwood et al 2000, Department of Health 2002a). Therefore, once a client has begun to reduce use or attained abstinence, interventions should address the prevention of future relapses. The principles and strategies of relapse prevention in SUD documented by Marlatt & Gordon (1985) are mirrored by Birchwood et al's (2000) strategies on relapse signatures for SMI. Marlatt & Gordon's work advocates identifying triggers, cues and high-risk situations likely to precipitate relapse and developing coping strategies, which are rehearsed proactively. Attention is given to the development of action plans should the client return to substance use. Relapse prevention views any lapse as a slip from which important insights can be gained and vulnerabilities identified, rather than as a failure. Birchwood et al's (2000) work regarding relapse in SMI focuses on the identification of subtle changes in cognition or emotional state (a personal 'relapse signature') that precede the development of acute symptoms. Interventions centre on arresting these processes through early identification and psychological and pharmacological management of symptom changes.

The experience of relapse can undermine individuals' motivation and their belief in their ability to succeed. Given the likelihood of lapses, it is important for clinicians to utilise these events in a constructive way and motivational interventions include specific attention to affirmations and supporting self-efficacy to reinforce the client's self-belief. Progress and success is gauged against reductions in the frequency of relapses, or in their duration, rather than complete cessation (Carey 1995, Holland 2002). Relapse prevention strategies can begin as early as the persuasion stage if there is some reduction in substance use.

Family and carer involvement

From the outset, the needs of significant others (e.g. family, partners or carers) must be recognised. Substance use and mental health problems can engender considerable anxiety or other strong emotional reactions in these people (Graham & Maslin 1998, Coppello et al 2000). Overt expression of these emotions can affect the client's behaviours, making them more vulnerable to relapse of SMI, SUD or both (Barrowclough et al 2001, Drake et al 2001). Behaviours such as over-involvement or confrontational or critical comments can increase client distress and contribute to relapse. Other factors that can also have a negative impact are enabling behaviours and co-dependence. Early liaison with significant others to provide support can enhance the foundations for longer-term treatment (Barrowclough & Parle 1997). Interventions may include basic SMI and SUD education, communication skills, referral for a carer's assessment or facilitation of links into support services.

Case study – Lottie

Lottie had a 12-year history of mental health admissions to acute in-patient care for psychotic and behavioural disorders, and, over 21 admissions, had accumulated seven different mental disorder diagnoses. She had spent a short spell in prison in her late teens and, more recently, was detained under mental health law in the Regional Secure Unit. While detained she was assessed by a new consultant psychiatrist who made a definitive diagnosis of paranoid schizophrenia and concurrent polysubstance use disorder. Following this assessment and diagnosis, Lottie was transferred back to the local hospital, to the Intensive Care Unit, for stabilisation of her psychotic features on neuroleptic depot medication. Following transfer to the open ward, her section lapsed and was not renewed, as she was compliant with treatment and mentally stable. Because of her history of poor engagement, she was referred to the assertive outreach team (AOT) as part of proactive discharge planning. They began inreach visits to start building a relationship with Lottie before her discharge. Because of weight gain, and at her own request, depot medication was withdrawn and a new oral daily neuroleptic was successfully introduced.

After 7 months of in-patient care, Lottie was discharged to sheltered housing, sharing with other people with similar problems (i.e. SMI and SUD). After 8 months, Lottie began to use cannabis and inject heroin daily, which was not detected until she herself asked for help when she began to experience financial problems. The AOT care coordinator referred directly to the consultant nurse – dual diagnosis (CNDD) for assessment and treatment guidance regarding Lottie's opiate dependence and cannabis use.

The CNDD had worked successfully with Lottie in the past to help her stop using heroin and therefore had access to significant information about her and could build on their previous therapeutic alliance. A specialised re-assessment was conducted collaboratively over several weeks in Lottie's own home, updating facts and gathering new information regarding all areas of her life. A motivational interviewing approach was used to help to examine some of the problem areas and to build commitment to further treatment. In order to build foundations for change, aspects of change talk expressed during the assessment process were reflected and emphasised as well as particular areas of discrepancy.

Significant negative events Lottie identified were: the death of her father, to whom she had been very close; sharing accommodation with other dually diagnosed people, which had led to the resurgence of heroin use; and continued contact with old substance-using acquaintances. Significant positive events she identified were: the assertive treatment of her psychosis with new medication, which had tolerable side effects; practical help from the AOT, and daily support from the housing worker in the accommodation. She acknowledged a significant reduction in her psychotic symptoms of paranoid ideas and auditory hallucinations. She also noted two main problem areas – dependence on heroin and the impact of others' substance use in the property preventing her own abstinence. The AOT concurred with her view and also noted episodes of unpredictable behaviour that they felt might be due to hormonal imbalance.

Case study – Lottie (cont'd)

The areas for targeting were jointly identified by the AOT, CNDD and Lottie.
These are listed below, identifying Lottie's stage of motivation to each:

- ◆ **Heroin dependence**, *requiring substitute prescribing; daily, supervised consumption, followed by slow long-term reduction and eventual abstinence:* motivation stage – determination and action
- ◆ **Management of breakthrough psychotic symptoms**, *requiring education and medication and symptom management interventions:* motivation stage – determination and action
- ◆ **Accommodation**, *requiring pursuance of longer-term stable independent living without other drug users present:* motivation stage – determination and action
- ◆ **Hormonal disturbance**, *requiring monitoring, further referral and investigation for treatment:* motivation stage – contemplation
- ◆ **Social networks**, *requiring avoidance of known using contacts and development of drug-free social pursuits and networks:* motivation stage – contemplation
- ◆ **Cannabis use**, *requiring ongoing monitoring for adverse consequences and a motivational approach to promote a reduction in use:* motivation stage – precontemplation

In order to prevent further harm associated with heroin use, Lottie commenced a daily prescription of methadone, at a dose commensurate with clinical guidelines, to prevent withdrawal symptoms. This was dispensed daily and consumption was supervised by a community pharmacist. Lottie's motivation to stop using heroin was high and within 8 weeks she had achieved this, as confirmed by weekly urinalysis. A diary to enhance planning and keeping appointments, and a folder in which to keep records and notes about relapse prevention and monitoring work, were provided to aid her recall of sessions.

As her methadone prescription was of paramount importance to Lottie, and to aid engagement and monitoring, weekly appointments were negotiated at which she received each prescription and provided a urine sample. As Lottie was precontemplative regarding her cannabis use, monitoring the consequences of this was incorporated into the weekly appointments. Regular exploration of cannabis use, with ongoing reference to stabilisation of symptoms and lifestyle through methadone, proved invaluable in moving Lottie into contemplating reduction in use in the longer-term.

The AOT provided daily assistance, medication and social monitoring, as well as education and support to the housing team, who visited the accommodation daily. They were able to explore options for independent living on a long-term basis, providing input to areas of deficit such as budgeting and Lottie's lack of constructive social networks. Weekly liaison by phone or face-to-face contact at some joint visits, as well as regular integrated care programme approach reviews, ensured good communication and joint reviewing of target areas.

Regular open discussion of substance use and mental health symptoms gave consistent opportunities to emphasise selectively the role of substance use in

Case study – Lottie (cont'd)

everyday activities. Over time, continuous and focussed assessment elicited an underlying anxiety disorder previously overlooked because of paranoid ideas and the impact of central nervous system depressants. These feelings of anxiety had a crucial influence on all other target areas and a skills plan of sustained relaxation and anxiety management was implemented on a daily basis.

Another vital factor was taking a long-term view of both mental health and substance use. Regular use of cannabis was monitored for adverse effects and gradually reduced to a point where there was no impairment of daily living with use. The use of long-term methadone stabilisation prior to reduction allayed Lottie's own fears and gave other clinicians the chance to work with her while she was stable, and in a consistent manner, something neither they nor she had experienced before. Urinalysis was able to confirm her abstinence from heroin, thus affirming Lottie's own ability to maintain change and giving concrete evidence of progress to other clinicians.

Lottie is currently undergoing a stabilisation admission following a brief mental health relapse after using 'crack' cocaine and beginning to use heroin on alternate days to manage the after-effects of 'crack' use. She herself emphasised the interrelatedness of her substance use and mental health consequences and this is being empathically used to reinforce her motivation to change by all the care team. Lottie's subjective anxiety levels rose with the cessation of heroin; this has been assessed and a daily relaxation and anxiety management programme is being implemented, to be continued with community staff. The CNDD and AOT continue to visit weekly to monitor, assess and communicate with ward staff and Lottie, improving the relationship long-term.

Summary of practical strategies identified

◆ Substance use among individuals with SMI is usual rather than exceptional.

◆ Clinical outcomes for this client group are poor when compared with non-substance-using psychiatric clients.

◆ All clinicians have a duty to screen for substance use and initiate a specialised assessment if necessary.

◆ Self-report procedures, including standardised measures, laboratory tests and collateral data sources are methods for initial screening and detection.

◆ Specialised assessments generate data on substance use patterns and severity, and enable the clinician to understand the wider biopsychosocial context of use.

Summary of practical strategies identified (*cont'd*)

◆ Mainstream mental health services have a duty to address both substance use and mental health issues in an integrated way.

◆ Identification of appropriate treatment goals, and plans to pursue these, must be collaboratively negotiated with the client.

◆ Effective treatment requires the integrated delivery of concurrent substance use and psychiatric interventions by one service or care coordinator.

◆ Treatment planning is based on an assessment of clients' readiness to change and the use of motivational interviewing to enhance their commitment to change.

◆ The process of treatment moves through the four stages of engagement, persuasion, active treatment and relapse prevention, with each stage requiring different interventions.

◆ Clinicians should adopt a longitudinal view of treatment with their clients, expect and work with relapse, and maintain optimism about the possibility of change.

References

Abdulrahim D 2001 Substance misuse and mental health co-morbidity (dual diagnosis): standards for mental health services. Health Advisory Service, London

Alcohol Concern, Drugscope 2002 Assessment and management of risk of harm in clients with dual diagnosis. Alcohol Concern in association with Drugscope, London

Arseneault L, Cannon M, Poulton R et al 2002 Cannabis use in adolescence and risk for adult psychosis: longitudinal prospective study. British Medical Journal 325:1212–1213

Babor T, de la Fuente J, Saunders J et al 1989 AUDIT, the Alcohol Use Disorders Identification Test: guidelines for use in primary care. World Health Organisation, Geneva

Bachman K, Moggi F, Hirsbrunner H et al 1997 An integrated treatment programme for dually diagnosed patients. Psychiatric Services 48:314–316

Banerjee S, Clancy C, Crome I (eds) 2002 Co-existing problems of mental disorder and substance misuse (dual diagnosis): an information manual. Royal College of Psychiatrists Research Unit, London

Barrowclough C, Parle M 1997 Appraisal, psychological adjustment and expressed emotion in relatives of patients suffering from schizophrenia. British Journal of Psychiatry 171:26–30

Barrowclough C, Haddock G, Tarrier N et al 2000 Cognitive behavioural intervention for individuals with severe mental illness who have a substance misuse problem. Psychiatric Rehabilitation Skills 4:216–233

References (cont'd)

Barrowclough C, Haddock G, Tarrier N et al 2001 Randomized controlled trial of motivational interviewing, cognitive behaviour therapy, and family intervention for patients with comorbid schizophrenia and substance use disorders. American Journal of Psychiatry 158:1706–1713

Bellack A, Gearon J 1998 Substance abuse treatment for people with schizophrenia. Addictive Behaviours International Journal 23:758

Birchwood M, Spencer E, McGovern D 2000 Schizophrenia: early warning signs. Advances in Psychiatric Treatment 6:93–101

Blume A, Davis J, Schmaling K 1999 Neurocognitive dysfunction in dually diagnosed patients: a potential roadblock to motivating behaviour change. Journal of Psychoactive Drugs 31:111–115

Carey K 1995 Treatment of substance use disorders and schizophrenia. In: Lehman A, Dixon L (eds) Double jeopardy: chronic mental illness and substance use disorders. Harwood Academic, Chur, Switzerland

Carey K 1996 Substance use reduction in the context of outpatient psychiatric treatment: a collaborative motivational harm reduction approach. Community Mental Health Journal 32:291–306

Carey K B, Correia C J 1998 Severe mental illness and addictions: assessment considerations. Addictive Behaviours 23:735–748

Copello A, Orford J, Velleman R et al 2000 Methods for reducing alcohol and drug related family harm in non-specialist settings. Journal of Mental Health 9:329–343

Crome I 1999 Substance misuse and psychiatric co-morbidity: towards improved service provision. Drugs: Education, Prevention and Policy 6:151–174

Daley D, Zuckoff A 1998 Improving compliance with the initial outpatient session among discharged inpatient dual diagnosis clients. Social Work 43:470–473

Denison S 2003 Handbook of the dually diagnosed patient: psychiatric and substance use disorders. Lippincott Williams & Wilkins, Philadelphia

Department of Health 1999 Drug misuse and dependence – guidelines on clinical management. The Stationery Office, London

Department of Health 2001 Safety first: five-year report of the national confidential inquiry into suicide and homicide by people with mental illness. Department of Health, London

Department of Health 2002a The mental health policy implementation guide: dual diagnosis good practice guide. Department of Health, London

Department of Health 2002b Models of care for adult drug misusers. Department of Health, London

Drake R, Mueser K 2000 Psychosocial approaches to dual diagnosis. Schizophrenia Bulletin 26:105–119

Drake R, Noordsy F 1994 Case management for people with co-existing severe mental disorder and substance use disorder. Psychiatric Annals 24:427–431

Drake R, Essock S, Shaner A et al 2001 Implementing dual diagnosis services for clients with severe mental illness. Psychiatric Services 52:469–476

Gibbins J 1998 Towards integrated care for patients with dual diagnosis: the Dorset Healthcare NHS Trust experience. Mental Health Review 3:20–24

Gournay K, Sandford T, Johnson G et al 1997 Dual diagnosis of severe mental health problems and substance abuse/dependence: a major priority for mental health nursing. Journal of Psychiatric and Mental Health Nursing 4:89–95

References (cont'd)

Graham H, Maslin J 1998 The development of services for people with psychosis and a substance misuse problem: The COMPASS Programme. Northern Birmingham Mental Health Trust, Birmingham

Graham H L, Birchwood M J, Maslin J et al 2003 The combined psychosis and substance use (Compass) programme: an integrated shared-care approach. In: Graham H L, Copello A, Birchwood M J et al (eds) Substance misuse in psychosis. Wiley, Chichester

Handmaker N, Packard M, Conforti K 2002 Motivational interviewing in treatment of dual disorders. In: Miller W, Rollnick S (eds) Motivational interviewing: preparing people for change. Guilford Press, New York

Ho A, Tsuang J, Liberman R, Wang R et al 1999 Achieving effective treatment of patients with chronic psychotic illness and comorbid substance dependence. American Journal of Psychiatry 156:1765–1770

Hodgson S, Lloyd C 2002 Leisure as a relapse prevention strategy. British Journal of Therapy and Rehabilitation 9:86–91

Holland M 2002 Dual diagnosis – substance misuse and schizophrenia. In: Harris N, Williams S, Bradshaw T (eds) Psychosocial interventions for people with schizophrenia. Palgrave Macmillan, Basingstoke

Jeffrey D, Ley A, Bennun I, McLaren S 2000 Delphi survey of opinion on interventions, service principles and service organisation for severe mental illness and substance misuse problems. Journal of Mental Health 9:371–384

Kavanagh D, Young R, Boyce L et al 1998 Substance treatment options in psychosis (STOP): a new intervention for dual diagnosis. Journal of Mental Health 7:135–143

King M 1986 At risk drinking among general practice attenders: validation of the CAGE questionnaire. Psychological Medicine 16:213–217

Kipping C (in press) Drug and alcohol use. In: Norman I J N, Ryrie I (eds) Mental health nursing: delivering the national service frameworks and beyond. Open University Press, Buckingham

Lamb H 1982 Young adult chronic patients: the drifters. Hospital and Community Psychiatry 33:465–468

Ley A, Jeffery D, McLaren S et al 1999 Treatment programmes for people with both severe mental illness and substance misuse. In: The Cochrane Library, Issue 2. Update Software, Oxford

Marlatt G A, Gordon J R 1985 Relapse prevention: maintenance strategies in the treatment of addictive behaviours. Guilford Press, New York

Maslin J 2003 Substance misuse in psychosis: contextual issues. In: Graham H L, Copello A, Birchwood M et al (eds) Substance misuse in psychosis: approaches to treatment and service delivery. Wiley, Chichester

Menezes P, Johnson S, Thornicroft G et al 1996 Drug and alcohol problems among people with severe mental illness in south London. British Journal of Psychiatry 168:612–619

Mercer-McFadden C, Drake R, Brown N et al 1997 The community support programme demonstrations of services for young adults with severe mental illness and substance use disorders. Psychiatric Rehabilitation Journal 20:13–24

Miller W R, Rollnick S 1991 Motivational interviewing: preparing people to change addictive behaviour. Guilford Press, New York

Miller W R, Rollnick S 2002 Motivational interviewing. Guilford Press, New York

Mueser K, Fox M, Kenison L et al 1995 The better living skills group. New Hampshire-Dartmouth Psychiatric Research Centre, Concord, NH

References (cont'd)

Mueser K T, Drake R E, Wallach M A 1998 Dual diagnosis: a review of aetiological theories. Addictive Behaviours 23:717–734

Noordsy D L, McQuade D V, Mueser K T 2003 Assessment considerations. In: Graham H L, Copello A, Birchwood N J et al (eds) Substance misuse in psychosis. Wiley, Chichester

Osher F C, Drake R E 1996 Reversing a history of unmet needs: approaches to care for persons with co-occurring addictive and mental disorders. American Journal of Orthopsychiatry 66:4–11

Osher F C, Kofoed L 1989 Treatment of patients with psychiatric and psychoactive substance abuse disorders. Hospital and Community Psychiatry 40:1025–1030

Phillips P, Johnson S 2001 How does drug and alcohol misuse develop among people with psychotic illness? A literature review. Social Psychiatry and Psychiatric Epidemiology 36:269–276

Prochaska J, DiClemente C 1986 Toward a comprehensive model of change. In: Miller W, Heather N (eds) Treating addictive behaviours: processes of change. Plenum Press, New York

Repper J 2002 The helping relationship. In: Harris N, Williams S, Bradshaw T (eds) Psychosocial interventions for people with schizophrenia. Palgrave Macmillan, Basingstoke

Rollnick S, Mason P, Butler C 1999 Health behaviour change: a guide for practitioners. Churchill Livingstone, Edinburgh

Rosenberg S, Drake R, Wolford G et al 1998 Dartmouth Assessment of Lifestyle Instrument (DALI): a substance use disorder screen for people with severe mental illness. American Journal of Psychiatry 155:232–238

Selzer M 1971 The Michigan Alcoholism Screening Test. American Journal of Psychiatry 127:1653–1658

Siris S 1990 Pharmacological treatment of substance-abusing schizophrenic patients. Schizophrenia Bulletin 16:111–122

Sobell L C, Sobell M B 1996 Timeline followback user's guide: a calendar method for assessing alcohol and drug use. Addiction Research Foundation, Toronto

Van Os J, Bak M, Hanssen M et al 2002 Cannabis use and psychosis: a longitudinal population study. American Journal of Epidemiology 156:319–327

Zammit S, Allebeck P, Andreasson S et al 2002 Self reported cannabis use as a risk factor for schizophrenia in Swedish conscripts of 1969: historical cohort study. British Medical Journal 325:1199–1203

Zuckoff A, Daley D 2001 Engagement and adherence issues in treating persons with non-psychosis dual disorders. Psychiatric Rehabilitation Skills 5:131–162

Annotated further reading

Banerjee S, Clancy C, Crome I (eds) 2002 Co-existing problems of mental disorder and substance misuse (dual diagnosis): an information manual. Royal College of Psychiatrists Research Unit, London

Annotated further reading (cont'd)

This information manual was written to accompany the Department of Health Dual Diagnosis Good Practice Guide. It provides an overview of dual diagnosis and is organised into seven sections: conceptual and theoretical issues, problems in service provision, ethical issues and the Mental Health Act, assessment, interventions, organisational issues and information sources.

Denison S 2003 Handbook of the dually diagnosed patient: psychiatric and substance use disorders. Lippincott Williams & Wilkins, Philadelphia

This compact volume provides an excellent overview of specific mental health disorders, their relationships with specific substances and concordant treatments from a medical perspective. It contains many useful up-to-date references and is a handy resource for all professions.

Department of Health 1999 Drug misuse and dependence – guidelines on clinical management. The Stationery Office, London

Intended primarily for medical practitioners, these guidelines provide a valuable resource for all clinicians working with people with SUDs. They represent a consensus view of good clinical practice, which is presented across seven chapters that loosely follow the process of treatment. The guidelines are annexed with 19 appendices that cover additional issues including drug use and comorbid mental illness.

Department of Health 2002a The mental health policy implementation guide: dual diagnosis good practice guide. Department of Health, London

As well as setting out the direction in which the Department of Health requires services to develop, this guidance provides useful contextual information including the wider policy context, models of treatment for mainstream mental health services and other useful background information.

Graham H L, Copello A, Birchwood M J et al (eds) Substance misuse in psychosis. Wiley, Chichester

This book is an edited volume that brings together the most up-to-date writing of many of the key players in dual diagnosis. It is divided into five parts: social and psychological perspectives, integrated service models, treatments, special populations and the evidence base. It is an excellent resource for people wanting an in-depth knowledge based on current evidence.

Miller W R, Rollnick S 2002 Motivational interviewing. Guilford Press, New York

This new version of the seminal text on the theory and application of motivational interviewing skills to help people change includes significant updated research evidence. It provides useful examples of practice and includes a chapter on the relevance and application of these skills to working with dually diagnosed clients.

15

Working with people with severe mental illness who are angry

Paul Rogers and Andrew Vidgen

KEY ISSUES

- Working with people who have a serious mental illness and who are angry
- Anger research and conceptualisation
- The relationship between anger and aggression
- The relationship between anger and serious mental illness
- The principles of working with such clients
- A pragmatic approach to the assessment and intervention of clients with anger and serious mental illness
- Strategies that will assist in the formulation of such clients' problems
- Intervention strategies for such clients

INTRODUCTION

This chapter examines the attitudes and skills required to help people with a severe mental illness who have anger problems. Because of the lack of research in this area, we will provide a text based on the limited available evidence, common sense and pragmatic ways of working *with* as opposed to working *against* people who are angry. In doing so, we will hopefully challenge some of the existing professional rhetoric and traditional practices used either with or against people who are angry.

Underpinning this chapter will be a cognitive–behavioural approach. A recent systematic review with meta-analysis of 50 studies incorporating 1640 subjects found that cognitive–behavioural therapy approaches are clinically effective in reducing anger and that the participants were relatively homogeneous across studies (Beck & Fernandez 1998). Anger is a common emotion, which we all experience frequently, and one that people have reported experiencing several times a week (Averill 1983). Ekman (1972) found that anger is one of the six emotions with identifiable facial expressions across cultures. Furthermore, historically, the power of anger is well documented (see Kemp & Strongman 1995), and well known: 'The Lord is full of compassion and mercy: long-suffering, and of great goodness. He will not always be chiding: neither keep his anger for ever' (Psalm 103, v. 8). Yet, despite early recognition of the power of anger and its long textual history (Kemp & Strongman 1995), it remains one the most understudied of human emotions (DiGiuseppe et al 1994). Furthermore, Deffenbacher (1996) notes that diagnostically 'there is no group of disorders for which anger is the primary defining characteristic (i.e. necessary for a diagnosis), even though there are well defined groups of anxiety and depressive disorders'. A number of authoritative researchers into anger have repeatedly called for a new 'anger disorder' to be included in the Diagnostic and Statistical Manual (Novaco 1985, DiGiuseppe et al 1994, Deffenbacher 1996); however, to date this has not happened.

Definitional difficulties compound the study of anger. While we all know what anger means, the definition is fraught with difficulties and to date no consensus of agreement exists (Russel & Fehr 1994). However, do we really know what anger actually means as suggested by Russel and Fehr? We all know what anger means for us and how it makes us feel, but can we really lay claim to knowing what anger means for others? Undoubtedly, we have all at one time or another observed, or been on 'the receiving end' of, another person's anger that we have felt was unjust or unwarranted. Likewise, we may have therefore concluded that the angry person must be ill-informed, jumping to conclusions or unreasonable. Alternatively, we have probably also found ourselves agreeing with another person's reasons for being angry and their perceptions of injustice. Whichever of the above conclusions we draw, we are making judgements as to the validity of another person's 'right' to experience anger.

However, as mental health professionals we are often informed (through implication or training) to be non-judgemental, as judgements are inherently wrong. But 'being judgemental' is a common experience for us all. If we do not make a judgement about another person's right to experience and demonstrate anger, then how are we to respond? There are a number of clichés which have become common-place in mental health texts and practice. For example, when attempting to care for another person who is demonstrating their anger, the following non-judgemental responses are common: 'You're obviously quite outraged at what's happened to you' or 'I can see that you're feeling very angry right now'. These statements demonstrate that you acknowledge the person's anger but then what? Where do we go next? And how do we get there?

Furthermore, the above response statements are probably not that useful if something that you have done is the 'source' of the other person's anger. For example, imagine that someone at work tells you that a trusted colleague and friend has broken a close confidence, one that you didn't want others to know. On hearing that they have told other people, you would probably feel angry. Thereafter, you confront your friend and ask them how they could break your confidence. You're feeling betrayed and you expect an apology, a commitment to stop disclosing and an explanation as to why they have done this to you. However, if the response you receive is 'I recognise that you're feeling angry', then you are probably going to feel even more annoyed.

Making judgements is not in itself something that should be avoided; however, if you allow these judgements to affect your attitudes about another person and your consequent behaviour then you may have difficulties working with angry clients. It is all right to believe that an *action* is wrong, e.g. stealing or punching someone. But you should resist making generalisations about the *person* because of their behaviour – they are a thief, they are assaultive – as these are not helpful. Asking yourself questions about the behaviour is more useful: What function does stealing and punching serve? What were the circumstances at the time? What was the person thinking at the time? Sometimes as mental health practitioners we need to make judgements, we need to have a view as to the validity of another person's claim of being treated unfairly, or of being frustrated because of our own actions.

WHAT IS ANGER?

Definitions of anger are numerous and there is little consensus on one single definition. Nonetheless, many definitions share a number of components in common. For example, Kassinove & Sukhodolsky (1995) provide the following definition: 'a negative, phenomenological (or internal) feeling state associated with specific cognitive and perceptual distortions and deficiencies (e.g. misappraisals, errors, and attribution of blame, injustice, preventability, and or intentionality), subjective labelling, physiological changes and action tendencies to engage in socially constructed and reinforced organised behavioural scripts' (Kassinove & Sukhodolsky 1995, p. 7). The main theme underlying most definitions of anger is that it is an emotional state that consists of cognitions, behaviours and physiological arousal. A number of descriptive models of anger exist; however, the work of Novaco (1975, 1976, 1979, 1985) is probably the best known.

Novaco's model

Novaco proposes anger as a dyscontrol phenomenon made up from three loosely related components when activated by an aversive event or environmental stressor (Box 15.1).

This model proposes that anger is influenced by thoughts that are related to behaviours. Thereafter, faulty appraisals of the triggering behaviour and our own future expectations will determine the presence and strength of anger. Anger is viewed as one response to the demands of the environment (stress), and continual exposure to these without coping skills will induce physiological reactions. These reactions then affect psychological and physical well being.

Interventions based on this model aim to provide the client with the necessary coping skills in adapting to and managing stress and is based upon the treatment called stress inoculation training (Meichenbaum 1975). The first goal is to assist the client to develop the necessary coping skills to deal with stress and then expose the client to graduated levels of triggering stressors in order that they can practise their new skills. As with all cognitive behavioural treatments, it is a collaborative process between the client and the therapist.

Anger and aggression

As mentioned previously, definitions in the area of anger are fraught with difficulty. The same problem occurs for definitions of aggression. Nonetheless, it is important to realise the differences between different terms. Friedman & Booth-Kewley (1987) provide some clarification: anger is an immediate emotional arousal, hostility is a more enduring negative attitude and aggression is the actual act of or intention of harming another. We can be angry without becoming aggressive and we can also be aggressive without being angry (e.g. during war). Averill (1983) reported on the responses of 160 subjects when angry, with direct physical aggression or punishment occurring in only 10%

Box 15.1 Components of Novaco's model

◆ **Physiological arousal:** Activation in the cardiovascular and endocrine systems causing somatic tension and irritability

◆ **Cognitive structures and processes:** Antagonistic thought patterns such as attention focus, suspicion ruminations and hostile attitude

◆ **Behaviour reactions** such as impulsive reactions, verbal aggression, physical confrontation and indirect expression of the subjects as a result of anger. Furthermore, DiGiuseppe et al (1994), when reporting on their clinical experience of aggressive and angry clients, noted that only '2–5% of clients' angry episodes co-occur with aggressive behaviour'. Thus, it can be suggested that the vast majority of people maintain and use coping strategies in relation to anger and behavioural control.

Thus, anger and aggression are not the same but an association between anger and aggression does exist. This inferred relationship has consequences. Novaco (1979) notes that 'the association between anger and aggression engenders the belief that anger is negative or harmful because it is expected to result in harmdoing'. The problem of violence and aggression are all too real for all healthcare practitioners in today's services and the importance of having meaningful policies, training and support cannot be understated. However, too often the single focus of mental health practitioners is on either the prevention or physical control and management of the aggressive incident and the violent client (Lion & Reid 1983, Vousden 1987, Thorpe & Olsen 1990, Bjorn 1991, Cahill et al 1991, Carton & Larkin 1991, Visalli et al 1997). Little if no attention is paid to helping clients who are angry to develop new methods of managing their anger, especially those who also have a serious mental illness. While we do not mean to criticise individual mental health practitioners who are regularly involved in the day-to-day management of some very assaultive clients, we do believe that there is a lack of education, training and research formulating the problems faced by the violent client from a number of perspectives, one of which is anger.

ANGER AND SEVERE MENTAL ILLNESS

While it is recognised that anger problems can co-occur with other mental health disorders, post traumatic stress disorder being the best known (Gerlock 1994, Reilly et al 1994, Chemtob et al 1997a, b). The relationship between anger and severe mental illness has largely been ignored, with only a handful of publications on anger and severe mental illness available. A recent study examining the effectiveness of the anger control programme in reducing anger expression specifically in patients with schizophrenia found positive changes in anger expression and anger control for those patients in the anger control programme (Chan et al 2003). Additionally, some single case studies and discussions of anger and severe mental illness are available (Rogers & Gronow 1997, Rogers & Gournay 2001). For clients who have a serious mental illness, the impact that their illness has on their day-to-day lives is a potential trigger for anger. Potential areas where a client's experiences can cause anger include the following.

Symptoms

Auditory hallucinations/voice hearing, specifically, the often unpredictable nature of voices, i.e. their content, meaning, frequency, volume and duration, can cause anger. Even the most patient of us can become highly irritable when we are being constantly interrupted or are fearful that someone is making us look stupid by deliberately trying to annoy us.

Belief systems and their meaning can also cause anger. Delusional beliefs, while often fantastical to others, are held by some with great conviction of their validity and meaningfulness. Our beliefs are very personal areas of our lives, whether they are religious, political or moral. Ridicule of our beliefs or observing external events that are not congruent with such beliefs can trigger a range of emotions, not least anger.

The impact of symptoms on lifestyle

The impact of symptoms on a client's lifestyle has been well documented (see Chapter 4). However, the emotional effect of such impact has been less recognised. If clients are to face a life of impaired employment, poor finances, poor housing, etc., then there will be times when they feel frustrated, victimised through prejudice, irritated by slow progress and aggrieved due to the loss of autonomy and freedom of choice.

Being a patient and 'the psychiatric system'

The negative effects of being a 'patient' in the psychiatric system are well recognised, with issues such a disempowerment, lack of autonomy and loss of control all regular features. Furthermore, the strategies of control that can be used by 'the psychiatric system' – seclusion, restraint, sections, enforced aftercare, enforced medication, and so on – can have a significant impact on a client. These control strategies can affect clients' anger considerably.

PRINCIPLES OF HELPING PEOPLE WITH SEVERE MENTAL ILLNESS AND ANGER

In working with clients who have severe mental illness and anger, a number of guiding principles are required, without which the chances of a client continuing to work in collaboration are small.

Engagement: The need for collaboration and negotiation throughout cannot be emphasised enough. All work is based upon partnership and exploration of difficulties and potential solutions.

Flexibility: Throughout your work you must remain flexible. The assessment may throw up something important that has not been identified before, or the client's goal may change from week to week. Flexibility will assist in fully meeting the needs of the client.

Problem identification: All work must be based on accurate problem identification. The success of any intervention relies on its appropriateness to the problem identified. Therefore, unless you have the 'right' problem, your intervention may be delivered perfectly but may change nothing.

Goal focused: All work must be directed towards predetermined and agreed goals. These goals must be the client's and not yours. Goal-focused interventions involve the agreement of a long-term goal so that the client will know that, once this is achieved, their work has been completed. Furthermore, weekly goals will be agreed as homework, which will assist the client to gradually build towards the long-term goal.

Pragmatism: The focus of any work is based on pragmatism as opposed to the application of cognitive or learning theories. What matters is what works for the individual client.

Homework: All work will inevitably involve homework tasks that the client and you will have agreed in session. The hourly session focuses on looking at ways of solving the agreed problem and then deciding on what is the best way for the client to practise these in real-life situations.

Regular evaluation: The two main principles that underlie any successful therapy are that the problem assessment is accurate and that the interventions used are appropriate to the identified problem. However, even the most experienced therapists will sometimes make a mistake. Regular evaluation (e.g. every 4 weeks) will ensure that if the problem is not changing this is detected early. Thereafter, you can either re-assess the problem or implement an alternative intervention. It is important to note that everyone can make mistakes in the above two areas and regular evaluation guards against this. For example, without regular evaluation, you may be 6 months into a treatment plan only to find that the client is making little or no progress towards their identified goals.

Case management: When involved with clients who have anger problems, effective communication and multidisciplinary working are essential to enlist the support of other key professionals and, if appropriate, carers in order to aid accurate risk assessment and management.

Short-term: All therapeutic work should be short-term (less than 20 sessions). By the end of this time you will know whether your interventions are assisting the client. Often, therapy does not aim to treat the client from start to finish but instead to provide the client with new skills or approaches to situations that they can then practise and incorporate into their daily lives. It will often take a long time after therapy has ceased before these skills become routine for clients.

Engagement

The issue of engaging clients is the crux of all successful interventions with clients who are angry and have a severe mental illness. Unless you can develop a collaborative relationship that aims to work towards the client's goals, you will have little success. It is possible to work with clients who are angry without their cooperation; however, this work will be carried out on them as opposed to with them. Furthermore, working on clients' anger usually

---

Box 15.2 Engagement issues

◆ **Develop a collaborative relationship**: Be aware that, unlike with other clinical disorders, most clients do not feel that anger is their main problem.

◆ **Agree that a problem exists**: Try and identify and agree the correct one.

◆ **Agree the goals of the treatment**

Box 15.3 Positive attitudes/beliefs required

◆ **Normalisation**: Anger is a common emotion; it affects us all. Internal and external triggers cannot be assumed for any one person and its effects can be both positive and negative.

◆ **Coping**: Anger is powerful – it controls, frightens and intimidates. Giving this up can be threatening, especially if it is the person's main coping strategy.

◆ **Ability to change**: Motivation to work on problems fluctuates within us. People with anger problems are no different. Just because they may not want to change this week does not mean that they won't be interested next week.

◆ **Self-management**: Recognise that working with such clients can cause us a number of emotions, including anger, frustration, exasperation and annoyance. Clinical supervision specifically negotiated to discuss, manage and use these emotions positively is invaluable (see Case study – Mike).

◆ **Expectations**: You both may have a number of expectations about your relationship, the work you hope to do, when benefits will occur, and so on. These expectations may interfere with engagement and it is useful to discuss these at the beginning of any interventions and at regular intervals.

involves behavioural management, which will not generalise as well as treatment aimed at reducing the underlying problem. The main obstacle to overcome when engaging such clients is that often, unlike with other clinical disorders (e.g. phobias, depression, obsessive-compulsive disorder and post-traumatic stress disorder), they do not feel that their anger is a problem.

All too often clients will not engage because of a problem in one of the three areas identified in Box 15.2. To aid the engagement process, a number of positive attitudes/beliefs are required, as identified in Box 15.3.

Case study – losing Mike

When one of us (PR) was training as a nurse behaviour psychotherapist, the first client assessed with an anger problem was a 32-year-old male taxi driver (Mike), who was motivated to work on one area of his anger but not on another. Mike's anger affected him in two areas: at home, causing him to commit a number of assaults on his wife, and at work, causing him arguments with, but not assaults, on work colleagues. When discussing the goals of treatment Mike was very clear that he only wanted help to deal with his anger at work and refused to work on his aggression towards his wife. The therapist could not understand Mike's reluctance to work on his problems at home and, after 30 minutes of both parties disputing and disagreeing about what the focus of the work should be, Mike stopped the interview, stating 'It's my problem, not yours', and left.

Based on feedback at clinical supervision at the time and the benefit of hindsight some years later, it is clear that the therapist's insistence that Mike work on both areas was a major barrier to engagement. The therapist was attempting to get the client to agree the therapist's goals for treatment.

The case of Mike highlights a number of important areas. The therapist's insistence that Mike worked on his assaultiveness towards his wife led to him refusing treatment. Because he refused treatment, it is likely that Mike's aggressive behaviour continued. If the therapist had worked on the main problem as Mike saw it, he might have been more willing to work on his assaultiveness towards his wife some time in the future. Also, the skills that Mike would have learned through working on his main problems might have generalised across to the context of assaulting his wife. While these latter points are hypothetical, they highlight some of the issues involved when there is disagreement between therapist and client on the goals of intervention.

Case study – engaging with John

John was a 24-year-old man who was detained in a medium-security unit with a diagnosis of paranoid psychosis. He had intermittent bouts of anger, which were followed by physical aggression on approximately 50% of occasions. He was referred by his clinical team for anger management. On assessment, John denied that he had any problems with anger and insisted that his actions were justified. John was asked if he would be happy to discuss the circumstances surrounding the referral as there appeared to be a disagreement between John's and his clinical team's views of his problems. John agreed to this. On assessment, John explained that he became angry and violent because he was being given medication against his will. He did not believe that he was mentally ill and believed that his voices came from a benevolent spirit who was telling John whom he could and could not trust.

It appeared that John's violence was linked to his symptoms and to issues involving his detention and being medicated against his will. To offer him anger management would therefore have been inappropriate. However, the problem causing his anger and violence could be targeted for further work. This was that the clinical team and John had not come to an agreement about his difficulties, treatment and management. John did not have a clear understanding of these areas. However, he was ready to accept that this lack of collaboration between the two parties was a trigger for his anger and violence.

Initially, John said that his goal was to be let out and not to have to take medication. While this was important to John, it was unfeasible that this could be guaranteed, as such a decision was beyond the control of both parties. After negotiation his goal was restated as 'To live in the community, and fully engage with my aftercare arrangements, which both the clinical team and I will have negotiated, recorded and agreed prior to my discharge'.

Assessment

The process of assessment of anger in people with severe mental illness is of paramount importance, as any intervention will only be as good as the data it is based upon. The assessment process has five key structures: preparation, anger assessment, assessment of SMI, personal history and current circumstances.

1. Preparation

Prior to beginning any assessment, you will need to fully prepare. The aim of preparation is to identify the areas where you may need to particularly focus on and to plan the goals of the assessment (see Chapter 8). Preparation includes:

◆ a full review of the information already available
◆ discussion with significant others (care workers and where possible family and carers)

◆ identifying any issues which may affect engagement prior to the interview and planning strategies of how you can overcome these.

2. Anger assessment

The assessment process will usually take between two and four sessions but can vary depending on the client. The focus of assessment is to identify those domains of anger that are 'current'. For the purposes of treatment the anger must be current and predictable. Current means that the problem is currently affecting the client's lifestyle. Predictable means that triggers for anger can be identified across aspects of time, situations and social interactions. Specific areas to focus on when assessing anger are:

Behavioural What is the client's main problem? Where does the anger happen more or less? With whom does the anger occur or is lessened? What is the frequency of anger (hourly? daily? weekly?), intensity on a 0–8 scale (0 = calm, 8 = rage), and duration of anger?

Behavioural excesses can be identified through asking clients what things they do 'more of' when they are angry. These might include: verbal expressions of anger (shouting, screaming, swearing); physical expressions (smashing things, hitting out, throwing things); or cognitive events (plotting revenge or planning a future interaction that may involve violence).

Behavioural avoidances can be identified by asking clients what things they avoid because of their anger. These might include prior avoidances (having arguments, certain people, certain places) as they are likely to trigger anger. They may also include post avoidances (talking to the person they are angry with, being in the same place as the person), which occur after the angry event. By identifying behavioural excesses and deficits you will be able to identify how the person responds when angry and what strategies they use to cope.

Cognitive Once these behavioural triggers have been identified, you can then use them to identify the cognitions that are problematic. Take the triggers and ask the client what they think about when these occur. By exploring the client's explanations you will be able to identify what the cognitive triggers might be (e.g. 'The last time this happened to you, what were you thinking at the time?').

In the case study of Joe, such explanations give an idea of which of Joe's thoughts are affecting his anger. The first indicates that Joe does not like injections, but this by itself is meaningless. What helped was asking Joe which areas of having an injection he disliked the most and which areas he was least bothered about. Some clients dislike needles, some dislike the side effects of injections, while others always refuse injections requiring physical restraint. Such reasons are understandable and require validating first and foremost.

Any attempt at challenging these cognitions will result in alienation as opposed to collaboration. Joe said that his rights were being violated and that the chemicals were poisonous. He also said that he was no longer in control of his life.

Case study – Joe

Joe's anger was behaviourally triggered more when in hospital than when living in the community. This information provided an indication that Joe had angry thoughts about being in hospital. When asked 'Why do you feel your anger is worse in hospital?', Joe responded with a number of reasons:

1. *'I hate injections.'*
2. *'There is nothing wrong with me.'*
3. *'I'm unable to do the things that I want to, when I want to.'*

Autonomic　The physiology of anger affects different people in different ways. Interestingly, there are a number of sayings that describe the physiology of anger – 'It made my blood boil', 'I was fuming', 'He's a hot-head', 'He's hot under the collar' and 'He's letting off steam' are all indications of the physiology of anger and its relationship with the cardiovascular system. Other sayings, such as 'I was really wound up' and 'He's ready to explode' are indications of somatic tension. Asking clients what happens to their body when they are angry will give an indication of the individual's autonomic symptoms. You should then ask the client what is the first physical sign that they notice when they are angry, as this can be used to help them later to detect anger early on (early anger signs monitoring).

Functional analysis　The ABC analysis (as described in Chapter 9) is of paramount importance when assessing anger. It allows you to conceptualise how the previously assessed areas interrelate and affect each other and provides you with an indication as to the person's patterns of anger. Furthermore, it should tell you whether your assessment to date has included all the relevant areas brought up in the functional analysis. It is important to conduct an ABC analysis on as many anger episodes as possible. This will ensure that you don't just focus on one area of a client's anger as there may be more than one trigger, behaviour and consequence.

3. SMI assessment

The assessment of severe mental illness is described in Chapter 8. In relation to anger and severe mental illness, however, a number of specific areas will require further assessment.

The client's view of their problems   Issues such as the client's agreement or disagreement about whether they have mental health problems and whether they need treatment are crucial in the assessment. The authors have found that those clients who feel that there is nothing wrong with them and who do not want treatment are much more likely to become angry and assaultive. Such clients will often view the actions of mental health professionals as unwarranted and as an intrusion into their lives.

Symptoms   Do the client's symptoms of severe mental illness ever cause them anger? If so, which symptoms? In assessing any relationship between voices and anger, you will need to examine what the voices are saying and who the client believes the voices belong to, the reason why the voices are talking to the client and the client's engagement with the voices – does the client resist them or want them? Do the voices talk about others, or their intentions? Do they annoy the client? Do they make the client irritable? Do they distract the client?

In assessing beliefs, you will need to examine whether the client has delusional beliefs that may make them more prone to feeling anger. For example, clients who are paranoid that others are out to hurt them may be more prone to feeling angry with their perceived tormentors. It is also useful to examine whether clients discuss their beliefs with others, and the responses that they have had. Sometimes the belittling of a client's belief may make them angry. Furthermore, if a client believes 100% that they are about to be murdered in their sleep and others dismiss this, then they will obviously be frightened and possibly feel angry and therefore want to either hit out or get out, even if this means escaping from a secure unit.

Once these areas have been assessed, it is useful to conduct a further functional (ABC) analysis on the relationship between the client's anger and their mental illness. Again, as many examples as possible will aid you in understanding this relationship and any particular patterns that are unique to the individual.

4. Personal history

The assessment of personal history is described in Chapter 8. The main areas to explore when assessing a client's personal history are the client's exposure to anger or violence throughout their lives (social learning) and the positive and negative impact of anger on their lives – has their anger caused them major problems (police contact, court appearances, loss of freedom)?

5. Current circumstances

Obtaining the client's view of current circumstances helps to identify what life stressors may be contributing to the anger. Difficulties with finance, housing, neighbours, family members or employment may be causing the client excessive stress. Stress has a significant relationship with anger, as described by Novaco (1979), and the client may be finding that, while they can normally cope with their symptoms of SMI, extra stressors are too much to cope with and they become more angry.

Assessment measures

It is important to stress that the measures used should always be an aid to assessment and not the priority or a replacement. Furthermore, the indiscriminate use of measures without consideration of the client's abilities can sometimes adversely affect engagement. Therefore the measures should not be exhaustive or exhausting. Measures that are useful include:

- ◆ Problem and Target Ratings (Marks et al 1986)
- ◆ Work and Social Adjustment Ratings (Marks et al 1986)
- ◆ Reaction to Provocation (Novaco 1990)
- ◆ Beck Depression Inventory (Beck et al 1961)
- ◆ General Health Questionnaire – 28 (Goldberg 1972, Goldberg & Williams 1988)
- ◆ Cognitive Assessment of Voices: Interview Schedule (Chadwick & Birchwood 1994)
- ◆ Beliefs About Voices Questionnaire (Chadwick & Birchwood 1995)
- ◆ State–Trait Anger Inventory-2 (Spielberger 1999).

Formulation

Once you have conducted the above assessments the next stage is to formulate the maintaining factors for the client's anger problems. The formulation exercise is usually best completed as a separate session and sometimes may take two or three sessions to complete fully. During the formulation, a number of possible variations of relationships may arise.

In assisting the formulation stage, a 'relationship chart' is a useful exercise to follow (Fig. 15.1). The purpose of this exercise is to establish how the client's anger relates to the other variables assessed. By simply placing anger in the middle of the other variables, you can then decide which of the others are related to the anger and draw links between them as appropriate.

Once this has been completed you can then map out any anger patterns that have been identified (Fig. 15.2).

This process of formulation should be conducted with the client; together, you can begin to examine these relationships more closely. The more frequently you practise this exercise with clients the easier and more sophisticated it will become. It is often helpful for clients if they are given a copy of the formula-

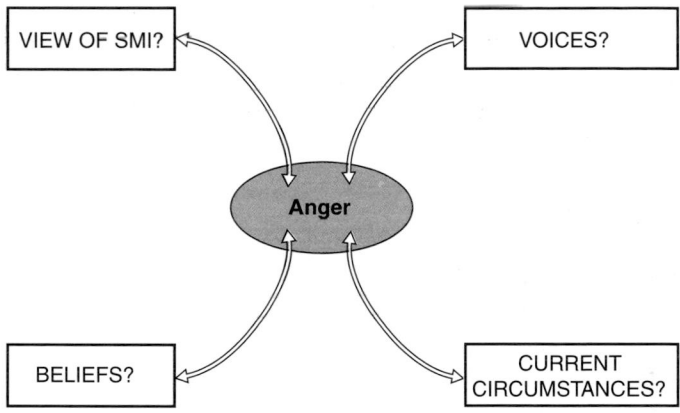

Figure 15.1   Example of relationship chart.

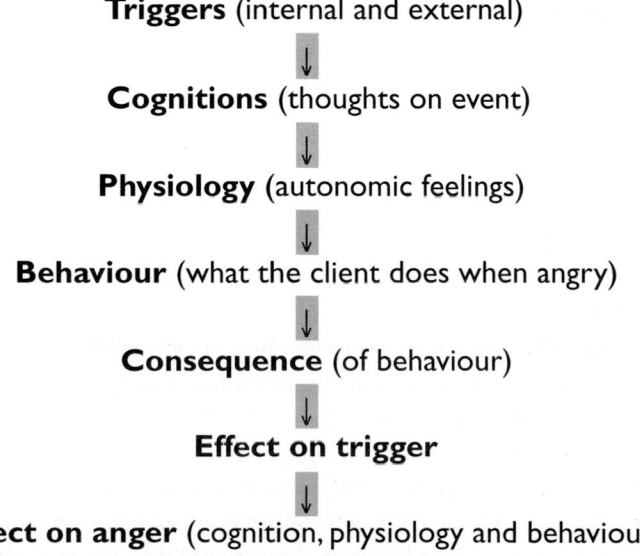

Figure 15.2   An anger map.

tion exercise to take away, either to look at further or to work on further if they wish to. This process of collaboratively looking at potential links can assist the engagement process and the focus of therapeutic work. Once the formulation exercise has been completed and agreed by both parties, the next step is to agree the problems and goals, as described in Chapter 9.

Interventions

So far we have engaged, assessed and formulated with our clients. The intervention(s) chosen will depend on the assessment and formulation. The application of the right intervention in the right place will greatly enhance the efficacy of the total treatment.

Self-monitoring

The first stage of most anger treatments involves varying degrees of self-monitoring. Self-monitoring aims to assist clients to assimilate their actual anger experiences into the formulation framework. A number of strategies are available to aid self-monitoring, the most common being the anger diary (Fig. 15.3). However, we have sometimes had to alter the method of self-monitoring. For clients who have difficulties with reading or writing, we have successfully employed a Dictaphone and then during sessions have used the Dictaphone record to elicit the details outlined in the homework diary.

When asking clients to record diaries, it is important to encourage them to fill out the details as soon as practically possible so that they don't forget. The anger diaries can then be used to further refine the formulation process and develop a collaborative treatment plan based on the themes that emerge. Intervention can involve a number of different treatment strategies that aim to break the cycle between behaviour, physiology and cognitions at varying levels. The crux of these interventions is that they are all solution-focused, practical and encourage the client to take active responsibility for carrying out their own treatment, thus encouraging self-efficacy and minimising dependence on the therapist.

Physiological strategies

Relaxation strategies aim to reduce the physiological component of anger and therefore have a knock-on effect on the client's cognitions and behavioural responses. Deffenbacher (1996) provides an excellent review of the evidence to date on relaxation strategies for anger. Deffenbacher suggests that 'the adaptation of anxiety management training be adopted in most cases. It is the most empirically supported relaxation strategy, and detailed procedure descriptions are available'. Deffenbacher references two such descriptions: Suinn

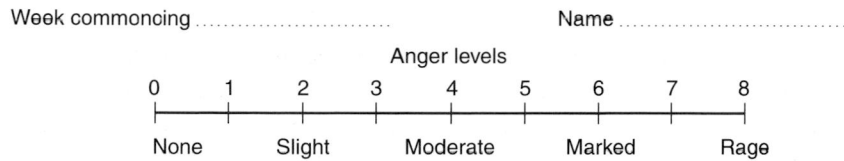

When		Trigger	Anger levels (0–8)			Thoughts	Behaviour	Outcomes
Date	Time and duration	What happened	Before	During	After	What were you thinking? Before? During? After?	What did you do? Before? During? After?	What were the positive benefits? What were the negatives?

Figure 15.3   An anger diary.

1990 and Suinn & Deffenbacher 1988. The process of applied relaxation will not be described in this text, as many descriptions are available. However, we have found that relaxation can be an effective and powerful method of engaging clients with the therapeutic process prior to moving on to some of the more challenging work (cognitive interventions) and if clients achieve some success in this stage their belief in the credibility of subsequent therapy can be enhanced.

Behavioural strategies

'Pre-anger' strategies   These focus on identifying anger cues/triggers and then developing strategies with the client as to how these cues can be avoided or better managed. This can often be helpful for clients who feel 'out of control' or whose lack of control is potentially about to cause significant problems in terms of offending. In our clinical experience, we have found that the greater the range of avoidance strategies the client has to hand, the more they can choose methods to suit themselves. For example, one client who had a strong and overwhelming anger towards an employer was fearful that in his rage he would seek out his employer and assault him. The client was frightened that he would not be able to control his anger once started, so agreed to attend his local police station as a last resort should all other strategies fail. This was never actually required, but it did give the client a sense of relief to know that he had this option of external control in case the self-control strategies proved ineffective, and meant he did not have to view his self-control strategies as 'all or nothing'.

'Current' anger strategies   These involve identifying behavioural methods that the client can use once their anger has been activated. These are more successful if the strategies are tailored to the individual, and may include:

◆ once angry, immediately leaving the scene and retiring to a place where the client can calm down without interruption
◆ interrupting the anger response by identifying an alternative behaviour that 'competes' with the usual anger response.

The client should generate these strategies wherever possible. One extreme but highly effective strategy that we used for one client who was becoming increasingly difficult to manage was 'undressing when in his room'. This client, with severe mental illness, was an inpatient in an intensive care unit within a medium-secure unit, suffering from post traumatic stress disorder after being raped in prison. Every time he had flashbacks he became immediately aroused and tended to smash up the ward, and had once assaulted a member of staff who had attempted to intervene. After this event he felt very guilty and wanted an immediate strategy to stop him assaulting staff again. He identified that if he were not fully clothed then he would not be able to come out of his room, and set his homework as going to his room and stripping off some of his clothes as soon as he identified the first signs that he was becoming angry.

Assertion training   In some cases, clients' anger may be directly related to an inability to assert themselves with other people who have transgressed against them (Frederiksen et al 1976, Deffenbacher et al 1987, Rogers & Gronow 1997). Consequently, they find that their anger continues after the transgression and that they ruminate about it for long periods thereafter. We have found that assertion training or social skills training early on in therapy can have excellent results and as well as improving the client's behaviour also improves their self-esteem and motivation to continue.

Cognitive strategies

Since the development of cognitive techniques, the issue of how a person's thoughts can lead to anger and strategies to change these have been greatly developed. It is beyond the scope of this chapter to present the full range of cognitive strategies available, as many will require training and practice under good supervision. However, the general principles are as follows.

Identifying cognitions   Following assessment and through the use of the anger diaries, it is possible to identify which cognitions may be linked to anger. Also, this process of self-monitoring can help the therapist to assist the client in examining internal relationships to anger as opposed to purely external events. Novaco (1979) identifies two types of cognitive process that are related to angry cognitions: appraisals and expectations:

Appraisals: The way we appraise a situation greatly affects our responses, and differs significantly between individuals. For example, a senior manager mentions to two staff that he likes their ties. One readily accepts the compliment, while the other becomes annoyed and irritated, believing it to be a reference to the fact that he was not wearing a tie the day before. Thus, appraisals are the meanings that we attribute to events. Furthermore, they usually have a historical connection to previous events or meanings.

Expectations: Our expectations can often be a cause for anger. If we expect that something will happen or will be done in a certain manner, and later find that it isn't, we can become angry. However, we may blame the other person for something not happening when in fact it was our expectation that was the problem. For example, if two clients attend their GP's surgery without making an appointment, one may expect a delay while the other may expect to be seen immediately. The person expecting to be seen immediately is likely to become more irate at having to wait.

Interventions – special considerations

We would like to urge caution against attempting to challenge a client's faulty appraisals or expectations immediately. As in all cognitive behavioural therapy, the process of examining thoughts is a collaborative process, which both parties enter (Box 15.4). Sometimes, professionals suggest that they are using cognitive therapy when in fact they have assumed that they have identified a 'problem cognition' and thereafter 'go straight in' and attempt to challenge it in a confrontative manner.

The process of cognitive interventions for misappraisals and false expectations requires that these are first identified and the client's anger experience validated as upsetting and difficult. Through a style of treating the anger experience as an event to be explored in terms of what happened, and even

> **Box 15.4** Challenging cognitions – some cautions
>
> ◆ 'Problem cognitions' – don't jump straight in with identifying and pointing out faulty cognitions. Examine the thoughts collaboratively.
> ◆ Don't challenge faulty assumptions immediately. Looking at the evidence for appraisals or reasonableness of expectations may be counterproductive at this early stage. Map out the relationships between thoughts, affect and behaviour.
> ◆ Don't expect clients to see relationships immediately. It is more beneficial to assist the person to identify and examine his or her own cognitions.

mapping out on paper visually, you can assist clients to come to their own conclusions and decisions. Questions like 'What's the evidence for and against?' should be avoided and replaced by 'Let's map out what happened and then we can look at all the events more closely'. This process of 'mapping out' is useful in getting clients to think about and record their internal thoughts in relation to external events. Further questions that encourage clients to investigate what things influenced the anger event may help them to examine their own cognitions.

Do not expect a client always to be able to see the relationship immediately. However, after this exercise has been completed a few times and across different settings, clients may be more able to identify that the factor that remains constant is their expectations or appraisals, as opposed to the event, the other person, the time of day, and so on. Once this has been achieved then cognitive techniques can be easily incorporated into treatment.

CONCLUSION

In this chapter, we have examined the assessment, engagement and treatment of clients with severe mental illness who are angry. These clients can often be the most difficult to engage and the most frustrating to work with, and have the potential for many difficult and complex problems along the way. However, they can also be highly rewarding and, as time and therapy progress, the relationship and the understanding of each other's positions can greatly improve. Often, these clients are the most unattractive to work with for a multitude of reasons and your colleagues may at times suggest that they are unable to change. We have frequently come across such problems and believe that the way forward is to try and get colleagues 'on side' by helping them to understand the client better and by focusing on the potential benefits and the 'what ifs'.

This chapter gives only a brief outline of the stages involved but does offer a firm starting point. We strongly advocate that anyone working with such clients, whether 'novice' or 'expert', ensures that they have a suitable clinical supervisor at all times.

References

Averill J R 1983 Studies on anger and aggression: implications for theories of emotion. American Psychologist 38:1145–1160

Beck A T, Ward C M, Mendelson M et al 1961 An inventory for measuring depression. Archives of General Psychiatry 4:561–571

Beck R, Fernandez E 1998 Cognitive-behavioral therapy in the treatment of anger: a meta-analysis. Cognitive Therapy and Research 22:63–74

Bjorn P R 1991 An approach to the potentially violent patient. Journal of Emergency Nursing 17:336–338

Cahill C D, Stuart G W, Laraia M T, Arana G W 1991 Inpatient management of violent behaviour: nursing prevention and intervention. Issues in Mental Health Nursing 12:239–252

Carton G, Larkin E 1991 Reducing violence in a special hospital. Nursing Standard 5(17):29–31

Chadwick P, Birchwood M 1994 Cognitive assessment of voices: interview schedule. In: Chadwick P, Birchwood M, Trower P (eds) Cognitive therapy for delusions, voices and paranoia. Wiley, Chichester, pp 195–200

Chadwick P, Birchwood M 1995 The omnipotence of voices II: the Beliefs About Voices Questionnaire (BAVQ). British Journal of Psychiatry 166:733–776

Chan H Y, Lu R B, Tseng C L, Chous K R 2003 Effectiveness of the anger-control program in reducing anger expression in patients with schizophrenia. Archives of Psychiatric Nursing 17:88–95

Chemtob C M, Novaco R W, Hamada R S, Gross D M 1997a Cognitive-behavioural treatment for severe anger in post-traumatic stress disorder. Journal of Consulting and Clinical Psychology 65:184–189

Chemtob C M, Novaco R W, Hamada R S et al 1997b Anger regulation in combat related posttraumatic stress disorder. Journal of Traumatic Stress 10:17–36

Deffenbacher J 1996 Cognitive-behavioural approaches to anger reduction. In: Dobson K S, Craig K D (eds) Advances in cognitive-behavioural therapy. Sage, London, pp 31–62

Deffenbacher J, Story D A, Stark R S et al 1987 Cognitive-relaxation and social skills interventions in the treatment of general anger. Journal of Counselling Psychology 34:171–176

DiGiuseppe R, Tafrate R, Eckhardt C 1994 Critical issues in the treatment of anger. Cognitive and Behavioural Practice 1:111–132

Ekman P 1972 Darwin and facial expression: a century of research in review. Academic Press, New York

Frederiksen L W, Jenkins J O, Foy D W, Eisler R M 1976 Social skills training to modify abusive verbal outbursts in adults. Journal of Applied Behavioural Analysis 9:117–125

Friedman H S, Booth-Kewley S 1987 The 'disease-prone personality': a meta-analytical view of the construct. American Psychologist 42:539–555

Gerlock A A 1994 Veterans' responses to anger management intervention. Issues in Mental Health Nursing 15:393–408

References (cont'd)

Goldberg D P 1972 The detection of psychiatric illness by questionnaire. Oxford University Press, London

Goldberg D, Williams P 1988 A user's guide to the General Health Questionnaire. NFER-Nelson, Windsor

Kassinove H, Sukhodolsky D G 1995 Anger disorders: basic science and practice issues. In: Kassinove H (ed) Anger disorders: definition, diagnosis and treatment. Taylor & Francis, Washington DC, pp 1–26

Kemp S, Strongman K T 1995 Anger theory and management: a historical analysis. American Journal of Psychology 108:397–417

Lion J R, Reid W H 1983 Assaults within psychiatric facilities. Grune & Stratton, New York

Marks I M, Bird J, Brown M, Ghosh A 1986 Behavioural psychotherapy: Maudsley pocket book of clinical management. Wright, Bristol

Meichenbaum D 1975 A self-instructional approach to stress management: a proposal for stress inoculation training. In: Spielberger C, Sarason I (eds) Stress and anxiety, vol 2. Wiley, New York

Novaco R W 1975 Anger control. D C Heath, Lexington, MA

Novaco R W 1976 The function and regulation of the arousal of anger. American Journal of Psychiatry 133:1124–1128

Novaco R W 1979 The cognitive regulation of anger and stress. In: Kendall P, Hollon S D (eds) Cognitive-behavioural interventions: theory, research and practice. Academic Press, New York, pp 241–285

Novaco R W 1985 Anger and its therapeutic regulation. In: Chesney M A, Rosenman R H (eds) Anger and hostility in cardiovascular and behavioural disorders. Hemisphere, Washington DC, pp 31–84

Novaco R W 1990 Reactions to provocation (NAS). University of California, Irvine, CA

Reilly P M, Westley Clarke H, Shropshire M S et al 1994 Anger management: critical components of post traumatic stress disorder and substance abuse treatment. Journal of Psychoactive Drugs 26:401–407

Rogers P, Gournay K 2001 Nurse therapy in forensic mental health. In: Kettle A, Woods P (eds) Therapeutic interventions for forensic nursing. Jessica Kingsley, London

Rogers P, Gronow T 1997 Turn down the heat. Nursing Times 92(43):26–29

Russel J, Fehr B 1994 Fuzzy concepts in a fuzzy hierarchy: varieties of anger. Journal of Personality and Social Psychology 67:186–285

Spielberger C D 1999 State-trait anger expression inventory – 2 (STAXI-2) Psychological Assessment Resources, Lutz, FL

Suinn R M 1990 Anxiety management training. Plenum, New York

Suinn R M, Deffenbacher J L 1988 Anxiety management training. Counselling Psychologist 16:31–49

Thorpe G, Olsen S 1990 Behaviour therapy: concepts, procedures and applications. Allyn & Bacon, Boston

Visalli H, McNasser G, Johnstone L, Lazzaro C A 1997 Reducing high risk interventions for managing aggression in psychiatric settings. Journal of Nursing Care Quality 11:54–61

Vousden M 1987 Are you safe? Nursing Times 83(26):29–30

16

Working with people with serious mental illness at risk of offending

Andrew Vidgen and Paul Rogers

KEY ISSUES

- ◆ Clinical and legal issues arising out of working with this client group
- ◆ Assessment issues relating to individuals who have committed offences, using a broad cognitive–behavioural and functional analysis approach
- ◆ Intervention approaches covering a range of options aimed at reducing offending

INTRODUCTION

This chapter provides an overview of the relationship between mental health and offending behaviour. Its focus is on more serious offences and the interface between symptoms, psychological functioning and offending behaviour. In order to be understood, this chapter is divided into two parts: the first part examines conceptual and theoretical positions whereas the second examines more clinical issues, for example engagement, assessment and treatment.

PART I – CONCEPTUAL AND THEORETICAL VIEWPOINTS: OFFENDING BEHAVIOUR AND SMI

The main problem for those who wish to unravel the available evidence on offending behaviour and diagnosis is that the literature is fraught with definitional problems. This hampers the study of the relationship between people with serious mental illness (SMI) and offending behaviour and often makes comparison across studies difficult. The points below highlight this anomaly:

◆ Mental illness is not defined in the Mental Health Act (Department of Health 1983)
◆ No single definition of criminality exists (Feldman 1993)
◆ Research definitions, even when operationalised, vary across studies.

In addition, offending by people with SMI often leads to them being involved with at least two formal systems: criminal justice and mental health. This is important: to understand the relationship between SMI and criminality we *must* consider more than the causal relationship between them (Blackburn 1993). Their relationship is also influenced by social factors within and between the mental health and criminal justice systems. For example, historically, homosexuality has been considered to be both criminal and a symptom of mental illness (Herek 1994).

This complexity can extend from ideas about this relationship to actual provision and planning of services for both the population and the individual. Examples of this confusion can be shown in considering the following questions:

◆ Are persons with SMI who offend 'criminals' or not?
◆ Who makes this decision?
◆ How generalisable are such decisions?
◆ If care is needed, who should provide it and where?
◆ If the SMI is in remission, should the person move from a care to a custodial setting or back to the community?

Historical, social and high media profile responses have also undoubtedly influenced the view of politicians and providers of mental health policy. In addition, these have helped frame the general public's view of mentally ill people, which one could argue also has an influence on mental health policy decisions. The following are well known assumptions expressed with regard to people with SMI:

◆ They are dangerous and commit violent crimes (Ritchie 1994)
◆ They are unpredictable – a risk to themselves and others
◆ They are 'untreatable' – so why not just lock them up and throw away the key? (Hall et al 1993, Hiday 1995, Levey & Howells 1995).

Although these views would indicate that the stereotypical viewpoint has no difficulty linking SMI and offending, the exact nature of the relationship between 'mental disorder' (including serious mental health problems) and 'crime', especially violence, remains controversial (Monahan & Steadman 1983, Blackburn 1993, Monahan et al 1994). Studies that have attempted to examine the relationship have often been challenged as being methodologically flawed because of their reliance on hospital and prison populations (thus introducing selection biases, see Walsh et al 2002) and have invariably lacked suitable comparison and/or control groups (Wessely & Taylor 1991, Shah 1993, Taylor & Hodgins 1994, Hiday 1995, Brennan et al 2000, Walsh et al 2002, Taylor 2003).

Nevertheless, it has been argued that people with diagnoses of mental illness are more likely to commit offences compared with the general population and that a significant proportion of these crimes involve offences against others (Côté & Hodgins 1992, Mulvey 1994). However, it is important to acknowledge that people with serious psychiatric disorders may be statistically over-represented in committing more serious offences such as murder. For example, in the UK, psychiatric disorder has been implicated in approximately 30–40% of murders over the last century (Blackburn 1996). However, when examining the mental states of 600 English prisoners, Gunn et al (1978) found that rates of depression and anxiety were higher than rates of schizophrenia. Spry (1984), when reviewing occurrence rates of schizophrenia in offender populations, found an incidence of only 1%, which is comparable to that found in the general population. Other studies have indicated that if this association exists at all then the relationship is weak and dependent upon the nature of both the mental disorder and the criminal behaviour in question (Brennan et al 2000, Taylor 2003).

Although it could be argued that the vast majority of this group are no more likely than members of the general public to commit serious offences, it remains difficult to draw any firm conclusions, especially if consideration is given to the following factors, which introduce bias in the number of persons with SMI appearing in statistical analyses:

◆ **The Home Office (1990) circular 66/90, Provisions for Mentally Disordered Offenders**: advises that offenders with a recognisable mental disorder should be diverted *away* from the criminal justice system.
◆ **Police detection and arrest rates**: 'Compared with "mentally stable" offenders this group may "choose more difficult targets, plan an offence less carefully or carry it out less skilfully – all failings increase the risk of detection, arrest and official statistics". The police may arrest or charge a disturbed person more readily than others' (Feldman 1993).

These factors indicate that we should be very careful in our formulation of the relationship between SMI and offending as there are particular biases inherent in the system.

Working with this client group

When working with people with SMI and offending behaviour it is all too easy to assume a direct causal relationship between the person's mental state/ psychiatric diagnosis and the offending behaviour. That is, to assume that their mental disorder *caused* them to offend. In our experience, this is particularly so within specialised mental health secure facilities where some of the more extreme ends of the mental illness spectrum receive services (stereotypically this would include the paranoid schizophrenic who has committed a very serious offence against a member of their family or the general public). It should also be noted that the committing of offending behaviour or entry into the criminal justice system may be associated with the development of mental illness (Taylor 2003).

However, we need to assume that a large degree of variation exists between people's mental health and offending behaviour. When working with this client group a comprehensive and careful assessment is essential to ascertain the nature of people's mental health in relation to their offending history (and risk of committing future offences). Also, it is insufficient to treat an individual's psychiatric problems solely (with medication) without directly addressing offending behaviour and psychological functioning. It is useful to bear in mind that people commit offences for a variety of reasons, including for financial gain, when angry, when influenced by peer or group pressure, when under the influence of drugs and/or alcohol or as a result of behavioural responses to hearing voices or beliefs regarding the victim (some of which may be delusional). Furthermore, attention must be paid to previous offending and age (McCord 1990). Obtaining a person's full criminal history is particularly useful when predicting future risk areas. Focusing on a person's range of criminal activities will add to the validity of the assessment as well as providing a number of pointers for risk management. For example, someone's offending behaviour may be exacerbated by drug taking; by addressing specific offences such as violence there may be scope to intervene at the level of the substance misuse. A further point to bear in mind is that criminal behaviour is versatile. Indeed, 'those who steal and commit burglary are pretty much the same people who engage in violence, vandalism and drug abuse, who drink excessively, drive recklessly and commit sexual offences' (Stephenson 1992). Thus, as mental health workers we should not automatically assume that a causal relationship exists between clients' mental health problems and their offending behaviour but look also at the offending behaviour and its relationship with mental health functioning.

It is also important to recognise that people with psychotic disorders are not a comparable group. Diagnosis alone does not clarify why a particular individual has committed an offence. In addition, the variety of current symptoms that people experience – hallucinations and idiosyncratic patterns of thought – have traditionally been seen as increasing the risk of offending. Indeed, over the past decade, there has been an increased interest in the phenomenology of symptoms and how these relate to people's experiences and offending behaviour (Wessely et al 1993, Taylor & Hodgins 1994, Junginger 1995, Chadwick et al 1996, Johnson et al 1997, Rogers et al 2002). For example, Wessely et al (1993) found that approximately 50% of their inpatient sample ($n = 88$) had acted on delusional beliefs on at least one occasion; however, violent behaviour was uncommon. To examine further the relationship between type of delusion and subsequent behaviour, a subsample of this group (approximately 10%) was studied. The researchers found that delusions of catastrophe were significantly associated with aggression. Interestingly, no association was found in those people experiencing other types of delusion, including those of reference, religion, jealousy, persecution, grandiosity, guilt or with a sexual content. However, this demonstrates only that some delusions may facilitate certain behaviours, not that certain delusions are more likely to be acted upon. Attention also needs to be paid to the type of hallucination that the client experiences. It is a common, but mainly unsubstantiated, assumption that people experiencing command hallucinations are at risk of committing violent acts. Indeed, it has been found that the presence of auditory hallucinations per se is not associated with violence towards others (Bjorkly 2002, Rogers et al 2002).

The need to pay attention to the content of hallucinations in order to formulate the relationship between them and behaviour (including offending) has recently been noted (Chadwick et al 1996). This can be done in two ways: first, by referring to the events preceding a person's offence(s) and, second, by gaining an understanding of the types of situation where people experience hallucinations (e.g. voices), as well as their beliefs about voices and their behavioural responses to them. In our opinion, too much attention is paid to voices as triggers for behaviour. The importance of environmental and/or psychological triggers has been neglected. The advantage of paying attention to such antecedents of voice hearing is that it provides another level for possible intervention. The following case study helps to illustrate this point:

Case study – Joan

Joan, a 19-year-old woman, had threatened staff with a knife in the local supermarket. She was admitted to hospital for assessment under the Mental Health Act. Joan was given a preliminary diagnosis of paranoid schizophrenia, her primary symptoms being auditory hallucinations (a male voice telling her to get a knife) and paranoid beliefs regarding members of her family (that they were trying to poison her). Joan's risk of violence increased when she heard the 'male voice' instructing her to obtain

Case study – Joan (cont'd)

a knife. On the ward, Joan reported hearing this voice on a number of occasions. Further assessment indicated that these experiences increased either after her mother departed having visited Joan or when she telephoned to say that she would be unable to visit. This left Joan feeling vulnerable and lonely. Thus, although Joan's risk of threatening others did increase when she was experiencing her voice, it was also significantly related to her mother leaving or informing Joan that she could not visit.

Traditionally, mental health practitioners were taught to distract clients when they experienced voices or when they wished to discuss their beliefs. This approach was largely influenced by the jasperian view that delusions cannot be altered by discussing them (Allen & Kingdon 1998). The framework of behaviourism lent support to this view, when it was demonstrated that, if nurses did not respond, clients were observed to state their delusional beliefs less frequently (Allyon & Haughton 1964). However, a reduction in the verbalisation of a belief does not equate with a reduction in its strength or frequency, or the client's preoccupation with it. This view has been very difficult to shift and it is only recently that the validity of such an approach has been fully challenged. Taking such a dismissive approach undoubtedly affects the engagement process, especially when clients become aware that their most distressing experiences are being actively avoided (Allen & Kingdon 1998). Indeed, while such practices continue it will remain difficult to develop trust and demonstrate genuine concern for a person's distress, and in this context potential risk areas will go undetected (see Ch. 10).

PART 2 – ASSESSMENT, INTERVENTION AND RELATED ISSUES

Working with people in secure environments

When examining offending behaviours in people with SMI in a secure setting there are a number of points worth consideration. Below are some of the more regular issues faced.

Engagement issues

Disclosure can affect disposal

Close consideration must be paid to general and more specific factors that may influence engagement. Clients learn fairly soon how a system works and its pros and cons. One of the main problems facing them is that disclosure of an offence can (and usually will) influence final disposal. This is particularly apparent in people who have been transferred from prisons to secure units. Disclosure of symptoms in a prison environment can often lead to transfer to a secure health facility. However, once this has occurred, 'not disclosing symptoms' can often lead to people moving through the system, especially if the index offence has been largely attributed to a person's mental health status.

Faking good and faking bad

As mentioned above, there may be global reasons why people would alter their presentation of symptoms within a secure environment. However, there may be blocks to therapeutic engagement on a more specific level. People may overaccentuate symptoms or psychological distress as a way of minimising their involvement in, and responsibility for, their offending behaviour (faking bad), in the same way that some offenders attribute the responsibility for their actions to being intoxicated at the time of their offence. To present a more favourable picture of themselves, people can also underplay the role of psychological factors (faking good).

Confidentiality

This can be one of the major blocks to engagement. Whether working in a clinical team or with outpatients, it should be made explicit that the information discussed will be disclosed if it impacts on the safety of others or of clients themselves, or has direct relevance to their clinical care. This does not mean that you have to disclose the exact details of your work; however, the main themes, issues and content of sessions may be available to a wider audience than can normally be agreed within a therapeutic relationship.

Labelling

Assessment should consider the role of the 'labelling process' in relation to engagement. The negative stigma attached to people who offend and have a SMI may block therapeutic work. Indeed, this can also be affected if clients do not hold the same views of their current mental health status as their clinical team. Also, careful consideration has to be paid to the language used when addressing issues that the assessment process has raised. A brief case example serves to highlight this.

Case study – Robert

Robert (26) had a diagnosis of paranoid schizophrenia that had responded well to medication. However, on the ward he was observed to be quiet in social situations and avoided approaching staff to meet day-to-day needs. The clinical team made a referral to one of the authors for an assessment of Robert's social skills and 'weaknesses'. Following assessment it was suggested that Robert would benefit from social skills training. However, Robert did not consider himself to have any problems in this area despite the clinical team's opinion that he would benefit from this work. Robert did not engage with this intervention and now believes that others see him as having a major psychiatric condition and social skills deficits.

There is often disparity between what an individual believes they need and what the clinical team believes they need. Engagement requires a full assessment of the client's difficulties and then, in conjunction with the clinical team, will require working on the priorities of the client in order to build trust. This may open the door for potential future work on 'wider issues' of psychological functioning, interventions and risk management.

Mental illness = offending

As mentioned, it is a common assumption that offending behaviour is a direct result of mental illness. This has two implications for engagement. First, this position is often reinforced by healthcare professionals and by the criminal justice system, in that clients may receive a health service disposal owing to their mental state at the time of their offence. Consequently, having observed such 'system rules' clients may not wish to engage (even at assessment level) because they fear that, if they continue to disclose symptoms, this will influence their clinical team's decision making and their treatment and disposal. Secondly, future engagement may be hampered by those professionals who rely solely on psychotropic medication to settle a person's mental state and leave clients believing that the major cause of their offending behaviour has been addressed – 'I'm not going to offend because I'm no longer ill'.

Professional overinvolvement early on

It is usual practice, irrespective of the setting, that, following a person's admission, there is a flurry of activity from a number of professionals (nursing, psychiatry, psychology, social work, occupational therapy, probation, etc.), all attempting to assess the person's presenting problems, mental health, offending behaviour, risk areas and current functioning. It should therefore not come as a great surprise if this 'bombardment' of questioning and scrutiny meets with some resistance from the person being assessed. Thus, we have to achieve a balance between the fulfilling of professional requirements and the need to be sensitive regarding time and the amount of information the person is required to provide at the time of admission.

Paranoia, voices and delusions

It can be very difficult to engage with clients when they are actively experiencing voices or hold beliefs that induce feelings of paranoia or vulnerability. Also, clients' beliefs about their voices (see Ch. 11) may hamper the assessment process – for example, if they believe the source of their voice to be extremely powerful or omnipotent, or if they believe that disclosing information about the source of the voice will lead to harm coming to themselves or 'significant others'. For additional material on engagement issues see the following.

- Chadwick et al (1996) discuss some issues in engaging with people who are experiencing voices, delusions and paranoia as well as strategies to overcome these
- Gresswell & Kruppa (1994) provide a number of strategies to enhance engagement, communication and the assessment process in relation to working in secure environments
- Perkins (1991) looks at working specifically with sex offenders in secure environments.

Assessment

In essence, the underlying guiding principles that should enhance the engagement process are those where both client and practitioner collaborate, are flexible and where the practitioner communicates understanding. These are detailed in Box 16.1.

Box 16.1 Attitudes and skills to enhance engagement

- **Collaborative:** Both parties agree the goals and processes involved.
- **Empathic:** Including providing feedback when you do and do not understand.
- **Short, frequent:** Work in manageable chunks with the person. Do not attempt to cram a full assessment into two interviews.
- **Pragmatic:** Be willing to adapt your work to suit the person's interpersonal style, cognitive ability and, most importantly, you do not have to follow intervention strategies by the book!

Before meeting the client you will always need to review all relevant materials and obtain background information. As mentioned in Chapter 15, the purpose of assessment is to identify those areas that need particular attention and to plan the focus and goals of the assessment (Richards & McDonald 1990). Such preparation will include:

◆ review of previous case notes, including depositions of offences, where available
◆ review of relevant literature
◆ discussion with 'significant others' (e.g. family and previous professionals involved in care)

As well as those engagement issues outlined above, preparation will allow the identification of specific issues as well as strategies of how to overcome these.

Agreeing the problems and the goals of assessment

Agreeing the focus of problem assessment is paramount to a successful assessment (and, therefore, subsequent interventions). As previously discussed, if we attempt to discuss issues that we perceive to be central to the person's difficulties in the absence of the client 'owning them' or 'agreeing' with this perception then we will probably run into problems. Work has to be collaborative. Interventions should be broken down into manageable tasks, and goals should be identified for short-, medium- and long-term outcomes.

Assessment usually takes approximately three or four sessions, but may take longer if there are a number or range of offences.

Functional analysis

There are a number of models of functional analysis (FA), which largely have their underpinnings in behavioural theory (Sturmey 1996). Largely, these involve some form of analysis of both antecedents (A) and consequences (C, reinforcements and punishments) of an individual's behaviour (B). This is commonly termed an ABC analysis (see Ch. 9) (Table 16.1).

Although a considerable amount of controversy exists regarding FA (Samson & McDonnell 1990, McDonnell & Samson 1992, Owens & Jones 1992), FA remains a useful, widely used tool. It helps us to understand and conceptualise patterns of behaviour and how each element of the person's difficulties interrelates. FA can also help to:

◆ provide material to weigh up the pros and cons of clients' offending behaviour (in relation to consequences)
◆ provide clients with self-monitoring strategies in relation to their own offending behaviour.

Table 16.1 ABC analysis of offence

A = Antecedents	**Distal:** Offence history Early experiences (e.g. traumas) Significant life events Previous behaviour patterns **Proximal (prior to offence(s)):** Where? When? What? Whom? Thoughts Feelings Arousal level Physical condition (modifiers? alcohol/drugs?)
B = Behaviour	Detailed description of offence(s)
C = Consequences	**Positive/negative reinforcements:** Thoughts Feelings Material gains Avoidances **Positive/negative punishments:** Fine/sentence Loss of family contact Decrease in positive affect Increase in negative affect

In relation to offending, FA can be extended to include the following categories.

Behavioural These include the following questions:

◆ Which offence does the person see as most serious or more accessible to change?
◆ Did the person act alone or in a group?
◆ If there was a victim or victims, who were they?
◆ Was a weapon used?
◆ If a sexual offence, which offence were professionals or 'significant others' most concerned about?
◆ Why that particular victim?
◆ What were the chief motivations to offending?
◆ How do environmental events activate behaviour?

Cognitive These include:

◆ attitudes towards the offence
◆ thoughts prior to, during and following the offence
◆ justifications – including 'victim blaming' or perceiving the crime as victimless (as in the case of drug dealing or burglary).

In relation to sexual offending, beliefs which minimise the seriousness of the offence or blame the victim are usually termed 'cognitive distortions'. These can include general attitudes towards the role of women in society, rape myths (Burt 1980) or beliefs about children and sexuality. Asking them to talk through their offence(s) can access more specific beliefs regarding clients' victims. Prior to this, a review of the depositions may also highlight potential distortions to be followed up during face-to-face assessment. Attempts to challenge distortions at this point may impact on future engagement and trust and should be avoided.

At a more specific level, assessment can be made of beliefs prior to, during and following the offending behaviour. Benefits include:

◆ rich information obtained by thorough functional analysis
◆ (by focusing on the antecedents) – the potential to provide the person with preliminary indicators that certain thoughts are associated with offending behaviour
◆ the provision of a good opportunity to discuss the role of thoughts and their influence on behaviour within a cognitive–behavioural framework.

Affective   Gaining a clear idea of the mood of the person at each stage of the offence(s) will enhance your assessment and provide information related to the function served by the offence. For example, did the person report getting a 'buzz' from the offence? Also, pay attention to the affect displayed by clients when recounting their offence. For example, do they appear: aroused, angry, upset or indifferent?

Determining the relationship between mental health functioning and offending

As mentioned, there are a variety of reasons why someone with a mental health problem may commit an offence. Knowing clients' diagnoses may contribute somewhat to understanding why their offending behaviour has occurred; however, it will offer little information in relation to the function it serves for them. Nevertheless, there will be symptoms and psychological consequences of mental health problems that will influence motivation, planning, commissioning and consequences of offending (including detection as mentioned above). For the purposes of assessment, we have divided these up into primary and secondary factors.

1. Primary factors   Primary factors include symptoms directly associated with diagnosis (e.g. delusional beliefs, voices, etc.). Assessment should focus on whether and if symptoms influence the offending behaviour. Again, working within a framework of functional analysis helps focus the person's experience of these symptoms at the antecedent, behavioural and consequence levels. A person may hold specific beliefs about their victim that can

Table 16.2 ABC analysis of mental health and offending

	Leading to
Antecedents (e.g. voices)	Anger Beliefs about voices Anxiety/fear Isolation Difficulty gaining employment
Behaviour	Psychological experiences during offence, e.g. beliefs about voices
Consequences	Positive reinforcement – attention from services Decrease in feelings of isolation (negative reinforcement) Increase in medication (positive punishment) Loss of liberty (negative punishment)

be understood in terms of the diagnosis – for example, that the client's partner is having an affair, or a 'significant other' is poisoning the person, or that aliens have replaced a close family member.

2. Secondary factors These include psychological and emotional problems that are not part of the primary diagnosis but may contribute to the offending behaviour – for example, memory, attention and concentration problems, irritability and anger. Talking through the offence(s) with the person should 'tease out' these factors. Focusing on these factors during the assessment period also enables a broadening out of the factors that may contribute to offending, apart from those directly associated with diagnosis.

Thus people's symptoms may influence their offending at the antecedent, behavioural and consequence levels. Table 16.2 illustrates this.

Assessment measures

Questionnaires and measures should be used in conjunction with clinical interview to aid the assessment process and also to evaluate interventions. Apart from assessing mental health (see Ch. 8), some specific measures that are useful include:

◆ Sexual Fantasy Questionnaire (Wilson 1978)
◆ Reactions to Provocation Scale (Novaco 1990)
◆ Situations–Reactions Hostility Inventory (Blackburn & Lee-Evans 1985)
◆ Internal–External Scale (Rotter 1966).

Formulation

Formulation usually takes between two and three sessions to complete. The main purpose of formulation is to reach a shared understanding of the person's

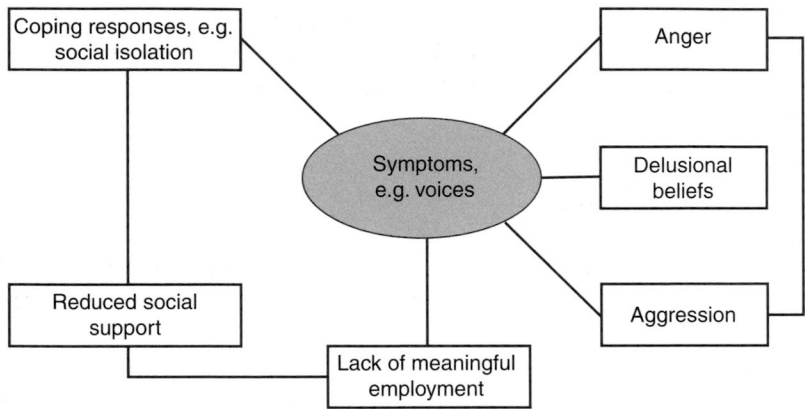

Figure 16.1 A relationship chart.

difficulties and functions served by their offending. Collaboration in this process facilitates ownership and will aid later engagement when intervening. Clients often have a view as to how their difficulties (offending and mental health) relate to each other, as well as an understanding of the development of, and reasons for, their offending. As discussed earlier (see Ch. 15), a relationship diagram (Fig. 16.1) is a useful tool for exploring these relationships, using either the client's mental health problems or their offending as a starting point.

Once this has been agreed with clients you can begin to identify which issues they feel are central to their understanding of their difficulties. It may happen that you, as a worker, will not share the same view as clients regarding the main influences on their offending behaviour or future risk. However, this is not entirely necessary; what is more important is that you both agree on which problems it would be practical and productive to work. Also, with sensitivity, your differences and reasons for these different viewpoints can be discussed.

Providing clients with a copy of the formulation is good practice and they can take it away with them and think about these potential relationships in their own time between sessions.

Interventions

As with the assessment procedure, intervention strategies have to be developed collaboratively. There is little point in getting straight in with a punishment schedule if the person does not agree with or own this process. General interventions regarding severe mental health problems are outlined throughout this book (e.g. Ch. 11). We will therefore outline only strategies pertaining to offending issues and relate these where applicable.

Offending behaviour does not occur in a vacuum. There are multiple influences on this behaviour and therefore there are a number of levels where interventions can take place, including arousal, cognitive, behavioural, interpersonal and social.

Cognitive–behavioural strategies

Cognitive–behavioural and behavioural strategies have been successfully applied to a variety of offences, including sexual offending (Laws & O'Neil 1981, Daniel 1987). There are a number of techniques available, including the following.

Stimulus control   The initial assessment should highlight some triggers to offending. Avoidance of these could be the first step to reducing the person's risk of committing future offences. Therefore, until a full assessment of the function of behaviours has been completed, it could be agreed that behaviours will be managed in this way in the interim.

Problem-solving strategies   A person's offending behaviour may relate to a particular problem (e.g. financial or interpersonal). Hence a person's risk of offending may be reduced through coaching in the skills of problem solving, including:

- identifying when problems arise
- generating alternative behaviours/strategies
- identifying steps to reach an alternative goal (e.g. getting money legally).

You can work with clients on generated solutions to problems, pre-empting triggers, predicting what is likely to happen in a high-risk situation and role-playing with them until they feel more confident that they have gained some of these skills.

Response cost strategies   This involves working with clients on identifying the consequences of their actions and has much in common with the problem-solving approach above. In other words, it involves agreeing what the client believes are appropriate consequences for risk taking or offending behaviours. For example, in mental health settings this may revolve around observation or parole status.

Offending behaviour chains   Any offence is a sequence of behaviours – from the planning stage to making off after the event. Work can be done on identifying this sequence and developing ways of disrupting it. This can be completed for a single offence or a range of offences.

Social skills and assertiveness training   Training should focus on verbal and non-verbal cues and behaviours. It should be comprehensive enough to include a variety of adaptive behaviours that a person can employ when circumstances and situations alter – for example, communication skills, anger management (see Ch. 15), problem-solving training and behavioural relaxation. A person may also benefit from more specific skills such as training in job interview skills.

Working on identified cognitions   Those cognitions identified during the assessment and formulation stages can be extended to using techniques such as diary keeping, enhancing awareness of habitual or automatic thinking and its influence on behaviour. From this, patterns of high-risk thinking and behaviours can be identified, for example:

◆ 'I feel lonely; I'll just go for a walk in the park' (sexual offending)
◆ 'This guy is taking me for granted; I'll sort him out' (violent offending).

There are a number of techniques available to alter cognitive distortions in sexual offenders. However, these are probably best addressed in a group setting where other difficulties can be explored, e.g. victim empathy training and relationship problems (Epps 1996).

Taking responsibility for offending   There are two main ways of working with clients' cognitions regarding their offending behaviour that may reduce the likelihood that they will continue offending:

◆ victim empathy awareness
◆ passive to active account of offending.

Victim empathy   The literature on sexual offending has been instrumental in raising awareness of the role of victim-blaming attitudes and cognitions and the part played by these in offending (Hildebran & Pithers 1989, Stermac & Segal 1990). Running through the offence(s) with clients and getting them to generate possible thoughts, feelings and experiences for their victim(s) is a way of raising awareness of the distress and damage caused by their actions. Even offences that are considered 'victimless', such as bank robbery, can be explored to highlight cognitions regarding the experiences of the victims and cognitions associated with offending, e.g. 'It's the bank I'm taking from – no one gets hurt and they can afford it'.

Passive to active accounts   Related to the above is the issue of passivity in clients' accounts of their offence. Moving the person from the notion of being a passive recipient to an active responsible participant is the goal of this intervention. Below are a few examples of passive and active accounts of sexual offending:

Passive:	'The kid sat on my lap. I tried to stop him.'
Active:	'I asked him to sit on me. I was horny.'
Passive:	'I started taking her blouse off and she never asked me to stop.'
Active:	'She was so drunk I could do what I wanted.'

In other words, such approaches attempt to help the client move from an external to an internal locus of control (Rotter 1966). This can be achieved by getting clients to talk through their offence(s) and recording those explanations and accounts that are passive.

Seemingly irrelevant (unimportant) decisions   Offending involves a number of behaviours that result in the final behaviour/offence. The literature on offending has been instrumental in highlighting those decisions in an offence chain that appear 'irrelevant' to the offending behaviour. To understand this concept, consider the following case study:

Case study

A person who is attempting to abstain from alcohol is walking through the city centre. He reaches in his pocket for his cigarettes and discovers that he has run out. He sees a pub in front of him and thinks, 'I'll just nip in here and buy some cigarettes'. He goes in and discovers that he has no change for the machine. He buys a half pint of beer to get change. Once he finishes this half pint, he buys another pint, takes his newspaper and settles down to read it.

This person has made a number of decisions in order to get to the stage where he is drinking alcohol in the pub. Working from the standpoint that offending follows the same pattern of seemingly irrelevent decisions/choices leading to the final act, targeting and changing these seems logical and essential to managing the risk of re-offending.

Challenging cognitions

On a one-to-one basis, direct challenging of cognitive distortions may be too confrontational if the timing is wrong. If this is the case (and getting it right is usually dependent upon experience and good supervision), getting clients to identify their own pro-offending attitudes and thoughts or working with the problems and contradictions that people's own belief systems present them with may be a more productive strategy. Another strategy is following the chaining of how cognitions can lead to behaviours that have serious consequences for clients as they see it, e.g. losing contact with family and friends.

CONCLUSIONS

This chapter has provided a brief outline of the issues faced when working with people with mental health problems at risk of offending. It is hoped that it has provided an introduction to stimulate further interest. The work is challenging; especially with clients who have committed very serious offences, which undoubtedly raise professional and personal issues. We have stressed the importance of obtaining supervision and working collaboratively with users, which includes not only agreeing problems and goals to focus on but also working on the difficulties as the person sees them.

Summary of practical strategies identified

◆ Negative stigma may block therapeutic work, therefore always endeavour to work on the client's priorities rather than your own or the team's.

◆ Don't rush the assessment process; plan to take it over 3–4 sessions or longer if there is a range or number of offences.

◆ Work on the problems as the client sees them. Both parties should agree the goals and processes involved.

◆ Using a functional analysis helps to frame, understand and conceptualise patterns of offending behaviour.

◆ Utilise cognitive–behavioural interventions as these have been successfully applied within a variety of offences.

References

Allen J, Kingdon D 1998 Using cognitive behavioural interventions for people with acute psychosis. Mental Health Practice 1:14–21

Allyon T, Haughton S 1964 Modification of symptomatic verbal behaviour of mental patients. Behaviour Research and Therapy 2:305–312

Bjorkly S 2002 Psychotic symptoms and violence towards others – a literature review and some preliminary findings. Part 2 Hallucinations. Aggression and Violence Behaviour 7:605–615

Blackburn R 1993 The psychology of criminal conduct: theory, research and practice. Wiley, Chichester

Blackburn R 1996 Mentally disordered offenders. In: Hollin C R (ed) Working with offenders: psychological practice in offender rehabilitation. Wiley, Chichester, p 128

Blackburn R, Lee-Evans J M 1985 Reactions of primary and secondary psychopaths to anger-evoking situations. British Journal of Clinical Psychology 24:93–100

Brennan P A, Grekin E R, Vanman E J 2000 Major mental disorders and crime in the community. In: Hodgins S (ed) Violence among the mentally ill. Kluwer, Dordrecht

Burt M R 1980 Cultural myths and supports for rape. Journal of Personality and Social Psychology 38:217–230

Chadwick P, Birchwood M, Trower P (eds) 1996 Cognitive therapy for delusions, voices and paranoia. Wiley, Chichester

References (*cont'd*)

Côté G, Hodgins S 1992 The prevalence of major mental disorders among homicide offenders. International Journal of Law and Psychiatry 15:89–99

Daniel C J 1987 Shame aversion therapy and social skills training in an indecent exposure. In: McGurk B J, Thornton D M, Williams M (eds) Applying psychology to imprisonment: theory and practice. HMSO, London, pp 245–254

Department of Health 1983 Mental Health Act. HMSO, London

Epps K 1996 Sex offenders. In: Hollin C R (ed) Working with offenders: psychological practice in offender rehabilitation. Wiley, Chichester, pp 150–187

Feldman P 1993 The psychology of crime. Cambridge University Press, Cambridge, p 172

Gresswell D M, Kruppa I 1994 Special demand of assessment in a secure setting: setting the scene. In: McMurran M, Hodge J (eds) The assessment of criminal behaviours of clients in secure settings. Jessica Kingsley, London, pp 35–52

Gunn J, Robertson G, Dell S, Way C 1978 Psychiatric aspects of imprisonment. Academic Press, London

Hall P, Brockington I F, Levings J, Murphy C 1993 A comparison of responses to the mentally ill in two communities. British Journal of Psychiatry 162:99–108

Herek G M 1994 Homosexuality. In: Corsini R J (ed) Encyclopedia of psychology, 2nd edn. Wiley Interscience, New York, pp 151–155

Hiday V A 1995 The social context of mental illness and violence. Journal of Health and Social Behaviour 36:122–137

Hildebran D, Pithers W D 1989 Enhancing offender empathy for sexual abuse victims. In: Hildebran D, Laws R (eds) Relapse prevention with sex offenders. Guilford Press, New York, pp 236–243

Home Office 1990 Circular no. 66/90: Provision for mentally disordered offenders. HMSO, London

Johnson B, Martin M L, Guha M, Montgomery P 1997 The experience of thought-disordered individuals preceding an aggressive incident. Journal of Psychiatric and Mental Health Nursing 4:213–220

Junginger J 1995 Command hallucinations and the prediction of dangerousness. Psychiatric Services 46:911–914

Laws D R, O'Neil J A 1981 Variations on masturbatory conditioning. Behavioural Psychotherapy 9:111–136

Levey S, Howells K 1995 Dangerousness, unpredictability and the fear of people with schizophrenia. Journal of Forensic Psychiatry 6:19–39

McCord J 1990 Crime in moral and social contexts. The American Society of Criminology, 1989, presidential address. Criminology 28:1–26

McDonnell A, Samsom D M 1992 Explanation and prediction in functional analysis: a reply to Jones and Owens. Behavioural Psychotherapy 20:41–43

Monahan J, Steadman H 1983 Crime and mental disorder: an epidemiological approach. In: Morris N, Tonrys M (eds) Crime and justice: an annual review of research. University of Chicago Press, Chicago, pp 1–19

Monahan J, Appelbaum P, Mulvey E et al 1994 Ethical and legal duties in conducting research on violence: lessons from the MacArthur Risk Assessment Study. Violence and Victims 8:380–390

Mulvey E P 1994 Assessing the link between mental illness and violence. Hospital and Community Psychiatry 45:663–668

References (cont'd)

Novaco R W 1990 Reactions to provocation. University of California (NAS), Irvine, CA

Owens R G, Jones R S P 1992 Extending the role of functional analysis in challenging behaviour. Behavioural Psychotherapy 20:45–46

Perkins D 1991 Clinical work with sex offenders in secure settings. In: Hollin C R, Howells K (eds) Clinical approaches to sex offenders and their victims. Wiley, Chichester, pp 151–179

Richards D, McDonald B 1990 Behavioural psychotherapy: a pocket book for nurses. Heinemann, Oxford

Ritchie J 1994 The report of the inquiry into the care and treatment of Christopher Clunis. HMSO, London

Rogers P, Watt A, Gray N S et al 2002 Content of command hallucinations predicts self harm but not violence in a medium secure unit. Journal of Forensic Psychiatry 13:251–262

Rotter J B 1966 Generalised expectancies for internal versus external control of reinforcement. Psychological Monographs 80 (no. 609)

Samson D M, McDonnell A 1990 Functional analysis and challenging behaviours. Behavioural Analysis 18:259–272

Shah A K 1993 An increase in violence among psychiatric inpatients: real or apparent? Medicine, Science and Law 33: 227–230

Spry W B 1984 Schizophrenia and crime. In: Craft M, Craft A (eds) Mentally abnormal offenders. Baillière Tindall, London

Stephenson G M 1992 The psychology of criminal justice. Blackwell, Oxford, p 11

Stermac L E, Segal Z V 1989 Adult sexual contact with children: an examination of cognitive factors. Behaviour Therapy 20:573–584

Sturmey P 1996 Functional analysis in clinical psychology. Wiley, Chichester

Taylor P 2003 NHS National programme on forensic mental heath research and development. Expert paper: Mental illness and serious harm to others. Department of Health. HMSO, London

Taylor P J, Hodgins S 1994 Violence and psychosis: critical timings. Criminal Behaviour and Mental Health 4:267–289

Walsh E, Buchanan A, Fahy T 2002 Violence and schizophrenia: examining the evidence. British Journal of Psychiatry 180:490–495

Wessely S, Taylor P J 1991 Madness and crime: criminology versus psychiatry. Criminal Behaviour and Mental Health 1:193–228

Wessely S, Buchanan A, Reed A et al 1993 Acting on delusions. I: Prevalence. British Journal of Psychiatry 163:69–76

Wilson G 1978 The secrets of sexual fantasy. Dent, London

Annotated further reading

Blackburn R 1993 The psychology of criminal conduct theory, research and practice. Wiley, Chichester

Comprehensive coverage of mental health and psychological functioning in relation to offending.

McMurran M, Hodge J (eds) The assessment of criminal behaviours in secure settings. Jessica Kingsley, London

Provides an excellent coverage of assessment techniques and issues in relation to secure settings. Especially see Chapter 2: Special demands of assessment in a secure setting.

Sturmey P 1996 Functional analysis in clinical psychology. Wiley, Chichester

Bolton D, Hill J 1996 Mind, meaning and mental disorder: the nature of causal explanations in psychology and psychiatry. Oxford University Press, Oxford

Excellent but extended philosophical discussion of causal explanations of behaviour, including psychiatric diagnosis.

17

Managing medication

Jacqueline Sin and Cliff Roberts

KEY ISSUES

- ◆ Neurochemistry and brain function
- ◆ The role of neuropharmacology and antipsychotics
- ◆ Typical and atypical antipsychotics
- ◆ Illustrative case study

INTRODUCTION

Healthcare professionals are often inadequately prepared to address practical issues such as understanding and managing medication. We need to be honest about the lack of pharmacological knowledge many healthcare workers have and the even greater divide between theory and its application to practice (Banning 2003).

This chapter aims to review some basic neurophysiology and its relationship to mental health and psychiatric disorder. From a pharmacological perspective it will examine the psychopathology associated with schizophrenia, its signs and symptoms and approaches. Because of current medication choices, the present preference for atypical over typical antipsychotic medication will also be examined. The chapter ends with a case study to demonstrate how the theories and knowledge in relation to psychopharmacology can readily be incorporated into clinical practice. Throughout the case study, a few contemporary issues in the area of medication management will be explored and discussed, such as assessment strategies, side effects management, polypharmacy and enhancing concordance.

INTRODUCTION TO NEUROPHYSIOLOGY

The study of brain chemistry and how neurons communicate with themselves is referred to as neurophysiology. The manipulation of brain neuronal pathways and communication by drugs is referred to as psychopharmacology. The study of psychopharmacology has informed our understanding of the human brain, in terms not only of its microstructure but also its function in health and disorder.

Substances that are ingested and have a discernible effect on mood are termed *psychoactive*. The most commonly used licit psychoactive substances are alcohol, nicotine and caffeine. Any substance that is psychoactive is liable to overuse or misuse and therefore very likely to be used as part of a coping strategy (Winger et al 1992).

There are of course many different groups of substances that are psychoactive but these can be placed into the following three groups:

◆ **Psychostimulants**: Cocaine, caffeine
◆ **Depressants**: Alcohol, opiates
◆ **Psychedelic (hallucinogens)**: LSD, mescaline.

The use of psychoactive chemicals in society, both licit and illicit, shows no sign of declining. It is perhaps not surprising, then, that many of our clients use psychoactive chemicals to deal with their experiences of life.

Neurophysiology/pharmacology

Psychoactive substances affect the nervous system, which is the communication system of the body. Nerve cells or neurons, which make up the nervous system, have special properties in that they are excitable cells and are capable of interacting with their internal environment. Nerve cells normally have one *cell body* from which an *axon* may give off many side branches, giving the ability to communicate with thousands of other neurons. Consequently, neurons tend to develop during embryological development into pathways or circuits. They conduct electrical impulses, sometimes over long distances, and are able to release *neurotransmitters* at their terminal.

A neurotransmitter is itself a very specific messenger. It will only be interpreted by specific nerve circuits and certainly not by all nerve circuits. These neurotransmitters are released into a cleft, the *synaptic cleft*, which is so small it can only be seen with an electron microscope. Once the chemical has been released into the synaptic cleft it has only a very small distance to move before it will come into contact with a *receptor* (Figs 17.1, 17.2). These receptors are located both on the nerve terminal from which the chemical was released and on the membrane of the next nerve cell, which lies on the other

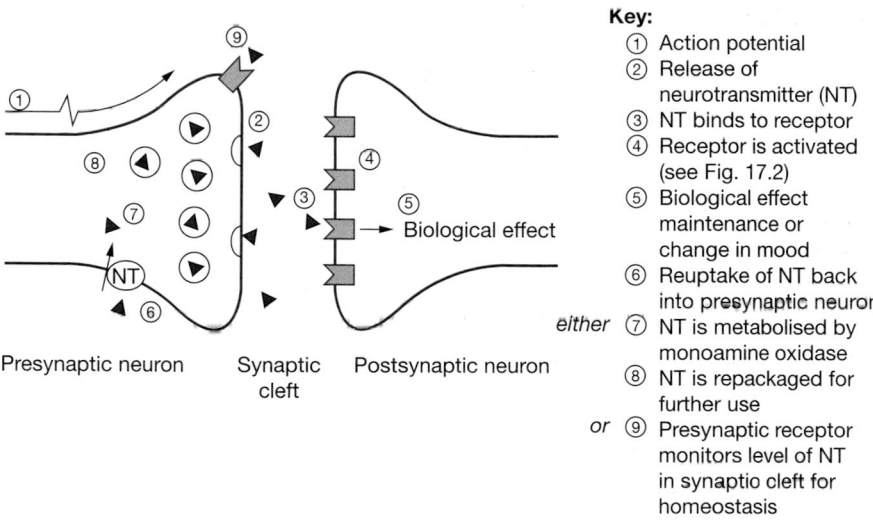

Key:
1. Action potential
2. Release of neurotransmitter (NT)
3. NT binds to receptor
4. Receptor is activated (see Fig. 17.2)
5. Biological effect maintenance or change in mood
6. Reuptake of NT back into presynaptic neuron

either 7. NT is metabolised by monoamine oxidase
8. NT is repackaged for further use

or 9. Presynaptic receptor monitors level of NT in synaptic cleft for homeostasis

Fig 17.1 Model of synaptic communication.

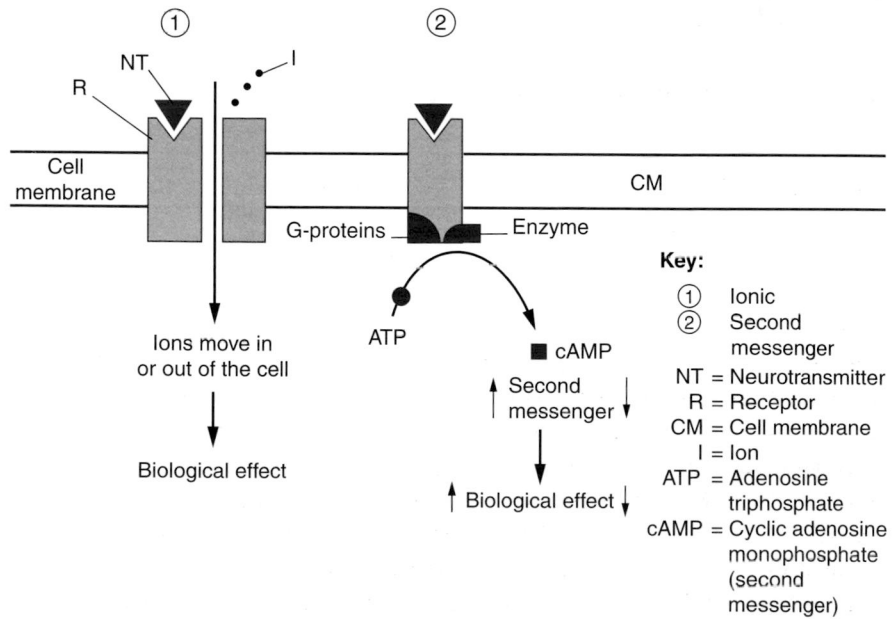

Key:
1. Ionic
2. Second messenger

NT = Neurotransmitter
R = Receptor
CM = Cell membrane
I = Ion
ATP = Adenosine triphosphate
cAMP = Cyclic adenosine monophosphate (second messenger)

Fig 17.2 The two types of receptor activity. Receptor activation may increase or decrease the turnover of cAMP, depending on the type of G-protein involved. This results in an increase or decrease of the biological effects respectively.

side of the cleft. Some examples of neurotransmitters are dopamine, serotonin (5-HT) and noradrenaline (norepinephrine). More than 40 transmitters have been identified at the present time.

Synaptic communication results in information transfer. Information transfer in the brain is made up of two processes. First, the chemical transmitter is released into the synaptic cleft (this is referred to as the *first messenger*). This chemical messenger binds with its specific receptor on the postsynaptic neuronal cell membrane and brings about a biological change in the postsynaptic neuron. Intracellular processes or enzymes (referred to as the *second messenger*) are altered, which changes the function of the postsynaptic neuron. As this activity is occurring in the brain the change in function could be, for example, a change of mood or alteration in level of alertness. The concept of receptors being the vehicle through which neurotransmitters and drugs produce a biological effect is central to the study of psychopharmacology.

SCHIZOPHRENIA AND PHARMACOLOGICAL STUDIES

Schizophrenia occurs in approximately 1% of the population. It is important to remember that the signs of schizophrenia are extremely varied and many of them are not exclusive to the disorder (see Ch. 7 for a discussion of signs and symptoms).

The dopamine hypothesis came about in a 'cart before the horse' situation when a drug was found to be efficacious in the management of psychotic symptoms but the action that allowed this was not known. Chlorpromazine was developed as an antihistamine but was found to have too sedative an effect. It was used to calm patients prior to anaesthesia and also to reduce allergic reactions sometimes caused by anaesthetic agents. The effects of chlorpromazine were described as inducing a 'beatific quietude'. The greatest advantage of this drug was that clients became manageable without being so heavily sedated that they fell asleep. Higher doses were used and resulted in clear improvements in psychotic symptoms. Initially the biochemical basis for this was unknown. Parkinsonian side effects were also noted. Parkinsonian effects are tremors brought about by dopamine depletion in the basal ganglia. Central mechanisms for dopamine release were implicated when antipsychotics were found to reverse amphetamine-induced abnormal behaviours.

As mentioned, the dopamine hypothesis arose from these findings and is the most prominent theory involving central transmitters. In its simplest interpretation the dopamine hypothesis suggests that schizophrenia arises as a result of excessive central dopaminergic neuronal activity. More recently, other neurotransmitters such as noradrenaline, serotonin, acetylcholine and gamma-aminobutyric acid (GABA) have also been suggested.

NEUROPHARMACOLOGY: ANTIPSYCHOTICS AND SCHIZOPHRENIA

Dopamine receptors are situated in central pathways (Table 17.1). Neuroleptic drugs have their effect on these pathways, and result in both *therapeutic* and *side effects*. Antipsychotics act as an antagonist at dopamine receptors (Fig 17.3). That is, they significantly interfere (antagonism) with the binding of dopamine to dopamine receptors. This results in a reduction in postsynaptic activity. As the dopamine hypothesis indicates that dopamine transmission in schizophrenia is hyperactive, antagonists of dopamine transmission will reduce

Table 17.1 Therapeutic effects and side effects of antipsychotics

Tract	Pharmacological effects
Mesolimbic and mesocortical tracts: Fibres originate in the ventral tegmental area and spread to the limbic system, frontal cortex and other regions	Therapeutic action of antipsychotics
Nigrostriatal tract: Fibres project into the caudate nucleus, the putamen and the basal ganglia	Extrapyramidal side effects such as parkinsonism, acute dystonias, akathisia and tardive dyskinesia
Tuberoinfundibular tract: Fibres originate in the arcuate nucleus of the hypothalamus and project to the median eminence (pituitary) (hypothalamic–pituitary axis, HPA)	Endocrine side effects such as gynaecomastia (enlarged breasts), amenorrhoea (absence of menstruation), weight gain, lactorrhoea (milk production from breasts), impotence and false-positive pregnancy tests

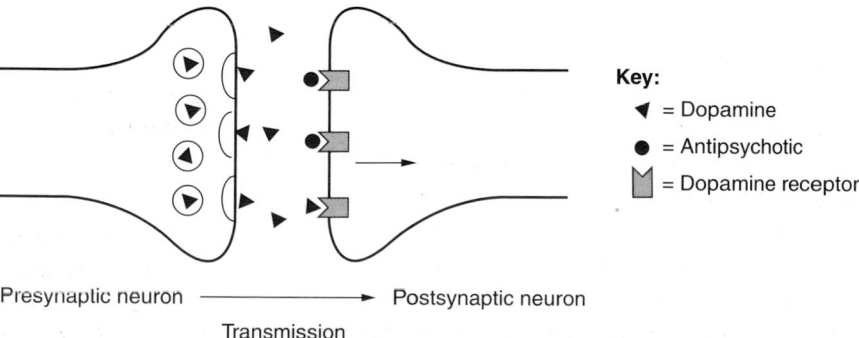

Key:
◀ = Dopamine
● = Antipsychotic
◘ = Dopamine receptor

Presynaptic neuron ──────▶ Postsynaptic neuron

Transmission

Fig. 17.3 Antagonistic effects of antipsychotics at dopamine receptors. This is a simple diagram: antipsychotics produce their effects through interaction at dopamine and other receptors such as serotonin.

this hyperactivity, thereby reducing the florid symptoms of schizophrenia. Unfortunately, as dopamine receptors are found in many pathways in the brain, the therapeutic effects are accompanied by side effects as well. Also, dopamine transmission may increase or decrease transmission in other transmitter pathways.

Neurotransmission of dopamine requires a specific receptor. However there is more than one dopamine receptor. At the moment there are known to be at least five, denoted by the letter D followed by the subscript 1, 2, 3, 4 or 5, i.e. D_{1-5}.

Clinical potency of antipsychotics, and in particular typical antipsychotics such as chlorpromazine, antagonise the normal effects of dopamine at D_2 receptors. In other words, typical antipsychotics block the binding of dopamine at dopamine receptors. Unfortunately this action is also responsible for side effects. Atypical antipsychotics have an antagonistic effect at both D_2 and serotonin 5-HT_2 receptors. The inclusion of activity at serotonin receptors achieves a therapeutic effect on negative symptoms in some people. It is unclear what role serotonin plays in the control of dopamine activity.

Major side effects are caused by the action of antipsychotics on a variety of dopamine, serotonin, acetylcholine and histamine receptors. This results in a number of potential side effects not necessarily attributable to dopaminergic antagonism.

It is impossible at the present time to design an antipsychotic that is therapeutic and has no side effects. The present problem is that a drug designed to have an antagonistic effect on dopamine receptors will antagonise most dopamine receptors to some degree. These receptors may be in brain pathways that have nothing to do with mood and behaviour.

Chemical groups used in the pharmacological treatment of schizophrenia

Antipsychotic drugs can be subdivided into typical (older) and atypical (new). Even on this point there is much controversy. These terms are only labels; they attempt to identify the individual drug's ability to bind with specific receptors, e.g. dopamine or serotonin.

Typical antipsychotic drugs

Typical antipsychotic drugs include chlorpromazine, haloperidol, trifluoperazine, thioridazine and flupenthixol. These drugs are also called major tranquillisers.

Typical antipsychotics are very good at treating the positive symptoms of schizophrenia but unfortunately induce extrapyramidal symptoms (EPS) such as parkinsonism, acute dystonic reactions, akathisia and tardive dyskinesia in

75% of clients. Results from randomised controlled trials indicate significant EPS effects from this 'group' (Table 17.2). Some 30% of clients with schizophrenia do not respond to typical antipsychotics or experience severe EPS (Gournay & Gray 1998).

Table 17.2 Identifying side effects and selecting an intervention

Side effect	Description/definition	Action/intervention
Extrapyramidal symptoms		
Parkinsonism	Parkinsonian symptoms can be mimicked by antipsychotic antagonism of dopamine transmission. Akinesia (slowing of movement and expression), rigidity, tremor	Administration of anticholinergic drugs and close monitoring
Acute dystonias	Fixed upward or lateral gaze. Torsion dystonia and torticollis (muscle spasms, particularly neck) may occur	Systemic administration of anticholinergic drug will restore the balance between dopamine and acetylcholine
Acute dyskinesia	Involuntary movements of head and neck. These symptoms are possibly caused by an imbalance of dopamine and acetylcholine in favour of the latter	As for dystonias
Akathisia	Motor restlessness, agitation, dysphoria (bad feelings and thoughts), leg shifting and/or tapping of the feet	Propranolol
Tardive dyskinesia	Involuntary movements of orofacial and buccal–lingual muscles. Uncoordinated movements of upper and lower limbs. Tics, abnormal postures, grunting and vocalisations may occur	Conflicting management strategies. Discontinuation of antipsychotic by gradual withdrawal provides better prognosis than continuation. Introduce clozapine as antipsychotics are withdrawn
Antipsychotic malignant syndrome	Hyperpyrexia (increase in temperature), severe rigidity, tachycardia (rapid heart beat), fluctuating level of consciousness. Complications such as renal failure can develop	Discontinue all antipsychotics, administration of dantrolene, or dopamine agonists L-dopa, apomorphine or bromocriptine

Table 17.2 Identifying side effects and selecting an intervention (*cont'd*)

Side effect	Description/definition	Action/intervention
Extrapyramidal symptoms		
Anticholinergic effects	Delirium, dry mouth, blurred vision, tachycardia (rapid heart beat), paralytic ileus (paralysis of the small bowel), constipation, erectile dysfunction and urinary retention	Many patients will develop tolerance to some of these side effects. If persistent and affecting quality of life, change to a more selective drug
α-adrenergic blockade	Orthostatic hypotension (positional fluctuations in blood pressure) and reflex tachycardia (rapid heart beat). Dizziness	During an acute episode, lie the client down and elevate their legs. Advise to rise slowly; tolerance may develop to these side effects
Antihistamine effect	Sedation	Can be beneficial, take medication at night if appropriate. Change to a more selective drug
Allergies	Jaundice, urticaria (rash), dermatitis, photosensitivity, optic neuritis, pigmentary retinopathy (visual changes in retina), agranulocytosis (lowering of white blood cells), aplastic anaemia (abnormally structured, non-functioning cells leading to blood disorder)	Careful monitoring of client for these symptoms is essential and discontinuation of the drug will be essential for a significant reaction

Atypical antipsychotics

Atypical antipsychotics include amisulpride, clozapine, risperidone, sertindole, olanzapine, and quetiapine.

In line with the widely recognised working hypothesis that antipsychotic drugs exert their effects through dopamine receptor blockade mechanisms and effects on cholinergic, alpha-adrenergic, histaminergic and serotonergic receptors (Rang & Dale 1991, King 1995, NICE 2002a), atypical (newer) antipsychotics command more complex receptor binding profiles than their conventional counterparts and thus carry with them a different if not superior side effects profile (Burkley 1997, Gray 1999). The evidence available indicates that atypical antipsychotics are at least as efficacious as the typical agents in terms of overall response rate and positive symptoms control (Kane et al 1988, Meltzer 1992, NICE 2002a). Furthermore, there is also speculation that atypical antipsychotics may produce better clinical outcomes in terms of control of negative symptoms and mood symptoms and prevention of relapse, largely because of their common pharmacological property of having a greater antagonism to 5-HT$_{2A}$ than to D$_2$ (Tandon & Jibson 2003). These clinical observations are very likely to be related to their lower risk of causing EPS, which in itself means a better quality of life for clients (NICE 2002b, Sin & Gamble 2003). However, in return for the lower risk of EPS and tardive dyskinesia (Tandon & Jibson 2003), there tends to be a higher propensity to cause weight gain and seizures, and an increased risk of ventricular arrhythmias according to clinical reports of the usage of clozapine and various atypical antipsychotics (NICE 2002a).

At the present time arguments are polarised over the therapeutic effects, side effects and costs of atypical antipsychotics, and the evidence from research trials. Some commentators (Geddes et al 2000) have questioned the present evidence for atypical over typical antipsychotics as the comparisons made were for higher doses of the older drugs than would have been therapeutically desirable. It is clear that, whatever the medication, consideration of how it suits the individuals who are taking it is essential.

CASE STUDY

The following case study encapsulates how systematic medication management can be used to monitor a client's medication needs.

Case study – Paul

Paul was diagnosed with schizophrenia at the age of 18. He had a satisfactory recovery from the first breakdown and returned to college 6 months afterwards. Later, he decided to stop taking his medication. Paul became unwell, was sectioned and readmitted after being violent to a number of people. Three years on, Paul has tried a variety of antipsychotic medication, including newer (atypical) antipsychotics, but unfortunately has reported only partial and limited therapeutic effects. Paul also experienced secondary depression and his presentation was dominated by negative symptoms, such as a lack of drive, concentration and poverty of speech, even when in remission.

Paul was keen to change his medication, as he derived little benefit from conventional antipsychotic therapy. He was therefore prescribed clozapine. Within 4 months, Paul had stepped up to 650 mg clozapine a day with therapeutic effects on psychotic symptoms. However, Paul experienced various serious side effects – urinary incontinence, seizures, hypersalivation, severe constipation and sedation.

Case study – Paul (cont'd)

Balancing the benefits and side effects of the medication, it was then decided that clozapine therapy should be continued at a lower daily dosage and augmented with sulpiride. Paul was also on antidepressants for the secondary and coexistent depression. At this stage, Paul's medication regime was: clozapine 100 mg OM and 200 mg nocte; sulpiride 800 mg bd; fluoxetine 40 mg OM; lorazepam 1 mg bd prn.

Source: adapted from Sin & Gamble 2003

Assessment process to inform and regulate medication regime

With the heralding of evidence-based practice, assessment should form the basis for proper adjustments of medication and is of crucial importance to clients receiving long-term medication (Bennett et al 1995b). A comprehensive and systematic assessment using research-based assessment tools is not only the beginning of the medication management but also underpins the process for monitoring and review over the course of management (Sin & Gamble 2003). The purposes of assessing Paul included obtaining baseline information of his side effects and the therapeutic effects of his current/pre-existing medication regime, understanding his subjective perception of the regime, identifying needs for psychoeducation, identifying needs for regime change or modification (e.g. changes of dosages and/or changes to another medication) and, last but not least, regular monitoring of his progress in response to medication (changes).

Nowadays, research-based assessment tools for detecting and measuring medication therapeutic and side effects are available for routine clinical practice. However, no assessment outcomes will be reliable or valid without practitioners being properly trained to master the tools and interpret the results. Bearing in mind that the chosen assessments will need to be repeated in a designated manner for monitoring and evaluation purposes during the medication management process, these tools need to be user-friendly as well as sensitive enough to detect minute changes.

In order to tailor-make the most effective and efficient assessment and monitoring programme, practitioners need to:

Measure the severity of client's current psychiatric symptoms to reflect the reaction to the medication and thus the therapeutic effects of the medication. The KGV Symptom Scale (Krawiecka et al 1977) is a recommended tool for

Table 17.3 KGV (M) summary of scores for Paul over a 6-month period

Item	Scores in first month	Scores in fifth month
Anxiety	4	2
Depression	3	2
Suicidal thoughts and behaviour	1	1
Elevated mood	0	0
Hallucinations	4	2
Delusions	0	0
Flattened affect	2	1
Incongruous affect	0	0
Overactivity	0	0
Psychomotor retardation	1	1
Abnormal speech	0	0
Poverty of speech	1	1
Abnormal movements	0	0
Accuracy of assessment	1	0

Source: adapted from Sin & Gamble 2003

this purpose and should be repeated at least every 4 months, or as indicated. Table 17.3 illustrates the KGV (M) Symptom Scale (Lancashire 1998) being used in Paul's case.

Monitor and assess side effects, as research has shown that intolerance of various side effects is the most common cause of clients discontinuing medication use (Taylor & Hardy 1997). Comprehensive side-effects assessments provide an overview of side effects experienced by the clients. The Liverpool University Neuroleptic Side Effect Rating Scale (LUNSERS; Day et al 1995) and the Side Effect Scale/Checklist for Antipsychotic Medication (SESCAM; Bennett et al 1995a) are choices worth considering here. LUNSERS can be a self-administered assessment tool and includes 41 known side effects of neuroleptics and 10 built-in 'red herring' items for a reference of reliability, with the total 51 items categorised into eight sectors of side effects (Day et al 1995). The updated version of LUNSERS has an additional level of distress scale of 1–10 (1 = not at all distressed to 10 = very much distressed) along all the items, which aims to yield information from the client's subjective viewpoint of suffering (Day et al 1995). SESCAM combines both the clinician's and the client's assessment of signs and symptoms of abnormal movements and other common side effects (Bennett et al 1995a). Most importantly, the SESCAM finishes its assessment with two global questions that explore the client's opinion of their medication (Bennett et al 1995a), which essentially opens the dialogue for joint decision-making on medication treatment (Tables 17.4, 17.5).

Table 17.4 Summary of LUNSERS scores for Paul

Extrapyramidal side effects	**Anticholinergic side effects**
Score = 10 (possible range 0–28)	Score = 7 (possible range 0–20)
Level of distress = 20 (possible range 7–70)	
Level of distress = 25 (possible range 5–50)	

Other autonomic side effects	**Allergic reaction**
Score = 5 (possible range 0–20)	Score = 0 (possible range 0–16)
Level of distress = 8 (possible range 5–50)	
Level of distress = 0 (possible range 4–40)	

Psychic side effects	**Hormonal side effect**
Score = 19 (possible range 0–40)	Score = 10 (possible range 0–16)
Level of distress = 28 (possible range 10–100)	
Level of distress = 20 (possible range 4–40)	

Miscellaneous	**Red herrings**
Score = 3 (possible range 0–16)	
Level of distress = 0 (possible range 4–40)	Score = 5 (possible range 0–40)
Level of distress = 2 (possible range 10–100)	

Overall score = 54 (possible range for men: 0–196)
Level of distress = 103 (possible range for men: 49–490)
Appropriate grade: Average

Source: adapted from Sin & Gamble 2003

Use specific side-effects or signs and symptoms assessment tools as indicated by clients' presentation and needs. For instance, if the changes in hallucinations in one client are the best reflection of the effectiveness of their medication treatment, the Hallucination Rating Scale (HRS; Haddock 1994) should be considered. Or, if the client's major side effects are movement disorder, including akathisia and tardive dyskinesia, the Abnormal Involuntary Movement Scale (AIMS) is a commonly used tool that provides a comprehensive assessment of involuntary movements of different body sites (Guy 1976, Lane et al 1985).

Review clients' insight into and attitude towards medication – finding out clients' awareness of their illness, and insight into their treatment needs, helps prepare a psychoeducation package about medication treatment; the Drug Attitude Inventory (DAI 30; Hogan et al 1983) is recommended for this purpose.

Table 17.5 SESCAM scores for Paul

Part I: Clinician rating: Rating: 0–4, mark shaded areas as indicated

	Parkinsonism	Akathisia	Tardive dyskinesia	Others
A. Face/mouth/neck				
1. Unchanging facial expression	1			
2. Dribbling	3			
3. Involuntary movements of mouth, lips or tongue			0	
4. Looks sleepy				4
5. Other (please specify)				
B. Extremities (Upper: arms, hands, fingers)				
6. Regular, resting or pill rolling tremor	0			
7. Other (please specify) Lower: legs, feet				
8. Tapping of feet/ restlessness (jogging on the spot)		0		
9. Other (please specify)				
C. Trunk/posture/gait				
10. Pelvic gyrations / or any writhing/rocking movements			0	
11. Rigid, shuffling gait	0			
12. Reduced arm swing	1			
13. Slowness and reduced spontaneity	3			
14. Other (please specify)				
Total	8	0	0	4
Reference Range	0–24	0–4	0–8	

Table 17.5 SESCAM scores for Paul (cont'd)

Part 2: Checklist: Please ask the patient the following questions and place a tick in the appropriate box

		Yes	No	If yes specify problem
1.	Do you have any of the following			
a.	Dizziness	√		Tolerable (related to lorazepam)
b.	Drowsiness	√		Afternoon only
c.	Sexual problems	√		No erection and ejaculation at all
d.	Constipation	√		I have Fibrogel and lactulose
e.	Urinary problems	√		
f.	Skin problems	√		
g.	Excessive weight gain	√		
h.	Blurred vision	√		Rarely
i.	Feeling restless	√		Rarely
j.	Lack get up and go	√		I find it difficult to motivate myself
k.	Other			

Further questions		**Yes**	**No**	**List reasons**
2.	Does the medication agree with you	√		The medication helps to a certain extent, but causes side effects, and not yet completely satisfactory
3.	Do you think this is the right medication for you?	√		I want to be on a medication which will aid my mental health and well being. For instance: an antidepressant that can lift my mood and an antipsychotic that 'matches my system and does not cause so much side effects'.

Source: adapted from Sin & Gamble 2003

Interpreting assessment results

Building upon the evidence-based assessment tools, a reliable and valid set of assessment results will inform specific interventions in terms of medication management for the client. Practitioners need to bear in mind that the medication side-effects assessment tools were not developed to assess known side effects commonly linked with atypical antipsychotics. Instead, they were designed to detect side effects commonly seen with older or conventional antipsychotics, such as tardive dyskinesia or photosensitivity. Moreover, some of the red herring items in LUNSERS are being recognised as side effects on further research into the area. For instance, 'running nose – common physical symptoms of rhinitis' (a red herring at present) has been reported to be associated with Risperidone (British Medical Association/Royal Pharmaceutical Society 2003). More research is needed to revalidate these tools, especially if the assessment tools are modified or updated. Meanwhile, practitioners need to exercise cautious discretion and take the client's individual presentation into consideration when interpreting the assessment results.

In the arena of severe and enduring mental illness, the phenomenon of poor physical health has been related to the higher vulnerability and propensity of developing side effects of individuals deemed treatment-resistant (Dev & Krupp 1995). In addition, poor diet, overuse of alcohol and heavy smoking further contribute to the picture. Recognition should also be paid to the fact that some clients find items on the assessment forms confusing, or the relationship between various items intriguing (Sin & Gamble 2003). In Paul's case, he had depression and experienced negative symptoms (as described earlier), which yield many similar signs and symptoms (Sin 2000) and largely echo the 'psychic side effects' assumed to be caused by antipsychotics within LUNSERS. Also, the subset of items aiming to detect hormonal side effects within LUNSERS ('flushing of face' and 'period problems') may produce false-positive results for menopausal women.

Managing adverse effects

If side effects/adverse effects are identified in the assessment process, clients should no longer be expected to endure them. Effective management and prevention of adverse effects, especially during the initial treatment phase, is an essential and relievable intervention for clients receiving antipsychotic medication (Taylor & Hardy 1997, Sin & Gamble 2003). Minimal medication side effects contribute to clients' perception of better quality of life (Sin & Gamble 2003) and concordance with treatment in the long term (Gray 1999).

Some suggested management strategies for a selection of common side effects found in treatment with atypical antipsychotics are illustrated in Table 17.6. As mentioned above, while the incidence of EPS has been lowered with the increasing popularity of atypical antipsychotics, weight gain, sexual dysfunction and sedation have recently been identified as topping the list of most troublesome side effects in clients' subjective experience (NICE 2002a). Unfortunately, the newer/atypical antipsychotics tend to be associated with this range of side effects.

Table 17.6 Managing adverse effects with Paul

Side effect	Receptors affected by antipsychotic*	Interventions/action
Hypersalivation (usually most pronounced during sleep)	Different receptors, including α and β adrenergic receptors and muscarinic receptors, located on the salivary glands	Anticholinergic agents are usually not indicated in clozapine-induced hypersalivation and may increase the risk of complications of cholinergic blockage (Dev & Krupp 1995) – do not use procyclidine. Clonidine, an α_2-agonist, can be used, e.g. perphenazine. Clients should be advised to prop themselves up on pillows at night and use towels to cover pillows if necessary.
Sedation/drowsiness	Histamine H_1 adrenergic receptors	Most clients develop a tolerance to sedation as treatment progresses. Otherwise, reduce dosage, or assign the majority of the daily dosage to night-time.
Seizure or convulsion	Relatively weak dopamine receptor blocking ability, combined with selectivity for mesolimbic D_1 receptors, reduced affinity for striatal dopamine receptors and significant anticholinergic profile may account for lowered seizure threshold (Silvestri et al 1998)	The risk of seizure can be prevented by using lowest possible dose and avoiding rapid dose increases. Discontinuation of clozapine may not be necessary. Co-administration of anticonvulsant, e.g. sodium valproate (not carbamazepine) to prevent further occurrences. Monitoring of clozapine plasma levels and use of electroencephalography, especially for high-risk clients.
Constipation	Antagonistic action on muscarinic receptors	Symptomatic treatment with stool softeners, laxatives, fibre supplements (e.g. Fibrogel and lactulose) and adequate fluid intake in addition to appropriate diet.

Table 17.6 Managing adverse effects with Paul (*cont'd*)

Side effect	Receptor effects of antipsychotic*	Interventions/action
Urinary incontinence (nocturnal urinary incontinence, increased frequency, urgency and retention)	Blockade of muscarinic receptors in the peripheral nervous system, as well as the sedative effects of clozapine causing pathophysiology – mechanism fails to indicate when bladder is full	Reviewing and reducing medication dosage. Use of imipramine (Lieberman et al 1994) or desmopressin (Taylor & Hardy 1997) in unresolved and severe cases has been suggested. Input from incontinence specialist may be valuable in advising any remedies and care alternatives in some cases.
Weight gain (can also affect a client's physical health because of the increased risk of cardiovascular problems and the potential development of diabetes)	Blockade of serotonin and histamine H_1 receptors	Regular monitoring of body weight. Psychoeducation about possible side effects and proper diet and exercise plan put in place prior to and/or together with commencement of medication treatment. Healthy diet advice. Any significant weight gain addressed promptly and measures reviewed. Ensure regular physical health check up if potential to develop physical problems is identified. If the above measures fail, consider change to a different atypical or a conventional antipsychotic (NICE 2002a)
Sexual dysfunction (e.g. period problems/ irregularity; galactorrhoea (secretion of milk); enlargement of breasts; impotence (failure of erection and ejaculation) tends to be under-reported	Drug-induced hyperprolactinaemia, associated with dopamine D_2 receptors	Dosage reduction or switching to an antipsychotic that does not raise prolactin levels, e.g. quetiapine (Gray 1999).

* See Fig. 17.2 for explanation of terms

The successful outcome of these strategies and interventions relies on effective multidisciplinary working and collaboration with the client. When there is a lack of understanding or knowledge about medication regimes, specialist pharmacological advice may need to be called in. In addition, multiagency collaboration is required when a client is discharged from hospital. For example, liaison between the GP, the clozapine clinic, outpatient follow-up and the day hospital are necessary to enable a comprehensive package of care that addresses the individual's clinical, emotional and social needs (NICE 2002b). Medication should be regarded as an essential component in helping to keep an individual stable enough for the possible benefits of all other treatments to aid progress towards recovery.

POLYPHARMACY

Schizophrenia is undoubtedly a complex and distressing illness that is still far from manageable with just medication. In the search for the ultimate resolution of every sign and symptom experienced, the prescription of more than one antipsychotic at the same time – so called polypharmacy – is frequently pursued (Taylor et al 2000). Polypharmacy problems increase with mixing typical and atypical antipsychotics on the same clients (NICE 2002a, b), as a growing body of research has found no additional therapeutic effects and little improvement in the side effects of both typical and atypical antipsychotics (Shiloh et al 1997). Therefore, the new prescribing guidelines issued by the National Institute for Clinical Excellence specify that concurrent use of antipsychotics should only be considered for short periods to cover changeover of medications. The only exceptional cases, such as are highlighted in the case study, should be those who have treatment-resistant schizophrenia and experience insufficient effectiveness with clozapine alone (NICE 2002a).

Practitioners should also be extra cautious that the concurrent use of two or more antipsychotics may result in the client being exposed to a high antipsychotic dose (High Dose Consensus Working Group, in press). Subsequently, polypharmacy may increase the propensity to cause various side effects, which may in turn jeopardise concordance and the client's subjective satisfaction.

Additionally, as each antipsychotic carries with it a specific profile of side effects, those under the polypharmacy regimen tend to be more complicated. Reviewing the prevailing literature and consulting the relevant experts, especially over the interactions of various drugs, and collaborating with multidisciplinary professionals form the essential basics in working out other potential management strategies and the most effective medication regime (Sin & Gamble 2003).

The presentation of side effects and therapeutic effects becomes even more complicated when polypharmacy involves mixing medication from different groups, e.g. the concurrent use of an antidepressant and benzodiazepine with an antipsychotic, as illustrated in the case study. Pharmacologically speaking, antipsychotics and antidepressants work in opposite ways within the brain; the interactions are much more complex than the interactions between similar medication from the same group and may even counteract or reinforce one another's actions/effects (for examples, see Rang & Dale 1991, King 1995, Taylor & Hardy 1997). Therefore, practitioners should be mindful when evaluating the purpose and ultimate benefits of concurrent use of multiple medications (i.e. combining typical and atypical antipsychotics). A more sensible approach is to try another antipsychotic, as an optimal medication regime is the simplest, most cost- and therapy-effective and easier for clients to follow (see Case study box below).

Case study – Paul (*cont'd*)

With Paul's regime, concomitant fluoxetine has been associated with elevated clozapine levels (Novartis 1999). At the same time, clozapine may enhance the central effects of alcohol, monoamine oxidase inhibitors and central nervous system depressants (including narcotics, benzodiazepines and antihistamines) (Novartis 1999). The sedative effects of benzodiazepines may also be increased if they are taken in conjunction with clozapine, and result in increased risk of circulatory collapse. Therefore, Paul's plasma clozapine level should be monitored carefully, as the continuous use of fluoxetine is identified as necessary. Lorazepam was replaced and stopped gradually. Alternative treatments for anxiety, e.g. cognitive–behavioural therapy for Paul's situation, were sought.

Source: adapted from Sin & Gamble 2003

ENHANCING CONCORDANCE AND OPTIMISING THE MEDICATION REGIME

The British National Service Framework for Mental Health (Department of Health 1999) has recommended that compliance therapy be incorporated into the routine clinical practice of practitioners with its proven benefits in improving treatment adherence and clinical outcomes in schizophrenia (Kemp et al 1996, 1998, Gray et al 2002, Haynes et al 2002). Psychoeducation on medication, both for therapeutic and side effects, has also been proved as beneficial in improving users' knowledge and increasing insight, even in acutely ill groups (Kavanagh et al 2003). Coupled with good medication management, which strives to optimise the treatment regime to its most tolerable, this will improve concordance rates and hopefully prevent relapses.

The key principles of psychoeducation on medication and work on concordance borrow largely from motivational interviewing (see Ch. 14 for detailed account), the cognitive–behavioural therapy and educational approaches (Gamble & Hart 2003, Kemp 1997, Kemp et al 1996, 1998), which allow clients to make an informed choice as to their treatment and to consider their own benefits and risks in taking and maintaining the medication. Some key principles and techniques in medication concordance work are:

◆ assessing clients' knowledge, understanding and stance towards medication treatment: undertaking an illness timeline; the Knowledge about Schizophrenia Interview (KASI), adapted version for clients' use, has a specific section on eliciting clients' knowledge on their prescribed medication, how long they will need to stay on it, possible side effects, etc. (Barrowclough & Tarrier 1995)
◆emphasising personal choice and responsibility
◆creating a non-blaming atmosphere in order for mutual discussion to take place
◆focusing on eliciting clients' concerns: by collecting and discussing evidence for and against medication; drawing up a balance sheet for pros and cons of taking medication
◆using and respecting clients' opinions: reviewing clients' experience of treatment using relevant assessment tools, e.g. LUNSERS, SESCAM
◆supporting self-efficacy – devising a medication problem-solving plan aiming for the client to devise measures to 'stay well'.

The prescription of antipsychotic medication should be preceded by a joint-decision made by the individual and the clinician responsible for treatment, based on an informed discussion of the relative benefits of the drugs and their side-effect profiles (NICE 2002a). If clients are encouraged to have treatment choice, they need to be knowledgeable about the different recommended treatment choices before they can commit themselves. Knowing and understanding possible side effects and prognosis usually predicts better concordance as preparation for side effects and therapeutic effects from both clients and carers are the prerequisite for commitment to long-term treatment regimes (Burnett 1994). Essentially, clients must be presumed to be competent to make decisions about their medication, unless proven otherwise. Unmanaged side effects of antipsychotic medication treatment and the stereotypical attitude of assuming that clients are either incompetent or insightless can only help in alienating clients. The collaborative medication management process described can address how practitioners and clients can work together to overcome this.

CONCLUSION

Instead of being regarded as a 'cure' for psychosis, 'antipsychotic therapy should be initiated as part of a comprehensive package of care that addresses the individual's clinical, emotional and social needs' (NICE 2002a, p. 19). An optimal regime of medication treatment should aim for maximum benefits in symptom control, minimal side effects and a simple regime to allow clients to maintain a stable mental state for further interventions to improve coping and functioning. This makes many demands of practitioners and those who educate them. Mastering the evidence-based tools will mean nothing if we do not care enough to rectify the identified side effects; asking clients for their opinion will be meaningless if we do not listen and adapt accordingly.

References

Banning M 2004 The use of structured assessments, practical skills and performance indicators to assess the ability of pre-registration nursing students to apply the principles of pharmacology and therapeutics to the medication management needs of patients. Nurse Education in Practice (in press)

Barrowclough C, Tarrier N 1995 Families of schizophrenic patients: cognitive behavioural interventions. Chapman & Hall, London, ch 11

Bennett J, Done J, Harrison-Read P, Hunt B 1995a A rating scale/checklist for the assessment of the side-effects of antipsychotic drugs. In: Brooker C, White E (eds) Community psychiatric nursing: a research perspective, vol 3. Chapman & Hall, London, pp 1–19

Bennett J, Done J, Hunt B 1995b Assessing the side effects of antipsychotic drugs: a survey of CPN practice. Journal of Psychiatric and Mental Health Nursing 2:177–182

British Medical Association/Royal Pharmaceutical Society 2003 British National Formulary 45. London: Royal Pharmaceutical Society of Great Britain

Burkley P 1997 New dimensions in the pharmacologic treatment of schizophrenia and related psychoses. The Journal of Clinical Pharmacology 37:363–378

Burnett S 1994 A new lease on life. Nursing Times 90(30):57

Day J C, Wood G, Dewey M, Bentall R P 1995 A self-rating scale for measuring neuroleptic side-effects. British Journal of Psychiatry 166:650–653

Department of Health 1999 A national service framework for mental health. The Stationery Office, London

Dev V J, Krupp P 1995 Adverse event profile and safety of clozapine. Review of Contemporary Pharmacotherapy 6:197–208

Gamble C, Hart C 2003 The use of psychosocial interventions. Nursing Times 99(9):46–47

Geddes J, Freemantle N, Harrison P, Bebbington P 2000 Atypical antipsychotics in the treatment of schizophrenia: systematic overview and meta-regression analysis. British Medical Journal 321:1371–1376

Gournay K, Gray R 1998 The role of new drugs in the treatment of schizophrenia. Mental Health Nursing 18:21–24

References (cont'd)

Gray R 1999 Antipsychotics, side-effects and effective management. Mental Health Practice 2:14–20

Gray R, Robson D, Bressington D 2002 Medication management for people with a diagnosis of schizophrenia. Nursing Times 98(47):38–40

Guy W 1976 ECDEU assessment manual for psychopharmacology, revised edn. US Department of Health, Education and Welfare, Washington, DC

Haddock G 1994 Auditory Hallucinations Rating Scale. Unpublished scale, University of Manchester

Haynes R B, Montague P, Olier T et al 2002 Interventions for helping patients follow prescription for medication (Cochrane Review). In: Cochrane Library, Issue 5. Update Software, Oxford

High Dose Consensus Working Group (in press) Revised draft of high dose consensus statement. Royal College of Psychiatrists, Royal College of Nursing, Royal Pharmaceutical Society, London

Hogan T P, Awad A G, Eastwood R 1983 A self-report scale predictive of drug compliance in schizophrenics: reliability and discriminative validity. Psychological Medicine 13:177–183

Kane J, Honigfeld G, Singer J et al 1988 Clozapine for the treatment-resistant schizophrenic (a double-blind comparison with chlorpromazine). Archives of General Psychiatry 45:789–796

Kavanagh K, Duncan-McConnell S, Greenwood K et al 2003 Educating acute inpatients about their medication: is it worth it? An exploratory study of group education for patients on a psychiatric intensive care unit. Journal of Mental Health 12:71–80

Kemp R 1997 Compliance therapy manual. Bethlem and Maudsley NHS Trust, London

Kemp R, Hayward P, Applewhaite G et al 1996 Compliance therapy in psychotic patients: randomised controlled trial. British Medical Journal 312:345–349

Kemp R, Kirov G, Everitt B et al 1998 Randomised controlled trial of compliance therapy: 18-month follow-up. British Journal of Psychiatry 172:413–419

King D (ed) 1995 Seminars in clinical psychopharmacology. Royal College of Psychiatrists, London

Krawiecka M, Goldberg D, Vaughan M 1977 A standardised psychiatric assessment scale for rating chronic psychotic patients. Acta Psychiatrica Scandinavica 55:229–308

Lancashire S 1998 KGV (M) Scale. Unpublished scale. Institute of Psychiatry, London

Lane R D, Glazer W M, Hansen T E et al 1985 Assessment of tardive dyskinesia using the Abnormal Involuntary Movements Scale. Journal of Nervous and Mental Disorders 173:353–357

Lieberman J A, Safferman A Z, Pollack S et al 1994 Clinical effects of clozapine in chronic schizophrenia: response to treatment and predictors of outcome. American Journal of Psychiatry 151:1744–1752

Meltzer H Y 1992 The importance of serotonin-dopamine interactions in the action of clozapine. British Journal of Psychiatry 160 (suppl 17):22–29

NICE 2002a Guideline on the use of newer (atypical) antipsychotic drugs for the treatment of schizophrenia (no 43). NICE, London

NICE 2002b NICE guideline on core interventions in the treatment and management of schizophrenia in primary and secondary care. NICE, London

Novartis 1999 Clozaril – summary of product characteristics: UK-specific. Novartis, Surrey

References (cont'd)

Rang H O, Dale M M 1991 Pharmacology, 2nd edn. Churchill Livingstone, Edinburgh

Shiloh R, Zemishlany Z, Aizenberg M et al 1997 Sulpiride augmentation in people with schizophrenia partially responsive to clozapine (a double-blind, placebo-controlled study). British Journal of Psychiatry 171:569–573

Silvestri R C, Bromfield E B, Khoshbin S 1998 Clozapine-induced seizures and EEG abnormalities in ambulatory psychiatric patients. Annals of Pharmacotherapy 32:1147–1151

Sin J 2000 One step at a time: negative symptoms. Mental Health Care 4:97–101

Sin J, Gamble C 2003 Managing side-effects to the optimum: valuing a client's experience. Journal of Psychiatric and Mental Health Nursing 10:147–153

Tandon R, Jibson M D 2003 Efficacy of newer generation antipsychotics in the treatment of schizophrenia. Psychoneuroendocrinology 28:9–26

Taylor D, Hardy S 1997 Psychopharmacology. In: Thomas B, Hardy S, Cutting P (eds) Stuart and Sundeen's mental health nursing principles and practice. Mosby, St Louis, MO

Taylor D, Mace S, Mir S, Kerwin R 2000 A prescription survey of the use of atypical antipsychotics for hospital inpatients in the United Kingdom. International Journal of Psychiatry in Clinical Practice 4:41–46

Winger G, Hofman F, Woods J 1992 A handbook on drug and alcohol abuse: the biomedical aspects. Oxford University Press

Annotated further reading

Julien R 1995 A primer of drug action – a concise nontechnical guide to the actions, uses and side effects of psychoactive drugs. Freeman, New York

As its title promises, you can have a concise non-technical guide into all the scientific and dry aspects of psychopharmacology with this book. It gives a very good review of synaptic transmission, pharmacokinetic and pharmacodynamic actions of various drugs on various receptors with some clear and useful diagrams.

Taylor D, Hardy S 1997 Psychopharmacology. In: Thomas B, Hardy S, Cutting, P (eds) Stuart and Sundeen's principles and practices of mental health nursing. Mosby-Wolfe, London, pp 411–440.

This chapter provides an easy-to-read and -understand introduction to psychopharmacology for all non-medical mental health workers (actually, not just for nurses, as its title suggests). It is particularly good in bridging the theories and knowledge of psychopharmacology into clinical practice in terms of assessing and managing side effects, providing psychoeducation and promotion of concordance with the medication regime, drug interactions, etc.

18

Integrated approaches to relapse prevention

Jo Denney and Eric Davis

KEY ISSUES

◆ Integrated approaches to relapse prevention
◆ Rationale for intervention
◆ Review of idiosyncratic and common early warning signs
◆ Relating how approaches can be integrated into routine clinical work

INTRODUCTION

The development of psychosocial approaches to psychosis has proceeded rapidly over the past decade, expanding the range of effective interventions, which previously relied on medication alone. Research demonstrates that treatments in early episode psychosis, including family interventions, are useful in reducing the risk of relapse and improving prognosis. However, the evidence base, which guides choices about interventions, may fail to provide guidance about the integration of a variety of approaches within clinical practice and may not take full account of the priorities expressed by users and carers in providing the rationale for treatment selection.

This chapter has three aims. The first is to present a case that illustrates the provision of a comprehensive approach to relapse prevention within a routine clinical setting. The study shows casework underpinned by the evidence base but also demonstrates flexibility in meeting the needs of a service user (Adrian) and his mother (Charlotte) that is informed by the philosophy of recovery. Anthony (1993) describes services delivered within this framework as conversant with strategies not only designed to reduce symptoms but also aiming to limit dysfunction in task performance, disability in role performance and disadvantage because of restricted opportunity. The philosophy recognises the episodic nature of mental illness but also acknowledges the ability of service users to recover from relapse and to gain mastery over the interference of symptoms. Recovery models further identify the mental health services as only one of a range of options that may be helpful to service users in recovery. Of equal importance are resources, including family support and access to non-mental health environments. Both the family work and early interventions for psychosis in the case study can be seen to include goals in accordance with such a philosophy.

The second aim of the chapter is to review idiosyncratic and common early warning signs, using the intervention with Adrian, and the third is to identify how to construct a relapse prevention plan that is transferable and can be used for early and chronic psychosis.

EARLY INTERVENTION FOR PSYCHOSIS

Recently, a growing body of research has suggested that the early years of psychosis may constitute a 'critical period' influencing the long-term course of psychosis, and that delays in first treatment increase early relapse (Macmillan et al 1986). This pioneering work in the UK led to increased optimism, so that other researchers and clinicians began to explore not only the concept of early intervention but also whether it might indeed herald better outcomes (Birchwood et al 1992, McGorry et al 1996). They found that early intervention in the clinical setting can improve long-term outcome in important ways such as increased social functioning and starting or recommencing employment.

Essentially, early intervention comprises two approaches: first, the early detection and treatment of psychosis and, second, the provision of treatment and psychological intervention during the 'critical' early phase (Birchwood 2000, IRIS Research Group 2000). Birchwood, in his review of recent research, suggests that aggressive social and psychological deterioration occurs in people thought to be experiencing first-episode schizophrenia or psychosis. He suggests that these deleterious effects have largely been completed by 3 years after the onset of illness. Therefore it logically follows that treatment should be assertively targeted within this 3-year timescale. It is thought that intervention efforts following the 'plateau of morbidity' (after 3 years) will face greater challenges than those efforts implemented during the first episode.

From the research literature, two further specific variables are thought to be of key importance in terms of their relationship to the 'critical period'. The first is duration of untreated psychosis (DUP). On average, this is very long, usually between 1 and 2 years (Keshavan & Schooler 1992, Larsen et al 2000). Larsen and colleagues suggest that lengthy DUP is associated with poorer global outcome and that reducing DUP represents an important challenge for service providers.

In addition to DUP, certain researchers have advocated that an even more proactive stance is required so that clinical intervention commences in the pre-psychotic stage (Thompson et al 2000, French & Walford 2001). Thus Thompson and colleagues describe their work in the personal assessment and crisis evaluation clinic. They report that it is possible to identify young people at ultra-high risk of developing psychosis and to monitor them both prior to and during the onset of psychosis. Various clinical criteria in use have helped detect those at risk of psychosis, allowing future treatment to delay or prevent psychosis, besides reducing DUP.

Case study – Adrian

Adrian is a young adult still engaged with the higher education system. He first experienced psychological difficulties in his mid-teens, which led to support from the local child and adolescent mental health services. The problems subsided and Adrian progressed to university, where he successfully completed his first 2 years as an undergraduate. His lecturers and peers then began to notice early, subtle changes in his personality and psychological functioning. He became more irritable, dispirited and began to display a 'haunted' look. Gradually this gave way to further overt behavioural changes. He became physically aggressive towards his peers and eventually damaged property. This culminated in a referral to a consultant psychiatrist, who organised hospitalisation and further psychological work with the author (ED).

When Adrian became ill he was unable to return to university at the end of the holidays. He therefore stayed at the family home on discharge from hospital, with his mother Charlotte who works part-time. Adrian's parents are divorced and his siblings have left home; they live some distance away. During recovery, in addition to psychological work, Adrian attended day hospital at a Community Mental Health Resource Centre, where he participated in the occupational therapy programme, in preparation for his goal of return to university.

Treatment approach

The general approach with Adrian was within a cognitive–behavioural therapy framework. A more specific aim was to construct a highly detailed working model of the psychological experiences and changes that Adrian had undergone. Studies have found that changes in domains such as thoughts, feelings and behaviours precede the onset of psychotic episodes. Such prepsychotic changes are known as prodromal changes. The nature of such changes is recognised as idiosyncratic, leading to the concept of a 'relapse signature' in

Table 18.1 Early warning signs of psychotic relapse

Thinking/perception	Feeling	Behaviours
Thoughts are racing	Afraid of going crazy	Difficulty sleeping
Senses seem sharper	Sad or low	Speech comes out jumbled
Thinking you have special	Anxious and restless	and filled with odd words
powers	Increasingly religious	Talking or smiling to
Thinking you can read	As if you're being watched	yourself
other people's minds	Isolated	Acting suspiciously, as if
Thinking other people	Tired or lacking energy	being watched
can read your mind	Confused or puzzled	Behaving oddly for no
Receiving personal	Forgetful or far away	reason
messages from the	In another world	Spending time alone
TV or radio	Strong and powerful	Neglecting your
Having difficulty making	Unable to cope with	appearance
decisions	everyday tasks	Acting as if you are
Experiencing strange	As if you are being	somebody else
sensations	punished	Not seeing people
Preoccupied with one or	As if you cannot trust	Not eating
two things	other people	Not leaving the house
Thinking you might be	Irritable	Drinking more
somebody else`	As if you do not need	Smoking more
Seeing visions or things	sleep	Movements are slow
others cannot see	Guilty	Unable to sit down for
Thinking people are		long
talking about you		Behaving aggressively
Thinking people are		
against you		
Having more nightmares		
Having difficulty		
concentrating		
Thinking bizarre things		
Thinking your thoughts		
are controlled		
Hearing voices		
Thinking a part of you		
has changed shape		

Additional examples of idiosyncratic early warning signs
◆ Wearing all-black clothes
◆ Teasing a pet
◆ Spending larger amounts of money
◆ 'Having a funny look in your eye'
◆ Preoccupation with the media
◆ Changing appearance

Source: Birchwood et al 2000

which the pattern of such psychological changes, taken together and often occurring in a predictable sequence, indicates a potential further psychotic episode (Birchwood et al 2000, French & Walford 2001; see Table 18.1 for general and idiosyncratic examples). Birchwood et al describe a five-stage intervention that provided a framework for construction of such a relapse signature with Adrian.

Engagement and education

The first stage of work began with specific attempts at engagement, together with the provision of relevant education. The early sessions explored Adrian's attitude towards his illness. A normalising rationale was used, in which psychotic experiences are viewed as existing on a continuum with normality, and the view is that given enough stress it is likely that most people would experience certain psychotic phenomena (Nuechterlein & Dawson 1984). The aim was therefore to emphasise commonality with (rather than difference from) others.

It was at this stage of the individual intervention that work with Charlotte was introduced. The weeks preceding admission had been difficult for her and, as Adrian's main source of support on discharge, it was thought that her needs as a carer required consideration. In addition, there is a robust evidence base to suggest that family work significantly reduces the risk of relapse in schizophrenia (Pilling et al 2002). This has led to recommendations for the provision of family interventions for psychosis in both the clinical guidelines for the management of schizophrenia (National Institute for Clinical Excellence 2002) and as a key element in provision of service for carers and families (Department of Health 2002; Box 18.1).

Family Intervention

A family intervention approach of the type described elsewhere in this volume was adopted. Adrian agreed to participate in the family work but expressed some unease about the possible blurring of subject matter that he was only comfortable discussing in an individual setting with family discussion. To prevent this possible rupture to the working alliance that Adrian had formed with his psychotherapist, two occupational therapists from the community mental health team were enlisted to facilitate family work – the author (JD) and a staff member involved with Adrian's day hospital programme.

Assessment

Initial assessment of Charlotte's needs using the Relative Assessment Interview (RAI; Barrowclough & Tarrier 1997) provided information about her perspec-

> **Box 18.1** Discussion – does a combination of successful psychosocial approaches lead to a better outcome?
>
> Given the advantages conferred by the addition of either early interventions or family work to routine care, it would be reasonable to suppose that supplying both interventions might increase the positive effects on relapse rate still further. Unfortunately there is little clinical evidence to support this theory: individual studies (Linzen et al 1996) have shown no 'added value' in providing family work alongside an individual psychosocial intervention, a finding endorsed by meta-analysis (Pitschel-Wals et al 2001). However, although the clinical evidence for the benefits of a combined approach is weak, research into the needs and preferences of the families of service users in early episodes demonstrates a requirement for support, beyond brief psychoeducation, that is provided in the home environment (de Haan et al 2001). This finding is endorsed by Rethink (2002), which states the importance of psychological therapies for individuals but also describes the needs of carers for inclusion, involvement and support from services to carry out their valuable role in the recovery process. A needs-led response, informed by all the relevant aspects of the evidence base, should therefore guide choice of intervention.

tive on Adrian's recent relapse, including her own distress at the recurrence. It also detected renewed thoughts that family changes prior to Adrian's first episode might have caused his schizophrenia.

The interview indicated Charlotte's expertise in the early stages of relapse in identifying an escalation of changes in Adrian's behaviour and mood that she clearly attributed to the onset of illness. This awareness, and the sympathy she described herself feeling for Adrian as he had struggled to contain the effects of symptoms, alerted the family workers to the possibility of Charlotte's later involvement in explicit relapse prevention strategies. This perception was strengthened by the outcome of the Knowledge About Schizophrenia Interview (Barrowclough & Tarrier 1997). Charlotte scored highly (4) on the categories about diagnosis, symptoms and medication because she had received helpful information in the past but also because of her own skill in locating reliable information about schizophrenia. She was less aware of ways to manage current tensions and those that had arisen during relapse, and identified avoidance of communication (as a way of avoiding confrontation) as the family's principal coping style.

The initial aim was therefore to:

◆ update the information already obtained
◆ identify specific current stressors and develop coping strategies

◆ develop problem-solving skills
◆ consider opportunities for participation at the 'staying well' phase.

It was hoped that the successful achievement of these aims would contribute towards Adrian's goal of return to university and resumption of his third year of study.

The psychoeducational element of family work was focused on updating and expanding the current information that Charlotte had identified. This stage proved unexpectedly problematic, as the family workers underestimated Adrian's discomfort about contributing his own experience of symptoms to the discussion. Previous positive experiences of service users contributing willingly to family work in an expert capacity had led to an assumption that all would be willing to do so. Inadequate engagement with Adrian by the lead family worker, who was unfamiliar with him before family work began, prevented a proper appreciation of individual need from correcting the belief that this was the method of choice. Given Adrian's determination to look forward and the fact that his behaviour during relapse had been painfully uncharacteristic of his usually warm relationship with Charlotte, it should have been predictable that sharing some of his experiences would be very difficult for him.

The educational material provided was therefore general and discussion based on literature (rather than Adrian's experience) was more acceptable. Charlotte was able to share her perspective on the relapse in a non-blaming way. This stage was also useful in facilitating clear statements of support for Adrian's goals from Charlotte and an expressed desire to be involved in supporting both rehabilitation strategies and relapse prevention measures.

The current stressors within the family environment were clarified by use of a problems, strengths and needs table. It was evident that many present problems were driven by anxieties about the future. The family wanted to be proactive in adopting coping strategies that would increase Adrian's chances of completing his studies but were unsure how to go about this. Principal subjects included Charlotte's need to identify and provide the most helpful base from which Adrian could rebuild his academic career; Adrian's anxiety about his ability to prepare himself adequately for a return to study and a recognition from both that reintegration would require planning, which (aside from the academic demands) would incorporate elements of stress management aimed at areas such as competency in activities of daily living and social reintegration.

Simply promoting a forum for communication assisted in the goal of stress reduction. Charlotte had previously considered moving to Adrian's university town, a considerable disruption that would have necessitated sale of the family home and loss of employment. Adrian was surprised to hear of this possibility and was able to reassure her that it would not be necessary. A timely reminder of the need for time apart for family members (Kuipers et al 1992), coupled with awareness of current tensions around Adrian's lack of participation in household management, built the case for recognising Charlotte's helpful intent but acknowledging the drawbacks of this option for achieving the original goal.

Consideration of alternative ways to approach this issue led to a focus on the development of problem-solving strategies as a relapse prevention measure. This was initially modelled by the family workers, who withdrew guidance as the family gained skills. This part of the intervention used the six-step problem-solving strategy described in Chapter 13 to construct an analysis of problems; an example is given in Box 18.2 applied to the problem 'Lack of exercise'. The example has been chosen because it demonstrates the incorporation of stressors that were current but also contained a 'future' component pertinent to Adrian's successful reintegration at university. It therefore illustrates how techniques learnt at an early stage of the intervention for management of symptoms and their outcomes can usefully be adapted later on in recovery to include the service user and their family in developing positive life experiences.

Box 18.2 Six-step problem-solving in recovery

Step 1: What exactly is the problem?

◆ **What is the problem?** Lack of exercise

◆ **How is that a problem?** More would be good for mental health: lack of exercise contributes to low self-confidence; when unfit Adrian is anxious about his physical health because of some familial vulnerability; lack of challenges maintains lack of interest, social isolation and low motivation, all viewed as contributory to relapse by Adrian.

◆ **Where is it a problem?** At home and at university.

◆ **Why is it a problem?** Hard to get to facilities. Lack of money. Low motivation.

◆ **Who is it a problem for?** Adrian, for the above reasons. Charlotte, because it increases Adrian's time spent inactively at home.

Steps 2 and 3: Possible solutions and their evaluation

◆ **Cycling**: Disadvantages – Can't do it and doesn't know of any clubs, the preferred environment, which would increase opportunities for meeting people and having fun. Advantages – Healthy, cheap, would solve transport reliance on irregular buses or lifts from Charlotte.

◆ **Dancing**: Disadvantages – silly, silly costumes, not much rhythm. Advantages – none!

> **Box 18.2** Six-step problem-solving in recovery (*cont'd*)
>
> ◆ **Kick boxing**: Disadvantages – perception is, it is aggressive. Might attract people very dissimilar to Adrian. Advantages – Adrian would feel less threatened. It is social and the advertisement looked fun.
>
> ◆ **Fencing**: Disadvantages – little opportunity to try it in home town. Advantages – feel motivated to try, inexpensive at university, new skill would boost confidence; you can learn it quite quickly; might attract like-minded people, provides a social environment.
>
> **Step 4: Choosing the best solution**
> Cycling is the most realistic choice for the current situation and would be transferable on return to university. Fencing, the most attractive option, would become possible on return to education.
>
> **Step 5: Plan implementation – goals**
> Adrian would go bicycle riding with his day hospital therapist as part of his programme. Once sufficient skill was attained he would cycle to the day hospital.
> Adrian would make a plan to locate the university fencing club during freshers' week, when they would be advertising and representatives would be available for Adrian to judge their compatibility with his needs.
>
> **Step 6: Review progress**
> Family work sessions were used as the forum for monitoring bike riding progress. Adrian felt this was quite slow but eventually achieved his goal of riding to the day hospital. This was one of a number of goals that led to additions in Adrian's day hospital programme and demonstrated the use of involving staff already facilitating the rehabilitation process. In addition, it located the responsibility for skills development partially outside the home, with the possibility of negotiated practice at home if it was required. This reduced tension around the allocation of domestic responsibilities at home.

Delivery of relapse prevention strategies

Family work progressed to the stage where development of 'staying well' strategies would form the next phase. Given the high level of Charlotte's awareness and enthusiasm one possibility would have been to approach identification of the relapse signature at least in part through family work and joint discussion. However, Adrian's negative experiences of discussing personal experience of symptoms during psychoeducation prompted open discussion about how to elicit the level of idiosyncratic detail required for an accurate relapse prevention plan while also accessing Charlotte's knowledge. The most acceptable solution was to identify early warning signs through individual work with Adrian and Charlotte separately. Having achieved its aims, family work was terminated after 5 months.

Identification of the relapse signature

The second part of the individual prodromal work was used to construct a hypothesis about Adrian's individualised relapse signature. Information from Adrian and Charlotte was used to construct the relapse signature. For Adrian this process began with assessment using the KGV scale (Krawiecka et al 1977), otherwise known as the Manchester Scale. It has recently been radically revised by Stuart Lancashire at the Institute of Psychiatry. It is a semi-structured psychiatric assessment tool that uses a phenomenological battery of questions to elicit rich clinical information, which can then be tailored for more specific purposes such as relapse signature formation leading to psychological formulation. Information from Charlotte elicited from the RAI was incorporated that provided further valuable material regarding Adrian's prodromal signs and symptoms.

The time line exercise

Adrian was supported in constructing a time line of significant external events proceeding backwards in time from the date of referral to the mental health services. Various early warning signs were 'pegged' to two major life events: first the onset of an exam and second the break-up of his parent's relationship. The break-up had caused Adrian great distress and this event had probably played a major part in triggering his psychotic episode.

Early warning signs grid

The information gleaned from Adrian and Charlotte was, through carefully structured questioning (by use of the KGV and the RAI) integrated into the seven stage early warning signs grid (EWSG) devised by the author (ED). This is illustrated in Table 18.2. An alternative method of constructing an early warning signs plan is via the card sort exercise developed by Birchwood et al (2000).

The construction of the EWSG took place over a number of carefully focused sessions. These sessions were highly structured, with initial information from the assessments revisited in careful fashion. The EWSG was described as an attempt to devise a working model of Adrian's experiences that would be used proactively to circumvent emerging psychological difficulty. The use of open-ended reflective questions – guided discovery – and collaborative setting of work between sessions for Adrian to bring back to therapy were consistent themes of clinical work and are thought to be beneficial in constructing a formulation for both user and therapist (Liese & Beck 1997).

Table 18.2 Adrian's early warning signs grid

Relevant domains of change	Early Green	→ Amber	Late Red
Somatic	◆ Preoccupation with muscular stiffness ◆ Tingling and pins and needles (late green)	◆ 'Burning sensation in brain – not painful' ◆ Harder to move my eyes	◆ Preoccupation with internal organs malfunctioning – e.g. kidneys but especially heart (grandfather died of heart attack)
Interpersonal		◆ Empathy towards others decreases as psychosis progresses	◆ Difficulties with other people increases and social interaction is more arduous ◆ (Increasing paranoia)
Situational			◆ Lectures become difficult due to sensory overload ◆ Applies to other situations where groups of people are routinely found, e.g. town centre
Cognitive	◆ Early bodily stages of stiffness are like 'mummification' ◆ Other people experience this, but aren't worried about it (late green)	◆ People in Africa don't drink milk – therefore it's not normal ◆ Toxins are being ingested – and nutrition is adversely affected ◆ Exercise 'will connect me back together' ◆ Far Eastern religions are good and most of Western culture is bad	◆ 'My lecturers are Nazis' ◆ 'People are out to get me/harm me' ◆ Police cars and ambulances are monitoring me ◆ Other people are causing my present difficulties ◆ The caretaker is a cannibal ◆ Security guards are monitoring me – with intent

Table 18.2 Adrian's early warning signs grid (*cont'd*)

Relevant domains of change	Early Green	→ Amber	Late Red
			◆ At yoga – not flexible. This is because kidneys are not working well ◆ Parasites infest my blood ◆ I will be forcibly conscripted into the marines
Affective	◆ Low mood ◆ Decreasing concentration	◆ Irritability ◆ Agitation and fear	◆ Feelings of passivity ◆ Feelings of anger and hostility towards others ◆ Fear of God
Behavioural		◆ Selective as to cosmetics used (only use shaving foam and soap, avoid use of toothpaste and shampoo) ◆ Vigorous exercise ◆ Giving possessions to mother and charity shops ◆ Throwing possessions away ◆ Selective eating and drinking (avoidance of alcohol, coffee, milk, cereal)	◆ Active avoidance of others – and therefore greatly increased level of self-isolation

Development of a relapse drill

In this third stage of the process, the relapse drill considers three areas for intervention:

◆ Pathways to support (service contacts 24 hours per day, including weekends)

Table 18.2 Adrian's early warning signs grid (*cont'd*)

Relevant domains of change	Early Green	→ Amber	Late Red
Sensory–perceptual	◆ Other people's movements and facial expressions seem impossible (and annoying sometimes) (late green)	◆ Noise distortion ◆ Fridge humming sounds very loud ◆ Sometimes colours and images are more beautiful and vibrant (could be people) with positive associations. Sometimes could be uglier and as if frozen still, although changing with negative associations (e.g. contempt for Western culture) ◆ Figures 'bathed in light' move towards me	◆ Aural acuity increases so 'hearing becomes almost painful', e.g. lectures

◆ Service interventions (medication review, cognitive therapy, home treatment)
◆ Personal coping strategies.

Thus, discussion for Adrian and Charlotte centred upon clear support contacts within the town, should there be concern. Various options were carefully considered should it be thought that Adrian was moving towards prodromal signs and symptoms as delineated in the EWSG. Adrian had previously found that reducing social activity and increasing medication had helped in the past.

Rehearsal and monitoring

Adrian and Charlotte were provided with their copies of the relapse prevention sheet as the fourth part of the process. This was also disseminated among the workers involved in Adrian's care and used as a standard part of the Care Programme Approach. Monitoring and relapse prevention were viewed as a shared endeavour between service user, carer and mental health team. The relapse drill was rehearsed using personalised scenarios and also role-played so that Adrian would be more sure of his response should early warning signs be detected, particularly fear and despondency.

Clarification of the relapse signature and relapse drill

The fifth part of the process represents 'work in progress'. As further warning signs come to light through therapy, these are incorporated into Adrian's care plan. Further coping strategies are actively explored and cognitive intervention continues. Therefore, impending or even actual relapse is used as a positive opportunity to revise the relapse signature and improve the relapse drill, with the overarching aim being to increase control over the illness.

Reflection

Overall, the work with Adrian and Charlotte resulted in a clear relapse prevention procedure reinforced by appropriate psychosocial interventions. Although the activities and goals of the family work and other routine interventions in Adrian's care plan may have been less overtly labelled as relapse prevention measures than the individual treatment, the evidence base supports their effectiveness in contributing towards this end. One potential difficulty for individual and family work lies in the amount of time required to elicit highly detailed information that can be used in a productive fashion for service users and their carers. Also, clinicians need to feel confident that they can practise such techniques, which have demonstrable benefit to service users but which require appropriate training (Davis & Coupland 2000).

WIDER IMPLICATIONS

In terms of the work regarding duration of untreated psychosis, further research is required. This concept possesses an appealing simplicity but DUP will benefit from randomised controlled trials to further establish clinical effectiveness (Norman & Malla 2001). DUP also needs to be investigated more specifically with regard to relapse rates, negative symptoms and cognitive functioning, among other variables. The potential effectiveness of family interventions to reduce the risk of relapse in schizophrenia is well researched and supported. Further work is now required to determine its position within early interventions for psychosis specifically. There are some indications emerging from the research that both content and method of delivery may require adaptation of the current models at this critical developmental period (see, for example, Gleeson et al 1999).

The issue of which interventions are most clinically effective also requires further exploration. The national service framework (Department of Health

1999) and mental health policy implementation guide (Department of Health 2001) made it clear that early intervention services should be introduced as part of mainstream clinical delivery by 2004 in England, and DUP needs to be assessed in the context of routine early intervention clinical practice. The routine delivery and effectiveness of family work within this setting is similarly dependent on the establishment of such services.

The case example presents the possibility of delivering a complex intervention to an individual and his family within a routine setting, where lack of time and high case loads frequently prevail. However, to offer complex and time-consuming interventions themselves routinely is not yet a clinical reality for many mental health services. Early intervention teams may increase the opportunity to achieve this goal and at the same time incorporate the evidence specific to this clinical group. What is clear is that the requirement extends beyond the provision of a minority of professionals with the technical capability to deliver appropriate interventions. Working environments that can make planned provision for routine co-working and extended support for individuals, coupled with an appropriate training and supervision infrastructure (e.g. access to the Thorn programme), are also essential.

Summary

Both Adrian and Charlotte expressed high levels of consumer satisfaction with the combined effects of both individual and family work that was focused on recovery and relapse prevention. There remains a clear need to continue to implement such integrated approaches, and a redoubling of effort to adequately research such clinical work, particularly when used in a creative and user and carer focused fashion.

 Summary of practical strategies identified

- ◆ Engagement and use of a time line are vital components of relapse prevention work.
- ◆ Construction of an early warning signs grid by using the KGV assessment is an essential precursor to aid psychological management and formulation. Common early warning signs for users revolve around increased anxiety and depression and social withdrawal. However, more subtle idiosyncratic 'unique identifiers', as exemplified by the various symptoms unearthed for Adrian, should routinely be sought.
- ◆ A relapse drill should be routinely incorporated into care planning that identifies practical support and effective interventions (medication, cognitive–behavioural therapy, home treatment).

Summary of practical strategies identified (cont'd)

◆ The relapse drill and early warning signs grid are dynamic constructs that benefit from continuous review and input from user and carer together with mental health staff.

◆ Issues of adjustment and loss in early episode psychosis may require a more than usually flexible approach in family interventions. Pacing of the work and content should be carefully matched to the needs of those involved.

◆ Finally, the practical step-by-step strategies identified here for relapse prevention are transferable. They can be used for many clients of different ages and varied stages of psychosis although the emphasis here has been on early-in-the-course psychosis.

Cross references

Chapter 5 An introduction to and rationale for psychosocial interventions

Chapter 13 Working with families and informal carers

References

Anthony W A 1993 Recovery from mental illness: the guiding vision of the mental health service system of the nineties. Psychosocial Rehabilitation Journal 16:11–24

Barrowclough C, Tarrier N 1997 Families of schizophrenic patients: cognitive behaviour intervention. Stanley Thornes, Cheltenham, pp185–194 (RAI), 215–226 (KASI)

Birchwood M 2000 The critical period for early intervention. In: Birchwood M, Fowler D, Jackson C (eds) Early interventions in psychosis: a guide to concepts, evidence and interventions. Wiley, Chichester, pp 28–63

Birchwood M, Macmillan J F, Smith J 1992 Early intervention. In: Birchwood M, Tarrier N (eds) Innovations in the psychological management of schizophrenia. Wiley, Chichester, pp 115–145

Birchwood M, Spencer E, McGovern D 2000 Schizophrenia: early warning signs. Advances in Psychiatric Treatment 6:93–101

Davis E, Coupland K 2000 Having the last word. Mental Health Care 4:26–29

De Haan L, van Raaij B, van den Berg R et al 2001 Preferences for treatment during a first psychotic episode. European Psychiatry 16:83–89

References (cont'd)

Department of Health 1999 A national service framework for mental health. The Stationery Office, London

Department of Health 2001 Mental health policy implementation guide. Department of Health, London

Department of Health 2002 Developing services for carers and families of people with mental illness. Department of Health, London

French P, Walford L 2001 Psychological approaches to early intervention for psychosis: what it is and what it can achieve. Mental Health Care 4:158–161

Gleeson J, Jackson H J, Stavely H, Burnett P 1999 Family interventions in psychosis: In McGorry P D, Jackson H J (eds) The recognition and management of early psychosis – a preventative approach. Cambridge University Press, Cambridge, pp 376–406

IRIS Research Group 2000 Clinical guidelines and service frameworks in relation to early intervention in psychosis. Initiative to Reduce the Impact of Schizophrenia (IRIS). Available online at: www.iris-initiative.org.uk

Keshavan S, Schooler N R 1992 First episode studies in schizophrenia: criteria and characterisation. Schizophrenia Bulletin 18:491–593

Krawiecka M, Goldberg D, Vaughan M 1977 A standardised psychiatric rating scale for rating chronic psychiatric patients. Acta Psychiatrica Scandinavica 55:299–308

Kuipers E, Leff J, Lam D 1992 Family work for schizophrenia: a practical guide. Gaskell/Royal College of Psychiatrists, London

Larsen T K, Johannessen J, McGlashen T et al 2001 Can duration of untreated psychosis be reduced? In: Birchwood M, Fowler D, Jackson C (eds) Early interventions for psychosis: a guide to concepts, evidence and interventions. Wiley, Chichester, pp 143–165

Liese B S, Beck J S 1997 Cognitive therapy supervision. In: Edward W C Jr (ed) Handbook of psychotherapy supervision. Wiley, Chichester, pp 114–133

Linzen D, Dingemans P, Van Der Does JW et al 1996 Treatment, expressed emotion and relapse in recent onset schizophrenic disorders. Psychological Medicine 26:333–342

Macmillan J F, Gold A, Crow T J et al 1986 The Northwick Park first episodes of schizophrenia study III. British Journal of Psychiatry 148:128–133

McGorry P D, Edwards J, Mihalopoulos C et al 1996 EPPIC: an evolving system of early detection and optimal management. Schizophrenia Bulletin 22:305–326

National Institute for Clinical Excellence 2002 Clinical Guideline 1. Schizophrenia: core interventions in the treatment and management of schizophrenia in primary and secondary care. NICE, London

Norman R M G, Malla A 2001 Duration of untreated psychosis: a critical examination of the concept and its importance. Psychological Medicine 31:381–400

Nuechterlein K H, Dawson M E 1984 A heuristic vulnerability-stress model of schizophrenic episodes. Schizophrenia Bulletin 10:300–312

Pilling S, Bebbington P, Kuipers E et al 2002 Psychological treatments in schizophrenia: I. Meta-analysis of family intervention and cognitive behaviour therapy. Psychological Medicine 32:763–782

Pitschel-Wals G, Leucht S, Bauml J et al 2001 The effect of family interventions on relapse and rehospitalisation in schizophrenia – a meta-analysis. Schizophrenia Bulletin 27:73–92

References (*cont'd*)

Rethink 2002 Reaching people early. Available online at:
   www.rethink.org/reachingpeopleearly
Thompson K N, McGorry P D, Phillips L J, Young A R 2000 Prediction and
   intervention in the pre-psychotic phase. Journal of Advances in
   Schizophrenia and Brain Research 3:43–47

Annotated further reading

Edwards J, McGorry P D 2002 Implementing early intervention in psychosis:
a guide to establishing early psychosis services. Martin Dunitz, London

*Helpful manual offering guidance on both organisational and practice issues
related to early intervention. Includes useful information on models of delivery and
further reading on recovery.*

McGorry P D, Jackson H J 1999 The recognition and management of early
psychosis – a preventative approach. Cambridge University Press, Cambridge

*An innovative handbook that comprehensively covers all aspects of early
intervention for psychosis. Of particular interest is the focus on the possibilities for
a preventative approach and it is essential reading if you are interested in following
up DUP and its implications for the treatment of schizophrenia.*

Schaub A 2002 New family interventions and associated research in
psychiatric disorders. Springer, New York

*Eclectic presentation of the evidence base for working with families, using a variety
of theoretical perspectives to address a range of difficulties. Chapter 3 discusses
family work in early episode psychosis; chapters on family work with bipolar
disorder and in substance misuse and psychosis will also be of interest.*

19

Cultural issues

Avie Luthra, Dinesh Bhugra and Rahul Bhintade

KEY ISSUES

- Culture shapes all aspects of our identity
- In all cultures there is an interaction between illness and its culture
- Epidemiology shows us differences and similarities in incidence rates of schizophrenia across cultures
- Assessing clients must include an awareness and understanding of their background and culture
- Physical treatments, psychotherapy and indigenous therapies are all possible options but depend very much upon the treatment situation
- Care plans should take culture, treatment setting and family resources into account
- Service provision is a key area for future development as it presents options for developing care tailored to the needs of specific ethnic minorities.

INTRODUCTION

Culture influences an individual's functioning in several ways. It defines the sick role and help-seeking, and where individuals get support from. The role of culture is paramount in making diagnoses and planning treatments, especially if the patients and clinicians come from different backgrounds (Bhugra & Bhul 1997a).

As this volume deals with severe mental illness, this chapter highlights some of the key problems in diagnosing and managing these illnesses, illustrating some of the key points through describing schizophrenia and depressive illness.

What is culture?

Culture refers to the many socially determined aspects of an individual's identity. Culture is broadly defined as a common heritage or set of beliefs, norms and values (Department of Health and Human Services 1999). It refers to the shared and largely learned attributes of a group of people. Anthropologists often describe culture as a system of shared meanings. It differs from ethnicity, which refers to a common heritage (including similar history, language, rituals and preferences for music and foods; Zenner 1996).

Race has a social meaning and overlaps with ethnicity but culture is applicable to groups of whites as well as same-profession groups or gangs (Department of Health and Human Services 2001). Clinicians need to be aware not only of the culture of the patient but also their own and of the relationship of mental health services with culture and society. Culture dictates not only the way people eat, sleep and function but also how people think and behave. It forms values and beliefs. Understanding illness is very culturally dependent. By this we mean that culture structures the way people perceive normal and abnormal health. It shapes how people appreciate the origins and mechanisms of illness and how medical and psychiatric services are used and accessed.

The advantage of understanding a client's culture is not to explain away certain trends or behaviours as simply 'cultural'. Further understanding of 'culture' functions as the means by which the primary goal of better care can be achieved.

VARIATION OF ILLNESS ACROSS CULTURES

Studies have shown significant epidemiological differences across cultures (World Health Organization 1973, Sartorius et al 1983, Jablensky et al 1992). There are striking disparities for minorities in mental health services and their underlying knowledge base. Racial and ethnic minorities have less access to mental health services than do whites. They are less likely to receive needed care and, if and when they get it, the quality of the care may be variable.

The Department of Health and Human Services (2001) reported that racial and ethnic minorities bear a greater burden from unmet mental health needs and therefore suffer a greater loss to their overall health and productivity. Even physical illnesses vary across cultures (MacMillan et al 2003). Undocumented migrants in New York's Chinatown showed a greater rate of hospitalisation and re-hospitalisation and lower treatment compliance and insight into illness (Law et al 2003). Thus, not only social disadvantage but attitudes, beliefs and migratory status play a role. Also, different generations of immigrant families have different levels of expressed illness within a given culture – so-called 'second generation' immigrants differ from the first generation (Bhugra &

Bhui 1998) and from refugees (Ager 1993). Each group therefore possesses its own characteristics, which shape illness behaviour. The following description of the research to date aims to discuss these differences, and their importance in the treatment and management of clients with serious mental illness.

Schizophrenia

One of the first key studies to ascertain whether schizophrenia exists across cultures, and what its symptomatology and outcome differences are, was the International Pilot Study of Schizophrenia (IPSS; World Health Organization 1973). The main aim of the study was to establish whether such a study was possible across cultures. Using nine centres around the world, World Health Organization (WHO) investigators were trained to a high level of inter-rater reliability. Several findings emerged that highlighted cross-cultural differences.

The key observation was that the core symptoms of schizophrenia (narrow-definition schizophrenia S+, according to the CATEGO programme of the Present State Examination) were broadly similar across cultures and the variation in rates was not very marked. The broad category of schizophrenia, on the other hand, showed marked differences – thereby suggesting that non-specific symptoms vary a lot. The outcomes at 2 years and 5 years were shown to be favourable in developing countries when compared with those in developed countries. The reasons for such a marked differential are many, and include family support, agricultural settings, low stigma, etc. The second important study that looked at the incidence rates of schizophrenia and other social factors was the Determinants of Outcome of Severe Mental Disorder study (DOSMD; Jablensky et al 1992). Having established the pattern in the IPSS, the WHO researchers then set out to study incidence rates in ten countries and 12 field centres (although, for purposes of carrying out incidence rates, Agra in north India and Ibadan in Nigeria were excluded).

The research instruments included PSE-9 (Wing et al 1974), the Psychiatric and Personal History Schedule (PPHS), diagnostic and prognostic schedules and follow-up PPHS along with the Disability Assessment Schedule. In addition, some centres included additional substudies – for example, expressed emotion was measured in Chandigarh in north India, Aarhus and Rochester, and life events were measured in nine centres. Disability and impairment were assessed in six centres and perceptions of illness in three centres. Not surprisingly, there were marked social–demographic differences across centres.

Annual incidence rates for narrow-definition schizophrenia in ages 15–54 varied from 0.7/10 000 population in Aarhus to 1.4/10 000 in Nottingham. Rates of broad-definition schizophrenia varied from 1.6 in Aarhus and Honolulu to 2.2 in Nottingham. By applying a uniform case definition and case-finding methodology, the study was able to demonstrate that there were no large differences in the manifestation rates of core schizophrenic disorders across cultures and geographical areas. Culture and ethnicity have been shown to influence the presentation of patients with schizophrenia.

The WHO studies, however, have been criticised by Cohen (1992) as well as others. Cohen's key argument is the emphasis by the researchers on similarities rather than differences – what the anthropologists would call the 'universalist view' rather than a relativist one. Better outcome in developing countries was shown to be the case and was attributed to low expressed emotion, as shown in north India (Wig et al 1987). However, looking at differences across cultures can introduce a range of variables that may cloud the picture; hence it becomes important to study rates of schizophrenia in the same culture but in different ethnic groups.

From the early 1960s there have been several studies in the UK that have reported high rates of schizophrenia in African-Caribbeans when compared with whites or Asians. These differences have been startling (Leff 1988).

Although some of the early studies had serious methodological flaws and sometimes relied on case-note data, even the more recent methodologically sound studies have upheld these findings (Harrison et al 1988, 1997, King et al 1994, Bhugra et al 1997). The finding that rates of schizophrenia among African-Caribbeans are much higher are robust and several possible explanations have been put forward (Harrison 1990). The rates of schizophrenia among Asians are not confirmed to be elevated. King et al (1994) reported that rates of all psychoses were raised among all migrant groups, although numbers in some of the groups were very small. Bhugra et al (1997), on the other hand, found that overall rates of schizophrenia were not elevated among all Asians but in older females only.

The outcome of schizophrenia has been shown to be generally poor in African-Caribbeans, except in one study (McKenzie et al 1995). The reasons for poor outcome have been hypothesised to be poor compliance, poor experiences of psychiatric services, social and economic deprivation, etc. The results of the long-term follow-up are not yet fully clear, but what is apparent is that different ethnic groups have different outcomes.

Depression

Depression has been notoriously difficult to classify. Different theories of depression have yielded different approaches to 'low mood', producing different classification systems (Kendell 1976). There has been so much variability within specific Western cultures that it is easy to see why examining depression across cultures is fraught with difficulty. Another interesting factor emerging is the role of globalisation and urbanisation in the likely increase of the rates of depression (see Bhugra & Mastrogianni 2004 for a review).

The 'depression' equivalent of the WHO IPSS is a study performed by the WHO in 1983 (Sartorius et al 1983). This looked at depressive symptoms across five centres – Basle, Montreal, Nagasaki, Teheran and Tokyo. The study employed specific inclusion criteria and used a schedule that included an open-ended component for culture-specific items. Overall, the most frequent symptoms seen were joylessness and sadness.

Cultural differences included fewer suicidal ideas in Tokyo and Teheran, with more feelings of guilt and self-reproach in Basle and Montreal and no psychotic depression recorded in Teheran. Comparisons within countries are equally varied.

The Indian subcontinent shows north and south differences in both prevalence rates and symptomatology (Wig 1980, Venkoba Rao 1987). Biological features of depression such as sleep disturbance, low libido and poor appetite are more common in the south than in the north, where loss of energy, loss of confidence and low self-esteem are more prevalent (Singh 1979).The colonial myth of low levels of depression within the 'happy savage' African population has been revealed for what it is (Wittkower 1969, Rwegellera 1981). Africa's complex mix of races and tribes, and the sheer size of the continent, opens the possibility of a wide range of presentations. A study from Ghana using the same WHO schedule shows a similar symptom profile to the other countries (Majodina & Johnson 1983). Guilt and suicide have been reported to be low in Nigeria (Binite 1975), atypical presentations higher in Senegal (Colomb 1965) and hysterical symptoms more common in Zambia (Bhugra 1996). Studies from the Middle East have been contradictory, and Far East studies reveal guilt to be as common among Japanese as among German Catholics (Bhugra 1996). Finally, work in the UK shows differences between ethnic minority groups. African-Caribbean studies suggest that first admission for affective disorders is slightly higher than in the white population (Hemsi 1967). This is more marked in English-born than Caribbean-born members of this group. Rates amongst Indians/Pakistanis are broadly similar to the white population. Correlates with depression in Asians include: length of time in the UK, speaking only another language, the experience of racial prejudice and the presence of children at home (Furnham & Li 1993).

Refugees also suffer increased levels of depression when compared with the general population. The factors behind this have already been mentioned (Ager 1993).

Other conditions

Rates of bulimia are particularly high in Asian females, and this has been linked to severe emotional deprivation. Rates of alcohol abuse are low in Asians and African-Caribbeans. Subpopulations such as Sikhs, however, have a high reported rate of alcohol abuse (Bhugra & Bhui 1998). Refugees have higher rates of post-traumatic stress disorder, which is linked to the experience of trauma (Ager 1993).

ASSESSMENT OF THE CROSS-CULTURAL CLIENT

Having discussed the importance of culture to mental illness, we shall now look at both assessment and management of the cross-cultural client.

The aim of assessment is to access the core of illness – that is, to peel away the layers of illness behaviour, and find the treatable centre. Those layers can be multiple and highly variable and are dependent upon both client and practitioner. The factors considered are both individual factors and general cultural factors. These are not mutually exclusive categories, just a convenient way of dividing the processes involved in the assessment of the cross-cultural client.

Individual factors

Individual factors relate to the practitioner and to the client. Practitioners should be aware of their position, which is not only their cultural and racial backgrounds but also their class, gender and professional roles. Identity is a shifting balance between these various elements, where at any time one aspect of identity is more relevant than another. Professional factors depend upon training and level of expertise. Important cultural factors include language and past experience of the other cultural group. With respect to the patient, there are extra aspects to be considered.

The practitioner observes not only the race/class/gender and culture of the client but also the specific experiences, which can be very different from those of the practitioner – e.g. racism, the process of seeking asylum, or linguistic difficulties. Appreciation of these without direct first-hand experience can be tricky.

A close relationship with the client is obviously highly beneficial, as is a good collaborative history. The family can often provide this history, acting as a rich source of cultural information (Bhugra & Bhui 1997a).

General cultural factors

These factors are wider than the individual factors, but the two areas overlap. 'World view' is the means of understanding events and situations. It is a product of culture. The North American world view is seen as individualistic rather than collaborative, focusing on self-actualisation and a linear interpretation of events. This generalisation is useful in providing practitioners with a background to the assumptions behind their own biomedical model – essential when treating clients from different cultures (Sue 1981). It is also important to remember that cultures shift and change. A migrant culture such as Indian culture in the UK may be engaged in a process of acculturation, which differs from generation to generation. Their world view therefore shifts accordingly. Identity is chiselled through acculturation and is shaped by family, peer groups, media and religion.

The period since migration and the reasons behind migration are very important in shaping this process. As each patient's needs are so unique, practitioners cannot expect to be experts in all these historical elements. Nevertheless, this broad principle should be kept in mind when working with the cross-cultural client.

The stigma attached to psychiatric illness depends very much on culture. This is one of the explanations put forward for somatisation, particularly within Asian culture. The expression of depression or anxiety as physical symptoms is less stigmatising in these cultures. Other explanations for somatisation exist, for instance that an internal psychological explanation of distress is an especially Western idiom, and non-Western cultures not based on such psychology prefer a physical model. In one study, Wang et al (2003) demonstrated that the clergy were more likely to be contacted than psychiatrists (23% vs 16%) for health care. Of those approaching the clergy one quarter were likely to have seriously impairing mental disorders.

Non-verbal behaviour differs between cultures as much as language. Eye contact and gaze avoidance may seem appropriate in certain cultures but threatening in others. The practitioner should always be aware of the power of such behavioural subtleties.

Finally, the standard mental state examination is open to much cultural shaping. The mental state examination investigates the signs and symptoms of the illness. Skills required include the non-verbal skills mentioned, interviewing skills and observation skills. Cultural points of view operate in all aspects: appearance and behaviours that seem unusual to the clinician may be of cultural significance; aggression and weeping are emotions especially sensitive to the client's cultural make-up; delusions and hallucinations are also very dependent upon culture.

In the last, misinterpretation can have several cultural routes. It could be a result of language miscommunication, producing misclassification of given phenomena as delusions/hallucinations. Or it could be the product of a lack of cultural knowledge. By definition, to understand a belief as delusional requires a knowledge of the mechanics of a culture. The explanation of an event as 'witchcraft' may be normal within Shona culture but is likely to be delusional in the West. To rescue ideas from the cultural mist, the practitioner should draw from the well of available information surrounding the patient.

This includes family and friends but also voluntary groups, user groups and support groups. Recording the beliefs verbatim and relaying them to these experts in the patient's culture is the most effective method of preventing misclassification (Bhugra & Bhui 1997a).

MANAGEMENT OF THE CROSS-CULTURAL CLIENT

The relationship between client and practitioner is the foundation of management. Trust has to be built for the client to follow mutual objectives towards therapeutic goals.

Many of the cultural ingredients of this relationship have been discussed in the section dealing with assessment, and these carry through for management. Migrant communities are heterogeneous in nature. Issues to do with access and treatment vary as much between generations as between migrant groups.

This heterogeneity makes treatment plans more complex in this client group. Planning is essential, as failure to recognise this complexity can perpetuate a misunderstanding that destroys trust. Management plans should be context-dependent – from inpatient, to outpatient, to community strategies. Therapeutic goals should be mutually understood within these contexts and, at a practical level, effort should be made to peel away specific cultural layers. For the practitioner this involves extra work – that is, finding interpreters and individuals to provide a cultural background and understanding details of cultural conflicts, ties and relationships. It should be remembered that any psychiatric assessment filtered through the perspective of a third party is fraught with difficulty. Third parties too close to the client (family or friends) can edit or sanitise for the ears of the professional. The converse – the use of interpreters unknown to the client – can bring out issues of sensitivity and confidentiality. It is easy to see why a client would not wish to reveal intimate personal information to a complete stranger for the purpose of translation (Bhugra & Bhui 1997a).

The rest of this chapter will focus on three aspects of management: first, the use of physical treatments across cultures, second, the role of various therapies with the cross-cultural client and third, the special needs and services required by this client group.

Physical treatments

Physical treatments include pharmacological and electroconvulsive treatment (ECT). Perceptions of the use of medication generally, and the use of psychiatric medication specifically, are very much culturally bound. Belief that medication should provide a quick response, poor communication of side-effects owing to linguistic barriers, and a lack of faith in the role of the practitioner per se all contribute to poor compliance (Westermayer 1989). Pharmacokinetics vary across cultures and races. This may be as much because of diet and social habits (smoking/drinking) as the physical make-up of the client. Specific examples abound (Bhugra & Bhui 1997b): Asians and black patients have shown greater blood levels of neuroleptics per milligram than caucasians. Asians develop extrapyramidal side-effects faster than do black or caucasian patients. Asians also have less need for high doses of tricyclic antidepressants, as blood and peak levels are reached earlier. Lithium displays highly variable blood levels, even within a single ethnic group: Taiwanese blood levels are lower than those of Hong Kong patients, which are lower than those of Chinese. Ethnicity has been shown to be a significant predictor of the type of antipsychotic that is prescribed.

Opolka et al (2003) found that African-Americans were more likely to be treated with conventional neuroleptics than atypical ones. Ethnic minority groups have lower rates of compliance and receive lower levels of specialist care (Algeria et al 2002) and were also less likely to receive psychotherapy both in primary and in secondary care (Lasser et al 2002).

Electroconvulsive therapy is controversial. This controversy lies not in its effectiveness – which is undoubtedly proven – but in the negative image it carries. This applies very much cross-culturally, and much effort should be made to explain the value and importance of this treatment. Evidence that ECT is given more frequently to African-Caribbeans, and the stereotype of it being an oppressive treatment, can only do damage to the trust between practitioner and this client group. Good communication is one means of overcoming such cultural barriers to a potentially life-saving treatment (Westermayer 1989).

Specific therapies

Among the specific therapies we shall look at psychotherapies and indigenous therapies.

Individual psychotherapy is very culturally biased. Western therapy has been described as ego-dependent and so can be at odds with cultures where the individual functions as an extension of a social or family unit. Such psychotherapies are not necessarily ineffective outside of Western cultural groups. An initial assessment can be useful in defining the needs of the client and whether or not psychotherapy will be effective. Examining the specific therapies, psychoanalysis is the most obviously culturally specific. The Oedipus complex and the concepts of the id, ego and superego all have clear European roots.

Also, the processes of countertransference and transference can be imbued with elements shaped by racism or language, adding a complexity when used cross-culturally that is not present with European clients. Conversely, behavioural therapy is very adaptable cross-culturally. This is because of the practical nature of this therapy – it requires little interpreter time, the therapy is specific and the results are clear. Cognitive therapy is also potentially beneficial, but remains to be tested cross-culturally (Sue 1981).

Finally, intercultural therapy has been developed as a means of tackling these issues. Nafriyat in north London is a good example of this. It is based on the psychoanalytical approach, and it involves challenging assumptions and assessing the patient's experience. The work deals with issues of race and the social consequences of racism, allowing discussion with both white and black therapists. A therapist of the same cultural or racial origin is not an essential element of the treatment, as therapeutic skills depend largely on the therapist. But for discussion of areas of sensitivity, such as racism, it is seen as beneficial. Thomas (1995) reports a 90% 'good outcome' from such therapy with a marked improvement in General Health Questionnaire score (Thomas 1995).

The use of indigenous therapies seems an appropriate way of bridging the cultural divide. This means drawing upon psychotherapies available in given cultures and adapting them to the Western context. Such adaptation can be very difficult as it is full of possible misinterpretation and dilution of the original effective treatment.

For example, Ayurvedic or Tibetan treatments of mental illness, which involve not only diet and herbal remedies but also a specific cultural–religious belief system, would require much reinventing to be transposed effectively to a Western city. Many reports exist, however, of specific therapies that have been adapted. Hatha yoga, meditation and acupuncture are widely available treatments for stress – although mainly as Western adaptations for predominantly Western clients. Other effective examples of adaptation include cuento therapy in Puerto Rican children in New York, and Japanese morita therapy in other parts of America (Fernando 1991). The fact that cross-cultural clients use a number of religious and non-medical healers, alongside Western doctors, shows the desire for several therapists. This remains fertile ground for development in the management of such patients.

Service provision

Service provision for cross-cultural clients with mental health needs is an area of much discussion. The aim is to provide specialised services for ethnic minorities based on their specialised needs. This involves setting up services de novo and modification of pre-existing services.

Bhugra & Bhui (1997b) propose an approach that emphasises clients' explanations of their symptoms, taking the focus away from psychiatric diagnosis. This approach should be the starting point for action and development. This is of value in all aspects of psychiatric care: inpatient, respite and long-term. Input from members of the community, non-statutory agencies and advocacy services belonging to a given cultural group is valuable. This approach also applies to forensic and liaison services, where ethnic minorities are over-represented in particular ways. Ethnic matching of patients and therapist has been put forward as one possible solution to increase compliance. In an interesting study, Ziguras et al (2003) demonstrated in Western Australia that those ethnic minority clients who were matched with bilingual case workers (when compared with those who had English-speaking therapists) were more likely to have longer and greater frequency of contact with community care teams and a shorter duration and lower frequency of contact with crisis teams. Patients of Vietnamese origin who had bilingual clinicians had a shorter annual mean length of hospital stay and a lower annual mean frequency of hospital admission than Australian-born clients. However, these findings need to be replicated.

A final mention needs to be made of user groups and non-statutory agencies. The user movement has a variable influence on psychiatric practice world-wide. It is particularly significant in Japan and America, where it broadens the scope of psychiatric care. Although there is no national user group for black people in the UK, individual agencies at a local level provide valuable input. If the practitioner is to develop a service for a client, then listening to that client's voice is crucial (Sassoon & Lindow 1995).

The same applies to voluntary agencies attached to the care of ethnic minorities. In London these include the Chinese Mental Health Association, the Brixton Circle and the African-Caribbean Mental Health Association. These agencies meet needs that cannot be met by statutory mental health services. Their position is both advantageous and unstable – the former because of their autonomy, the latter because of the variability of their funding. Collaboration between the statutory and voluntary sectors has been patchy, and how they fit together has yet to be determined. However, the grass-roots perspective supplied by voluntary groups is invaluable to the practitioner providing care for the cross-cultural client (Ahmed & Webb-Johnson 1995).

CONCLUSIONS

In this chapter we have discussed the key aspects of serious mental illness in the cross-cultural client. Culture is relevant to all illness behaviour and clothes disease with different presentations. Not only does this 'clothing' vary with different cultures but so too does the disease itself. These cultural differences have been discussed for schizophrenia and depression particularly. In order to get beyond the covering provided by culture, practitioners must have an understanding of the basics of assessment. This involves being aware of their position relative to the patient. Individual and general cultural factors operate with the cross-cultural client.

These include differences in world view and changes in cultural identity, stigma and somatisation. The standard mental state must also be scrutinised if it is to be used appropriately. Management of all clients involves planning and trust. These aspects are even more important in this group. The practitioner has to work hard to unpack the complexity provided by culture. This involves an awareness of how physical treatments and psychotherapies vary across cultures, and trying to adapt therapies for the client. A service for the cross-cultural client will be provided only if needs are assessed and measured, and then catered for. This means listening to clients closely and using as many organisations as possible in the client's care – including voluntary groups and user groups.

References

Ager A 1993 Mental health issues in refugee population: a review. Project on international mental and behavioural health. Harvard Medical School, Department of Social Medicine, Cambridge, MA

Ahmed T, Webb-Johnson A 1995 Voluntary groups. In: Fernando S (ed) Mental health in a multi-ethnic society. Routledge, New York, pp 74–88

Algeria M, Canino G, Rios R et al 2002 Inequalities in use of specialty mental health services among Latinos, African Americans and non-Latino whites. Psychiatric Services 53:1547–1555

Bhugra D 1996 Depression across cultures. Primary Care Psychiatry 2:155–165

Bhugra D, Bhui K 1997a Cross-cultural psychiatric assessment. Advances in Psychiatric Treatment 3:103–110

Bhugra D, Bhui K 1997b Clinical management of patients across cultures. Advances in Psychiatric Treatment 3:233–239

Bhugra D, Bhui K 1998 Transcultural psychiatry: do problems persist in the second generation? Hospital Medicine 59:126–129

Bhugra D, Mastrogianni A 2004 Globalisation and mental disorders. Overview with relation to depression. British Journal of Psychiatry 184:362–363

Bhugra D, Leff J, Mallett R, Der G et al 1997 Incidence and outcome of schizophrenia in whites, African-Caribbeans and Asians in London. Psychological Medicine 27:791–798

Binite A 1975 A factor analysis study of depression across cultures. British Journal of Psychiatry 127:559–563

Cohen A 1992 Prognosis for schizophrenia in the third world. Culture, Medicine and Psychiatry 16:53–75

Colomb H 1965 Assistance psychiatrique en Afrique: experience Senegalese. Psychopathologie Africaine 1:11

References (cont'd)

Department of Health and Human Services 1999 Mental health: a report of the Surgeon General. DHHS, Rockville, MD

Department of Health and Human Services 2001 Mental health: culture, race and ethnicity. DHHS, Rockville, MD.

Fernando S 1991 Mental health, race and culture. Macmillan, London

Furnham A, Li Y H 1993 Gender, generational and social support correlates of mental health in Asian immigrants. International Journal of Social Psychiatry 39:22–33

Harrison G 1990 Searching for the causes of schizophrenia: the role of migrant studies. Schizophrenia Bulletin 16:663–671

Harrison G, Owens D, Holton A, Neilson D, Boot D 1988 A prospective study of severe mental disorder in Afro-Caribbean patients. Psychological Medicine 18:643–657

Harrison G, Glazebrook C, Brewin J et al 1997 Increased incidence of psychotic disorders in migrants from the Caribbean to the United Kingdom. Psychological Medicine 27:799–806

Hemsi L K 1967 Psychiatric morbidity of West Indian immigrants. Social Psychiatry 2:95–100

Jablensky A, Sartorius N, Emberg G et al 1992 Schizophrenia: manifestations, incidence and course in different cultures. A World Health Organization 10 country study. Psychological Medicine Monograph (suppl 20)

Kendell R 1976 The classifications of depressions: a review of contemporary confusion. British Journal of Psychiatry 129:15–29

King M, Coker E, Leavey G et al 1994 Incidence of psychotic illness in London. British Medical Journal 309:1115–1119

Lasser K E, Himmelstein D, Woolhandler S et al 2003 Do minorities in the United States receive fewer mental health services than whites? International Journal of Mental Health 32:567–578

Law S, Hutton M, Chan D 2003 Clinical, social and service use characteristics of Fuzhounese undocumented immigrants patients. Psychiatric Services 54:1034–1037

Leff J 1988 Psychiatry around the globe: a transcultural view. Gaskell/Royal College of Psychiatrists, London

McKenzie K, Van-Os J, Fahy T, Jones P 1995 Psychosis with good prognosis in Afro-Caribbean people now living in the United Kingdom. British Medical Journal 311:1325–1328

MacMillan H L, Walsh C A, Jamieson E et al 2003 The health of Ontario First Nations people: results from the Ontario First Nations Regional Health Survey. Canadian Journal of Public Health 94:168–172

Majodina M Z, Johnson A F W 1983 Standardised assessment of depressive disorder in Ghana. British Journal of Psychiatry 143:442–446

Opolka J L, Rascati K L, Brown C M et al 2003 Ethnic differences in uses of antipsychotic medication among Texan medical clients with schizophrenia. Journal of Clinical Psychiatry 34:635–669

Rwegellera G G C 1981 Cultural aspects of depressive illness. Psychopathologie Africaine 17:41–63

Sartorius N, Davidson H, Ernberg G et al 1983 Depressive disorders in different cultures. WHO, Geneva

Sassoon M, Lindow V 1995 Consulting and expanding black mental health system users. In: Fernando S (ed) Mental health in a multi-ethnic society. Routledge, New York, pp 89–106

Singh G 1979 Depression in India: a cross-cultural perspective. Indian Journal of Psychiatry 21:235

References (cont'd)

Sue D W 1981 Counselling the culturally different: theory and method. Wiley, New York

Thomas L 1995 Psychotherapy in the context of race and culture. In: Fernando S (ed) Mental health in a multi-ethnic society. Routledge, New York, pp 172–192

Venkoba Rao A 1987 Depressive disease. ICMR, New Delhi

Wang P S, Berglund P, Kessler R 2003 Patients and correlates of contacting clergy for mental disorders in the United States. Health Services Research 38:647–673

Westermayer J 1989 Psychiatric care of migrants: a clinical guide. APA, Washington, DC

Wig N N 1980 Depressive illness in North India. In: Venkoba Rao A, Parvathi S (eds) Depressive illness. A V Rao, Madurai

Wig N N, Menon D K, Bedi H et al 1987 Expressed emotion and schizophrenia in north India. Distribution of expressed emotion components among relatives of schizophrenic patients in Aarhus and Chandigarh. British Journal of Psychiatry 151:160–165

Wing J K, Cooper J E, Sartorius N 1974 Measurement and classification of psychiatric symptoms. Cambridge University Press, London

Wittkower E D 1969 Perspectives in transcultural psychiatry. International Journal of Psychiatry 8:811–824

World Health Organization 1973 Report of the International Pilot Study of Schizophrenia, vol 1. WHO, Geneva

Zenner W 1996 Ethnicity. In: Levison D, Ember M (eds) Encyclopedia of cultural anthropology. Holt, New York, pp 393–395

Ziguras S, Klimidis S, Lewis J, Stuert G 2003 Ethnic matching of clients and clinicians and use of mental health services by ethnic minority clients. Psychiatric Services 54:535–541

Annotated further reading

Bhugra D, Bahl V (eds) 1999 Ethnicity: an agenda for mental health. Gaskell, London

This book covers a range of theoretical and clinical issues on diagnosis and management across different ethnic groups.

Bhugra D, Cochrane R 2001 Practice of psychiatry in multicultural Britain. Gaskell, London

Specialty-based chapters for practice of mental health care delivery in the UK.

Okpaku S O (ed) 1998 Clinical methods in transcultural psychiatry. APA, Washington, DC

From across the Atlantic, this book provides an overview of diagnostic and clinical management issues and education and training for different ethnic groups in the USA.

Tseng W-S 2001 Handbook of cultural psychiatry. Academic Press, San Diego, CA

Excellent source book on cultural psychiatry. American-focused.

Vaccaro J V, Clark G H (eds) 1996 Practicing psychiatry in the community. APA, Washington, DC

This book covers a range of clinical issues in community mental health. It is aimed at multidisciplinary teams.

Section 4

Considerations for effective practice

4

20

Ethical considerations

Paula Morrison

KEY ISSUES

◆ Ethical decision making
◆ Ethical theory: consequentialism, deontology, professional codes
◆ Autonomy
◆ Consent
◆ Confidentiality
◆ Non-maleficence and beneficence
◆ Developing ethical practice

Ethics (which contains the morality of decision-making) is often perceived as the exclusive domain of philosophical thinkers and those who are searching for the 'meaning of life'. In truth, everyone wrestles with ethical decision-making on a daily basis. All of us are faced with decisions and their consequences. All of us have to find answers to questions such as: 'Should I buy this product, as it pollutes the environment?', 'Should I report the misconduct of a colleague?' or 'Should I give an older person with dementia medication hidden in their food?'

Doubts and anxieties when faced with decisions can often make us uncomfortable. This is often compounded in professional practice as mental health care and treatment may, at times, infringe human freedom and dignity. Yet doubts and anxieties should not be feared but celebrated within our work, as it is from the subsequent reflection and analysis that ethical decisions are often made and practice enhanced.

So, what exactly is ethics? In a nutshell, ethics can be defined as the rightness or wrongness of human actions.

This chapter will introduce the reader to some of the main ethical theories. It will discuss principles that stem from those theories, which need to be developed by individual practitioners. Developing ethical decision-making skills is a lifetime challenge and this chapter will highlight only some of the issues. The reader may find they have more questions than answers by the end of the chapter. As Barker & Davidson (1998) point out, 'ethics as a state of being involves confronting our childlike self who is constantly looking for absolute answers'. Since life rarely has absolute answers we find ourselves facing many dilemmas in practice.

ETHICAL THEORY

Beauchamp & Childress (1989) state that a well-developed ethical theory provides a framework of principles within which a person can determine moral actions. The two types of ethical theory most cited to inform clinical practice are consequentialist theory and deontological (derived from the Greek word *deon* meaning 'duty') theory.

Consequentialism

This is the moral theory that actions are right or wrong according to their consequences rather than to any features they may have, such as telling the truth. The most prominent consequentialist theory is that of utilitarianism. David Hume (1711–1776), Jeremy Bentham (1748–1832) and John Stuart Mill (1806–1873) are most connected to this theory. Utilitarianism is often described in lay terms as 'the end justifies the means' and that we must 'promote the greatest good of the greatest number'. Alternatively, we could say that 'what is right is what is the most useful'.

An example of utilitarian thinking would be that to achieve the greatest benefit from mental health resources these resources should be targeted at serious mental illness. This act would be justified under utilitarianism if it produces more good than any other action. However, those who require services but who are not seen as seriously mentally ill might feel that this targeting means they lose out as individuals. There are many debates regarding targeting in the NHS, with people trying to decide what is the most moral way of apportioning resources to achieve the greatest benefit. The decisions are difficult and controversy often follows because particular groups often feel excluded. The ethical dilemma in Box 20.1 illustrates this.

Deontological

By contrast to consequentialist theory, deontological theories hold that some features of an act make it right or wrong for reasons other than its consequences. For many deontologists, deception is wrong independently of its consequences. An example of this would be giving a patient a placebo

---

Box 20.1 Ethical dilemma 1

You are employed by a large GP practice as an autonomous mental health professional. On assessing the case histories you realise that you can deal with all clients diagnosed with psychotic illness or all clients with obsessive-compulsive disorders, or a mixture of both, but do not have the resources for all people requiring a service.

How would you decide who receives your service and who does not? What factors would influence this decision?

---

without their knowledge. Deontological thinking would suggest that this is a non-moral act because deception is involved. Immanuel Kant (1734–1804) is regarded as the first deontologist.

The need for guidance with regard to what is right or wrong is often crucial within this framework. Some writers in religious traditions appeal to divine revelation, for example, the Ten Commandments, whereas others appeal to Natural Law, which they believe can be known by human reason. For example, the Nuremberg trials held that the holocaust was against Natural Law. The defence of 'obeying orders', given by those who carried out mass executions, was seen as indefensible because human reason would know that this was wrong and against humanity. In other words, the Natural Law was seen to be higher than any law of the land.

The ethical dilemma in Box 20.2 illustrates this.

One of the most prominent deontological theories in recent philosophy has been Rawls's theory of justice (1972). Rawls argued for the following principles of justice:

◆ the principle of equal liberty
◆ the difference principle, which permits inequality in the distribution of social and economic goods only if those inequalities will benefit everyone, especially the least advantaged
◆ the principle of fair equality of opportunity.

Box 20.2 Ethical dilemma 2

Let us say that you have specialist skills in a certain area of mental health care. A person comes to you who would benefit from your skills, but you know that this person is in an experimental control group and that to give active treatment would affect the research.

Do you see it as your duty to treat this person, or do you consider it your duty to support the research, which may help all people with this particular health issue? How do you decide this?

Rawls's theory has led to the development of equal opportunities as we see them today.

PROFESSIONAL CODES

Together with these ethical theories, public policy, formal guidelines and codes of professional ethics, such as those developed by the Nursing and Midwifery Council (NMC 1992a, b, 1996, 1998), have been developed in an attempt to introduce guides to ethical practice. However, Beauchamp & Childress (1989) argue that one of the major defects in contemporary theory in ethics is that it is distanced from clinical practice. They state that some professional codes oversimplify moral requirements or claim more completeness than they are entitled to. As a consequence, professionals may think that they have satisfied all moral requirements if they have simply followed the rules of the code.

It is therefore essential for clinical practitioners to develop their understanding of ethical theory and how to apply this in their practice. This goes well beyond the requirements of professional ethical codes.

Ethics in care involves:

◆ obtaining relevant factual information
◆ assessing its reliability
◆ identifying moral problems and mapping out alternative solutions to problems that have been identified.

This mapping entails presenting and defending reasons in support of one's decisions, while at the same time analysing and assessing one's basic assumptions and commitments (Beauchamp & Childress 1989) – for example, the assumption that people should be kept alive at all costs versus the commitment of a carer to relieving pain, which may also hasten death.

ETHICAL PRINCIPLES IN PRACTICE

As stated earlier, certain principles derived from ethical theory need to be developed in practice in order to care for people in a moral and human way. These principles are: respect for autonomy, non-maleficence and beneficence.

Principle of respect for autonomy

People are assumed to be self-determining, self-governing individuals who use reason and choice in their lives. This is described as 'autonomy' and professional ethics promote the idea of ensuring that people's autonomy is respected. Seedhouse (1988) describes autonomy as: 'a person's capacity to choose freely for himself, and to be able to direct his own life'.

This is sometimes questioned when applied to people with mental health problems as temporary constraints imposed on thinking, owing to the illness, can lead to diminished autonomy. However, even if someone has been determined as legally incompetent they may still be able to make autonomous decisions such as the right to refuse to see relatives or to permit any clinical information being given to carers. Roberts et al (2002) states that understanding clinical and ethical practices will help clinicians serve patients with mental health in their everyday clinical activities in a manner that is respectful, engenders trust and ultimately fosters optimal clinical care.

Promoting client independence and autonomy and seeing this as a prerequisite to any care provided is essential in mental healthcare practice. This recognises a person's capacities to make choices and take action based on personal values and beliefs. Promoting autonomy also includes enabling people to act autonomously to the best of their capacity. But what does this mean in reality? Kohner (1996) argues that if we respect the idea of autonomy this would demand that the following imperatives are followed:

◆ discussing any proposed treatment and care with the client
◆ being aware of power inequalities in the professional–client relationship
◆ determining the client's priorities and needs
◆ communication and sharing of knowledge
◆ listening
◆ honesty
◆ confidentiality
◆ dignity and respect for the client and the client's situation
◆ consent.

Conflicts often arise because clients competently refuse treatment that professionals think would be of benefit, or some clients act autonomously, placing themselves or others at risk. Determining mental capacity for autonomous decision-making in combination with risk assessment is therefore a skill to be developed. This has been addressed in previous chapters (see Chs 8 and 10).

Respecting the autonomy of others beside the client also needs consideration. Gillon (1994) describes respect for autonomy as: 'the moral obligation to respect the autonomy of others in so far as such respect is compatible with equal respect for the autonomy of all those potentially affected'. This is a difficult area in mental health, where conflicts often arise between respecting both clients' and their families' autonomy. For example, clients may refuse to permit information about their illness to be disclosed to family members, even though the family members are affected by the illness and are none the less expected to carry on caring without any information. The balancing of need and duty in this situation is itself an ethical dilemma (see Ch. 16).

Consent

Clients have a fundamental legal and ethical right to determine what happens to their own bodies. Valid consent to treatment is therefore absolutely central in all forms of health care, from providing personal care to undertaking major surgery. Seeking consent is also a matter of common courtesy between health professionals and clients (Department of Health 2001). There are certain responsibilities in regard to obtaining consent that need to be followed in order for the autonomy of any client to be respected (Barker and Baldwin 1991, NMC 1998):

◆ that competence for consent is present
◆ that information is disclosed and that the information is understood
◆ that the consent is given voluntarily
◆ that authorisation is given by the person to consent to treatment.

Assessing whether a client is competent depends on whether the client can understand and retain treatment information and can weigh it up to make an informed decision. This assessment of competence is an integral part of mental state examination, although rarely specified (see Ch. 5).

Assumptions are often made about the capacity to consent for those people with a serious mental illness. These assumptions detract from the autonomy of individuals. An example would be that clients are often given large doses of neuroleptic medication without the necessary information on side effects or long-term consequences. For this reason, consideration should be given to using trained advocates to assist clients in decision-making processes in order to protect their autonomy. This will be particularly important when clients' first language is not English or when they have other communication difficulties. Clear plans should exist on how these difficulties can be overcome, such as using an interpreter. The ability to provide informed consent should be conceptualised as a continuum that varies with each patient and may indeed be different for the same patient in different circumstances and at different phases of illness (Roberts et al 2002).

Confidentiality

Confidentiality is another cornerstone of respecting client autonomy, which is generally accepted by professionals but can be widely ignored in practice. Consider what clients would think about the fact that sometimes over 20 people may see their clinical records. Clients in a wide variety of settings stated a preference to be better informed about the ethical and legal dimensions of confidentiality, particularly regarding the limits of the concept and their recourse when they feel their rights have been violated (Roberts et al

2002). Clients may expect more rigorous standards and therefore the limits of confidentiality should be explained and reasons should be given for when that confidentiality will be broken. It is also important to explain the need to disclose to others in the team and what that entails. It is also generally accepted in mental health that confidentiality should be broken only in certain circumstances. Beauchamp & Childress (1989) state that breaking confidentiality should happen only when a higher obligation needs to be followed, such as to adhere to the law or to protect the client or the public.

The principles of non-maleficence and beneficence

Non-maleficence

The principle of non-maleficence is the maxim 'that above all do no harm' or 'one ought not to inflict evil or harm'. This is interpreted by Johsen et al (1986) as the moral requirement of health professionals:

◆ to strive to serve the well-being of their clients
◆ to promote standards of due care
◆ to carry out risk–benefit assessments that focus on risks of harm and determine detriment–benefit assessments that focus on the harms that occur at the time of procedure or benefit (see Ch. 10).

When considering 'doing no harm', omitting care is of prime importance. Many negligence claims are for omissions of treatment that subsequently caused harm. For instance, many public enquiries into crimes committed by people with mental health problems living in the community have stated omissions of care as one of the main reasons for the incidents happening.

Beneficence

The principle of beneficence proposes an obligation to help others to further their important values, beliefs and interests. It requires the provision of benefits and the balancing of benefits and harms. Therefore, promoting the welfare of clients, not merely avoiding harm, is the goal of health care (Beauchamp & Childress 1989).

However, beneficence confronts limited resources, and controversies abound on policy decisions that limit beneficence. For example, three people need psychosocial interventions; however, there are only two places, so how will the decision be made to be beneficent to all three clients?

When considering beneficence in mental health it is important to consider paternalism also. For instance, suppose that a client was suicidal and was deemed unable to make a reasoned decision on treatment. Professionals often act beneficently by protecting clients against the potentially harmful consequences of their own actions (e.g. not allowing the person to commit suicide), thus limiting clients' autonomy and acting paternalistically. The accepted wisdom on how to decide to act in a paternalistic fashion is that it is accepted by professionals if:

◆ a client is at risk of injury or illness
◆ the risks of the paternalistic action to the patient are not substantial
◆ the benefits outweigh the risks
◆ there is no alternative to the paternalistic action
◆ infringement to autonomy is minimal.

DEVELOPING PRACTICE

Understanding the stress and vulnerability of a person's situation, and insight into the ethical consequences of decisions made on behalf of the person, is the prime development need for mental health care providers. Lutzen et al (1997) have named this 'moral sensitivity'.

Moral sensitivity and the relationship with the client underlie all other mental health knowledge. Mental health practice in its widest sense as well as everyday interactions between clients and practitioners are in fact ethical; they happen in an environment of disproportionate power, especially that of the interpersonal relationship when the illness occurs (Pellegrino & Thomasma 1993). Clients rely on practitioners to make decisions that are in agreement with their value systems. The clinician, however, has the authority in some instances to make decisions for the client that may not always agree with the latter's value system (see Ch. 21).

Although trust is central in professional ethics, as well as being a basic ingredient in a therapeutic relationship, it can be either exploited or forfeited if patients do not understand or agree with decisions that are made on their behalf (Pellegrino & Thomasma 1993). Another characteristic of mental health ethics is the unpredictability and emergency of situations that can arise. There is no highway code of rules to adhere to; however, there are principles and guidelines, such as those already discussed, that clinicians can use to help in developing their ethical decision-making skills.

Lutzen et al (1997) state that this sensitivity can be developed through the following means:

◆ building a trusting relationship
◆ reflection on finding moral reasons for actions
◆ expressing beneficence – doing good
◆ knowing when to limit autonomy and understanding why limits are imposed

◆ experience of ethical dilemmas
◆ confidence in clinical knowledge.

Many clinicians rarely have opportunities to reflect on their experiences from an ethical viewpoint. Formulating and debating the specifically moral questions raised by particular experiences can help clinicians develop their awareness of the moral dimension of their everyday practice, their confidence in addressing ethical issues and their ability to think in ethical terms (Kohner 1996).

Opportunities to reflect on and discuss experiences of ethical difficulty can be created formally or informally within a work setting. Using Johns's (1993) model of structured reflection, for example, will guide practitioners through clinical experiences, their consequences, alternative approaches and the learning that has occurred. Debriefing sessions, case reviews, ward rounds, clinical supervision and CPA reviews already exist and can be used to discuss ethical issues, thus making the issues live, real and related to practice. Although classroom approaches can be useful to discuss philosophical theory and offer distance from the clinical area, which can be useful to reflect on what Kohner (1996) calls the moral maze of practice, it is in the practice arena where the biggest difference will be felt by clients.

It is also important to create opportunities to reflect on and discuss the ordinary events of practice, which are frequently ignored because of their ordinariness but which raise significant ethical issues. Clinical supervision, based on reflection and closely related to practice, offers an appropriate means of developing ethical thinking in a more sustained way around everyday events. Carlisle (1997) reports on a study carried out by Tower Hamlets Community Trust that showed that 77% of all care providers experienced one or more ethical problems a week at work and that 93% of these discussed them with colleagues. The most commonly cited problems were client rights, client autonomy, treatment decisions, resource allocation, client competence, confidentiality and client quality of life.

CONCLUSIONS

Everyone in clinical practice wrestles with ethical decision-making on a daily basis, which challenges us on choices of decisions and their consequences. Being able to walk a path through this decision-making is a foundation stone for effective clinical practice in mental health. Everyday realities will produce ethical dilemmas. This chapter can be used to introduce clients and practitioners to ethical theory, principles of ethics and approaches to developing practice in ethical decision making so that more 'moral' or more 'right' decisions can be attempted.

References

Barker P J, Baldwin S (eds) 1991 Ethical issues in mental health. Chapman & Hall, London

Barker P J, Davidson B 1998 Psychiatric nursing – ethical strife. Arnold, London

Beauchamp T L, Childress J F 1989 Principles of biomedical ethics, 3rd edn. Oxford University Press, Oxford

Carlisle D 1997 Moral maze. Health Service Journal 3 April:26–27

Department of Health 2001 Good practice in consent implementation guide: consent to examination or treatment. Department of Health, London.

Gillon R 1994 Medical ethics: four principles plus attention to scope. British Medical Journal 309:184–188

Johns C 1993 Professional supervision. Journal of Nursing Management 1:9–18

Johsen A R, Siegler M, Winslade W J 1986 Clinical ethics, 2nd edn. Macmillan, New York

Kohner N 1996 The moral maze of practice – a stimulus for reflection and discussion. King's Fund, London

Lutzen K, Evertzon M, Nordin C 1997 Moral sensitivity in psychiatric practice. Nursing Ethics 4:472–482

NMC 1992a Code of conduct for the nurse, midwife and health visitor. United Kingdom Central Council for Nursing, Midwifery and Health Visiting, London

NMC 1992b The scope of professional practice. United Kingdom Central Council for Nursing, Midwifery and Health Visiting, London

NMC 1996 Guidelines for professional practice. United Kingdom Central Council for Nursing, Midwifery and Health Visiting, London

NMC 1998 Guidelines for mental health and learning disabilities nursing. United Kingdom Central Council for Nursing, Midwifery and Health Visiting, London

Pellegrino E D, Thomasma D C 1993 The virtues in medical practice. Oxford University Press, Oxford

Rawls J 1972 A theory of justice. Oxford University Press, Oxford

Roberts L W, Geppert C M A, Bailey R 2002 Ethics in psychiatric practice: essential ethics skills, informed consent, the therapeutic relationship and confidentiality. Journal of Psychiatric Practice 8:290–305

Seedhouse D 1988 Ethics: the heart of health care. Wiley, Chichester

Annotated further reading

Barker P J, Baldwin S (eds) 1991 Ethical issues in mental health. Chapman & Hall, London

This book explores some of the key ethical issues affecting mental health workers. An emphasis has been placed on autonomy, therapeutic ideologies, treatment and therapy in relation to people with mental illness, learning difficulties and ageing.

Barker P J, Davidson B (eds) 1998 Ethical strife – psychiatric nursing. Arnold, London

This book explores the philosophical background to ethical dilemmas, the individual strategies that they generate for practitioners and some of the ideological conflicts in mental health care.

Beauchamp T L, Childress J F 1989 Principles of biomedical ethics, 3rd edn. Oxford University Press, Oxford

This book provides a thorough introduction to ethical theory for health professionals. Its practical purpose is a systematic analysis of the ethical principles that apply to biomedicine.

Kohner N 1996 The moral maze of practice – a stimulus for reflection and discussion. King's Fund, London

Nurses, midwives and health visitors tell stories of their experiences of ethical difficulty in their everyday practice. The stories are offered as material for reflection, with suggested discussion points and commentary on four themes – accepting and respecting the individuality and autonomy of the client/patient, the nurse–patient/client relationship, the nurse–family relationship and the role and responsibility of the nurse.

Roberts L W 2002 Informed consent and the capacity for voluntarism. American Journal of Psychiatry 159:705–712

This paper describes and discusses a framework for voluntarism in clinical and research consent decisions, focusing on developmental factors, illness related considerations, psychological issues and cultural and religious values, and external features and pressures.

21

The tip of the iceberg

Sharon Dennis

KEY ISSUES

- ◆ In order to deliver care, practitioners need to be appropriately trained, supervised and supported
- ◆ They also need to be able to work alongside users and carers
- ◆ To achieve this a massive cultural shift is required as well as ongoing investment in staff development, both individually and within teams
- ◆ Furthermore, managers need internal and external resources to facilitate and sustain change, while organisations need to have processes in place that support meaningful public and patient involvement

INTRODUCTION

The interface with service users and carers is usually at the point of delivery, with clinical practitioners and support staff. This is of course just the tip of the iceberg. In order to deliver care there must be a demand for it, criteria and systems of referral, the service needs to be available in suitable environments and the people delivering it need to have the skills and support to do the work. Figure 21.1 demonstrates the complexities of today's mental health services and the variety of situations in which service users and practitioners may meet. Most importantly this system needs to be acceptable to the recipient. This chapter examines the issues that affect the effective implementation of treatment and both at practitioner, sector and organisational level.

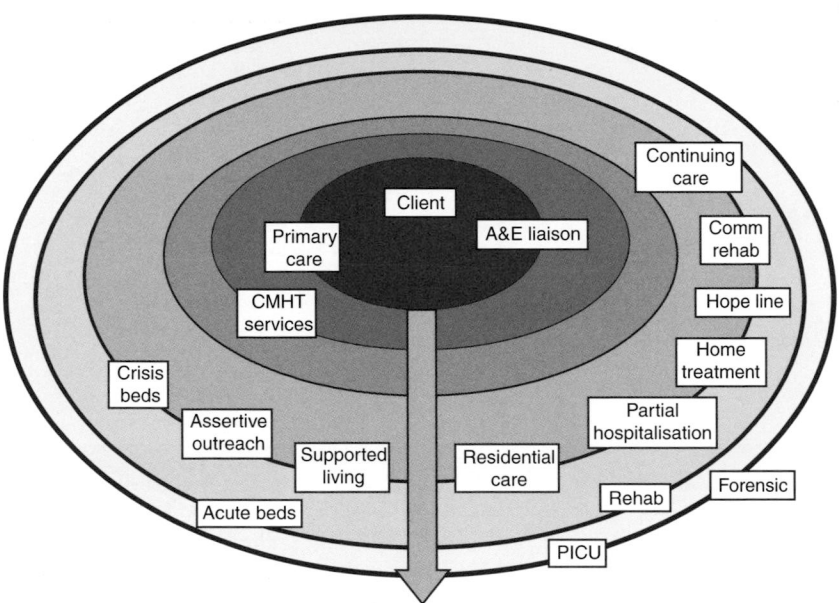

Figure 21.1 The complexity of modern mental health care services.

CONTEXT

It has been argued that mental health has never received greater focus than is on it right now. It is one of the National Health Service's four priority areas (Department of Health 1999a). This has been much welcomed, as has the investment the Department of Health has committed to mental health, which has long been seen as a 'Cinderella service'. However, with this focus comes much greater scrutiny and control than ever before as performance and outcomes are monitored, which directly relates to each Trust's reputation and potential for autonomy and income under the star rating system.

There have been many influences on the development of mental health care, which have shaped the tone and direction of modern mental health services. These are reviewed later. It is important to recognise that the entire NHS has been challenged with an ambitious modernisation agenda.

The NHS Plan (Department of Health 1999b) is a ten-year template that underpins this restructuring exercise. It outlines the need for more staff and new ways of working, and specifically describes clinical teams as the cornerstone of high-quality care delivery. The concept of multidisciplinary, now termed interdisciplinary working, while newer in wider health care, has long been a feature of mental health work. The achievements and tensions experienced by mental health and social care providers may well be lessons that colleagues in other specialties can learn from.

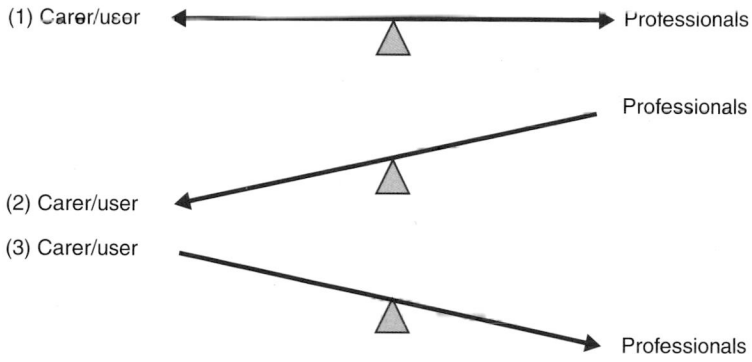

Figure 21.2   The 'power see-saw'.

The positive aspect of interdisciplinary working is the opportunity for clients to receive care influenced – and possibly provided – by many different professions. This is believed to improve both the quality and the diversity of the care offered. This view assumes that equity underpins the world of collegiate working. A huge reorientation is required for many practitioners to enable them to work successfully in this era of partnership and collaboration. While a recent review of staff roles has identified similarities between the skills of the various mental health professionals (Duggan et al 1997), practitioners experience differential levels of power, which vary according to the group they are in (see the power see-saw in Fig. 21.2). Many practitioners work in jointly managed teams and within trusts that cover several primary care trusts' catchment areas; they are well aware of the differences in health and social care policy and practices, terms and conditions, and 'acceptable' case load sizes within teams and across organisations.

Furthermore, at the time of writing, Agenda for Change (Department of Health 2003) has pilot status; this framework promises to acknowledge staff competence in terms of status and therefore pay. This should go some way to addressing inequalities between team members in terms of recognition.

POWER

Power is an important issue within mental health with regard to relationships both between users and staff and between staff groups. Price & Mullarkey (1996) suggest three types of power: (1) expert, by virtue of the role; (2) legitimate, as employees with certain responsibilities, and (3) referent, as a result of identification (and self-disclosure) with the service user.

Currently, it is evident that most professional groups are ignorant of the skills base of their colleagues and the contribution they make to client care (Gijbels 1995). One way to address this issue would be to introduce interdisciplinary education (Jackson 1994). This is being pursued to some degree at undergraduate level and there is now a move towards common learning for postgraduate staff. In addition, if team members explicitly express the skills they each contribute to everyday practice (including the philosophy underpinning these competencies), this would go some way to reducing misconceptions and difficulties born of ignorance.

Service users and carers are now firmly placed within the power struggle (Fig. 21.2). The survivor movement has influenced professionals and mainstream policy directives alike by highlighting the lack of power users have had over their own care, treatment and self-determination. An annual 'patient survey' has been introduced – although at the time of writing this is voluntary for mental health trusts. Trusts will have to demonstrate how the information from this is being used to change services. When statutory, the patient survey will ensure that organisations and practitioners alike 'work with ' not 'do to'.

Service users, by virtue of their role, will always be the most expert in relation to how they experience mental health problems and how they would like to be treated. Indeed, advance directives have now been included in the National Institute for Clinical Excellence Guidelines on Schizophrenia (National Institute for Clinical Excellence 2002) in recognition of this. Practitioners are aware of what services are available and have access to them, are privy to discussions that take place without the client and have all the information contained in medical records at their disposal. Therefore, to share power it is essential that information and choice on the pros and cons of each treatment option is provided. In addition, information on alternatives should also be supplied to facilitate informed decision-making and empowerment. Access to independent advocacy services must also be made available to support service users in their decision-making and so start to redress the power (im)balance.

Achieving a balance of power continues to rely on a practitioner's willingness to create the conditions in which the service user can act autonomously. While some older people's services have had a tradition of admiral nurses, whose role is to support carers, carer support has now been introduced for adult services (Department of Health 2002). Carers have the right to an annual assessment of their needs in relation to their caring role, and needs such as advice, advocacy, information, respite and access to interventions such as training have been suggested (Department of Health 2002).

Statutory mental health work is also complemented by the voluntary sector and other statutory agencies such as primary health care, housing and hostel workers. Professionals and managers are spending more time developing links with other players as mental health delivery increasingly uses a multi-agency approach.

However, a power discrepancy remains. On a macro level, one attempt at redressing the power differential is enshrined within the newly established

Commission for Public and Patient Involvement in Health. Their Patient Forums are planned to influence the Trust via the Patient Advice and Liaison Service and will also elect a member to work as a non-executive member of the Trust Board. Professionals have the responsibility of developing consultancy mechanisms that allow users' and carers' views to be canvassed. They need to be imaginative and systematic in gathering information and to target users who do not join organisations such as user groups.

Ideally, practitioners should be aiming for an equilibrium, as illustrated in position 1 of the 'power see-saw' (Fig. 21.2) and progressively fewer should experience the situation Sully (1996) describes where professionals who attempt to provide conditions in which service users are empowered encounter conflict from others who feel challenged by the service user exercising control. It is possible that positions 2 and 3 in Figure 21.2 will occur. In these positions, one party exercises power over the other. Professional power has already been discussed, but in scenario 3 there is a likelihood that the carer and user may opt out, as professionals are not perceived to have anything to offer.

It should also be acknowledged that the needs of the user and carer may well be different, hence the need for services that support each perspective. Increasingly, the voluntary sector is contributing to mental health service provision and, with the establishment of public protection panels, managers and practitioners are being challenged by conundrums such as balancing confidentiality and appropriate information sharing.

There are even threats to statutory services from within, as one survey (Sainsbury Centre 1997) indicated that service users value the input of support workers above all other groups of staff. This is sobering for those with 'professional' qualifications in mental health. It is often that very professionalism that has created difficulties, as users may experience it as a barrier that mitigates against the experience of warmth and empathy, which are therapeutically desirable. It is interesting to note that Menzies's (1984) classic work identified nurses as using task allocation to defend themselves from the emotional burden of the nursing role, but also stated that professional detachment is a necessary method of self-protection. Somehow, staff must balance warmth and engagement, which benefits the patient, with appropriate distance, which protects the practitioner. Advanced skills indeed.

In terms of legitimate power, professional groups do have certain responsibilities by virtue of their role and the professional codes by which they are bound. Paternalism – acting in another's best interests – for example, is inherent in the spirit of application of the Mental Health Act and its judicious use is an expectation of many professional groups; the acts that are required in order to exercise these duties may be at odds with the desires of service and carers alike. However, adhering to professional codes must always be at the core of practitioner's decision making.

MODERNISATION OF MENTAL HEALTH SERVICES

Some of the important influences that have paved the way for the National Service Framework documents *Acute Problems* (Sainsbury Centre 1998), *Modernising Mental Health Services* (Department of Health 1998), *Safety, Privacy and Dignity in Mental Health Units* (NHS Executive 2000) and *Not Just Bricks and Mortar* (Royal College of Physicians 1998) outlined the issues that adult services were facing and made recommendations in relation to care delivery, staff training and supervision, the physical environment, management, and retention and recruitment. All of these support the Care Programme approach (see Ch. 8), which is the system of care delivery in mental health. All services users screened and accepted for the Care Programme approach have the right to a health and social care assessment that includes risk, a care plan, regular review and a named care coordinator.

The National Service Framework (Department of Health 1999c) overarched these proposals and the follow-up *Policy Implementation Guide* (Department of Health 2001) has become a 'recipe' for adult mental health services, as it advises what types of team are required in modern mental health services, their role and function and the skills required by workers in these teams.

The *Policy Implementation Guide* describes community mental health teams as the mainstay of community work and acknowledges the need for a whole systems review in order to introduce these teams; in the past, new services have drawn staff from existing services, potentially destabilising these. With the prediction that 30 000 extra staff are required to deliver the National Service Framework and in the context of decreases in both the birth rate and the number of young people opting for health and social care courses, a focus on retention and recruitment is required like never before. Furthermore, mental health continues to be perceived as a less popular career option and there are concerns that staff who work in mental health services are stigmatised. A recent survey (Mentality 2002) reviewed the opinions of both staff and service users in relation to stigma. Interestingly, staff experienced this from colleagues as they 'accepted stigma was a real issue and its major impact professionally appeared to be between peer groups as opposed to amongst the general public' (Mentality 2002, p. 62).

The need for more staff more quickly has led to the creation of new non-professionally affiliated staff groups such as support time recovery and graduate workers. These have the potential to create confusion if careful management of their introduction is not employed. In addition, new roles for existing staff, such as therapy and nurse consultants, have been introduced. The development of any roles should be in the context of service need and as part of a whole-systems review. Tacking on new posts to existing systems with little regard for how these will function significantly reduces the likelihood of success, which is of course in no-one's interest.

The *Policy Implementation Guide* advocates a comprehensive review process to ensure services meet local needs (Department of Health 2001, p. 89; Fig. 21.3). However, this sound process might be at odds with achieving in terms of performance indicators and star ratings, which may in turn lead to mental health providers and commissioners deciding to establish new teams based more on public image than on local need.

New teams are likely to have some opportunity for training and development, both together and individually. However, established workers in

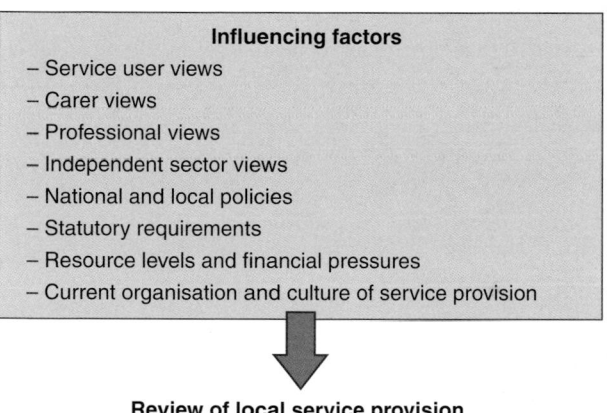

Influencing factors
 – Service user views
 – Carer views
 – Professional views
 – Independent sector views
 – National and local policies
 – Statutory requirements
 – Resource levels and financial pressures
 – Current organisation and culture of service provision

Review of local service provision

 • All elements in place/planned to be in place?
 • Sufficient service, staff and financial capacity?
 • Coordinated pathway for the service user and carer?
 • Quality?
  • Accessibility
  • Effective use of contemporary interventions
  • Service user and carer experience
  • Achieving desired outcome
  • Efficient use of resources

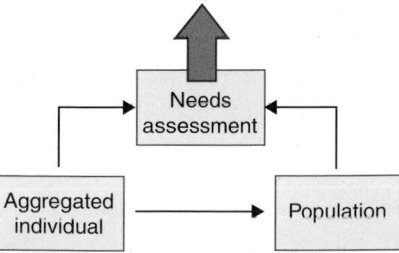

Needs assessment

Aggregated individual — Population

Figure 21.3 Comprehensive review process. (Source: Department of Health 2001. Crown copyright material is reproduced with the permission of the Controller of HMSO and the Queen's Printer for Scotland.)

inpatient units, community mental health teams and rehabilitation services, for example, must have the same opportunities to ensure that service users receive quality interventions from each part of the service and to prevent some teams being regarded by colleagues as elitist or special. In these days of limited resources skills-oriented, evidence-based education should take priority over other types of development. It should be further noted that reviews of those who have undertaken the Thorn psychosocial interventions course have shown that they have found it difficult to implement the skills they have learned (Jackson 1998). Managers need to fully consider the implications of training (time required per case versus overall case load, for example) to assist practitioners in establishing new ways of working. A SWOT analysis, use of project management techniques and ongoing audit would help newly trained practitioners to deliver and implement care using their new skills.

Findings from clinical governance reviews have found that trusts that have made good progress have the following attributes:

◆ lower vacancy rates
◆ good information and performance management systems
◆ cohesive visible leadership valued by staff and partners
◆ an infrastructure that supports clinical governance in directorates and corporately
◆ strong relationships between clinicians and managers
◆ good progress with regard to modernisation
◆ integration with social care.

SUPERVISION AND SUPPORT

Clinical supervision (Department of Health 1993) is described as 'a term used to describe a formal process of professional support and learning which enables individual practitioners to develop knowledge and competence, assume responsibility for their own practice and enhance consumer protection and safety of care in complex situations'. This arrangement therefore requires a person who is supervised and one who is the supervisor and it has become accepted within most professions within mental health. The interaction is aimed at the supervisee's growing independence and proficiency. Clinical supervision has been established longer in mental health than in other areas of health but its accessibility and acceptability in terms of quality and content is unknown at worst and patchy at best. Figure 21.4 describes the many functions of clinical supervision in terms of development, monitoring and support. Clinical supervision needs organisational commitment and an ongoing strategy to sustain it and ensure it is available to all practitioners.

Cooper (2003) reported that 60% of public sector staff cite stress as the principal cause of long-term sickness. The physical and psychological effects of too much stress are described as: anxiety, agitation, insomnia, irritability, low motivation, anger, frustration, poor concentration and difficulties in decision-making (Thomas 1997). Associated with these symptoms are lack of either fulfilment at work or enjoyment of social activities, increased absenteeism, domestic conflict and increased caffeine, alcohol, drug or tobacco intake. Long-term stress may also lead to burnout. Subsequently, those on the receiving end may experience a distant practitioner who avoids contact and lacks empathy. Tackling staff stress is therefore a concern for users, carers, practitioners and managers alike. The Royal College of Nursing (1992, p. 4) advocates the following organisational approach: 'recognising that stress exists, acknowledging the need for support, educating staff in the prevention and management of stress, providing adequate support services, creating a caring culture in the workplace and promoting good staff support practices throughout the system'. The NHS Plan (Department of Health 1999b) has formalised some of this advice by instructing all trusts to make counselling services and networks for black and ethnic staff available.

Managers are as challenged by the emerging landscape as practitioners and, as they are often required to facilitate change, they are key to developing services. The NHS Confederation (2003, p. 8) describes a key task as to 'lead, motivate and develop their staff' and 'focus on effective systems that enable clinicians to provide high quality care'. It is vital that professionals and managers work together using their complementary skills and incorporating the various influences from users, carers and other agencies to develop the service.

CONCLUSIONS

Collaboration is the key to providing a comprehensive mental health service. Practitioners and managers alike must have strategies in place that will facilitate use and carer empowerment both at individual and group levels.

The responsibilities inherent in mental health work are such that staff must be supported by the employer with procedures that are workable and opportunities for development that fit service and individual needs. By working together in an atmosphere of openness all parties can fully contribute to a service that delivers appropriate and effective care at the tip of the iceberg.

References

Cooper 2003 Feeling the pressure. Nursing Standard 17(49):12–13

Department of Health 1993 Vision for the future: the nursing, midwifery and health visiting contribution to health and health care. HMSO, London

Department of Health 1998 Modernising mental health services. Department of Health, Leeds

Department of Health 1999a Our healthier nation (White Paper). HMSO, London

Department of Health 1999b The NHS plan. Department of Health, Leeds

Department of Health 1999c A national service framework for mental health for adults of working age. Department of Health, London

Department of Health 2001 The Mental Health Policy Implementation Guide. Department of Health, Leeds

Department of Health 2002 Developing services for carers and families of people with mental illness. Department of Health, London

Department of Health 2003 Agenda for change – proposed joint agreement. Department of Health, London

Duggan M et al 1997 Pulling together. Sainsbury Centre, London

Gijbels H 1995 Mental health nursing skills in an acute admission environment: perceptions of mental health nurses and other mental health professionals. Journal of Advanced Nursing 21:460–465

Jackson S 1994 The case for shared training for nurses and doctors Nursing Times 92(26):40–41

Jackson C 1998 Thorn in a dilemma. Mental Health Care 2:86–87

Mentality 2002 Working well programme London Region. Mentality, London

Menzies I E P 1984 The functioning of social systems as a defence against anxiety. Tavistock Institute of Human Relations, London

National Institute for Clinical Excellence 2002 Guidelines on schizophrenia. NICE, London

NHS Confederation 2003 Management matters. NHS Confederation, London

NHS Executive 2000 Safety, privacy and dignity in mental health units. Department of Health, London

Price V, Mullarkey K 1996 Use and misuse of power in the psycho-therapeutic relationship. Mental Health Nursing 16:16–17

Royal College of Nursing 1992 A charter for staff support. RCN, London.

Royal College of Physicians 1998 Not just bricks and mortar. RCP, London.

Sainsbury Centre 1997 More than a friend. Sainsbury Centre, London

Sainsbury Centre 1998 Acute problems. Sainsbury Centre, London

Sully P 1996 The impact of power in therapeutic relationships. Nursing Times 92(41):40–41

Thomas B 1997 Management strategies to tackle stress in mental health nursing. Mental Health Care 1:15–17

22

Clinical support

Geoff Brennan and Catherine Gamble

KEY ISSUES

- ◆ Managerial and clinical support
- ◆ Structuring clinical supervision
- ◆ One to one supervision
- ◆ Group supervision
- ◆ Peer supervision
- ◆ The reflective process

Many of the chapters in this book contain case studies of psychosocial interventions carried out with clients. While it is necessary for the practitioners completing these case studies to be brief as to the nature of their work, it is clear in many of the studies that the process of the intervention is complex and often difficult. In some examples these case studies involve individual practitioners working in a manner that is not only collaborative but also places them at odds with other team or family members. As Vidgen and Rogers state in their account of working with individuals who are at risk of offending (Ch. 16) 'We have found that there is often disparity between what an individual believes they need and what the clinical team believe they need. By helping them to work on their priorities rather than the teams', clients are more willing to trust you' (p. 302).

This attitude seems counterintuitive if we consider the fear of 'splitting' between professionals and the often-quoted issue of consistency in the therapeutic relationship. With this regard Vidgen and Rogers are not talking about a secretive pact between the named client and the practitioner but an active and open process of therapeutic risk taking with clear understanding as to what is appropriate. However, for the practitioner to maintain this open attitude to therapeutic risk taking and client engagement they require clinical support in the form of organisational trust and organisational monitoring. In other words the organisation must both trust practitioners to work in the client's best interests and understand that the practitioner may need assistance to 'protect the client from the practitioner and the practitioner from themselves' (to paraphrase Barker 2004). Trust cannot and should not be blind. Implicit in this quote is the understanding that the interventions being used are safe, sound and supportive. Psychosocial interventions have a strong evidence base, yet little is described within the literature as to how they are supervised in clinical practice. Indeed, further research is needed to ascertain what skills, competencies and attributes are required by supervisors. However, in the role of supervisor it is our experience that the principles of the interventions mirror that of supervision. This will be reflected throughout this overview.

PROTECTING CLIENTS FROM PRACTITIONERS AND PRACTITIONERS FROM THEMSELVES

Working with clients and families consistently is difficult and often confusing. Moral and ethical dilemmas are commonplace in the working lives of mental health professionals. We have power and we have responsibility and yet we work in a system that can have many divergent needs and opinions at the same time. To add to our difficulties, we often have situations where there is little consensus as to the best course of action. Do we allow a patient autonomy with oral medication or do we advocate depot medication to ensure a therapeutic dose? There are pros and cons either way. Do we give a diagnosis of schizophrenia and risk outright denial or do we behave with caution and talk about monitoring for a period of time? In many instances our decisions are based on a mixture of experience and intuition in the absence of a definitive evidence base.

The chapter on ethical consideration in this book highlights some ways of thinking through the dilemmas evident in the previous paragraph. The remainder of this chapter is devoted to a consideration of structures that can be operationalised to assist practitioners to monitor their own practice and protect themselves and their clients.

CLINICAL SUPPORT STRUCTURES

At first sight there seems to be a plethora of clinical support structures for individual practitioners already in existence within mental health services. A few seconds thinking brings to mind phrases such as supervision, preceptorship, mentorship, appraisal, professional development and lifelong learning.

While the demand for the professional to remain updated and reflective is laudable, it does become confusing when we consider the range of terminology that surrounds supporting the practitioner. Part of this confusion is the mixing up of managerial agendas with the clinical agendas.

Table 22.1 shows a breakdown of four different types of structural system. While they are collectively concerned with maintaining and improving standards of care to clients through developing and monitoring practitioners, they approach this objective from different angles. Moving from the top to the bottom it is clear that there is a shift in the control of the process from the practitioner to the organisation in the person of the 'manager'. In this shift we can also see that the situation becomes more bureaucratic and operationally tighter. The reasons for this are self-evident as the organisation needs to monitor both what goes on in its name but also what the organisation should provide to allow the practitioners to perform. Hence the Personal Development Review and disciplinary situations should also contain some analysis of practical support offered to the practitioners to ensure they have the necessary resources to carry out their duties but will demand that these duties are carried out in a competent manner if the resources are or were available.

A further complication is the manner in which different professional groups perceive and value supervision. As already indicated above, there is a difference in terminology between the professional groups with regard to supervision. This is not just a semantic issue as the difference in terminology reflects deep differences in models of supervision and its value within professional cultures. This is demonstrated by Boud & Holland (1999) in Figure 22.1.

Psychosocial interventions require supervisors who have the capacity to step outside their particular professional culture and remain focused upon the client within a psychosocial framework, and to assist the supervisee, whoever the latter is professionally, to stay similarly focused. The key here is the acquisition and development of psychosocial skills to assist clients. At present supervision is perceived by some as a luxury and it is recognised that there can be conflict between a need for supervision within a professional or clinical structure as opposed to specialised psychosocial supervision. As we learnt in Chapter 5, follow-up studies of psychosocial trainees have indicated a difficulty in accessing appropriate supervision and, although this has not been analysed, it should not be underestimated how many of the dilemmas highlighted above contribute to the non-uptake and negativity in some quarters surrounding supervision and its value.

In many ways it is easier to see the managerial agenda as it deals with workforce through a public process with clearly defined objectives. In essence, practitioners are given a job description that sets out the details of their roles and the manager is a person who will practically assist with this and who will

Table 22.1 Four types of clinical support structure

	Who sets the agenda?	Level of confidentiality	Record-keeping	Information giving and advice	Challenging the supervisee	Level of support	Level of catalytic help
Clinical supervision	Supervisee	Total, except in the case of legal requirements*	Supervision agreement or contract agreed by supervisee. Record of attendance and content	Given to supplement supervisee's own expertise to enable them to see own options and make own decisions	Based on evidence given during supervision session	Supervisee encouraged to recognise and use their own expertise. No practical help given outside session	Establishing reflection on issues affecting practice. Planning, decision-making and reviewing
Management supervision	Line manager or delegated other	Not confidential	May be recorded by manager in personal file	Given to direct supervisee towards set objectives or training needs	Based on evidence gained/observed in work situation	Practical help may be given outside session	Manager elicits information on work done and standards achieved
Personal development review (PDR)	Policy/document	Not confidential	Copy of PDR. Portions may be sent to other organisational departments e.g. to access training	Given to direct worker towards PDR objectives	Based on evidence gained/observed in work situation	Practical help may be given outside session	Overall performance review and objective setting
Disciplinary interview	Investigating manager	Not confidential	Recorded by manager in personal file	Given to instruct and inform worker of process and possible outcomes	Based on evidence gained/observed in work situation	Practical help may be given outside session or this may be delegated to an independent advisor	Manager elicits information on the issues under discussion and sets goals

* Clinical supervision notes are actually the legal property of the employing organisation, but guidelines indicate that they can only be 'demanded' in a legal situation such as a court hearing

Source: adapted from Wheeler 2000

Diagram One   **Place Diagram One Here**

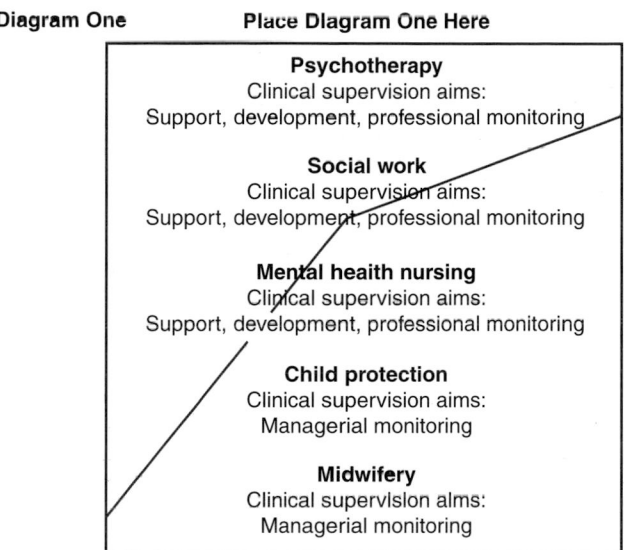

Psychotherapy
Clinical supervision aims:
Support, development, professional monitoring

Social work
Clinical supervision aims:
Support, development, professional monitoring

Mental heaith nursing
Clinical supervision aims:
Support, development, professional monitoring

Child protection
Clinical supervision aims:
Managerial monitoring

Midwifery
Clinical supervislon alms:
Managerial monitoring

Main aims of clinical supervision related to various professional cultures

Above the line, professions explicitly value therapeutic use of self as part oif the professional culture

Below the line, professions explicitly value management monitoring as part of the professional culture

Figure 22.1   Main aims of clinical supervision related to various professional cultures. (**Source:** redrawn from Bond & Holland 1999, p. 31.)

practically monitor progress against this job description. Ideally, duties are clear and we, as practitioners, know where we are going, what we need to get there and how to map out the route. Appraisal is a pit stop along the way to inform our manager if we are on track and take measures if we are not.

It is much harder to be definitive about the process of clinical supervision. In essence, clinical support is dependent on huge and powerful unknowns – the 'client' and the practitioner's relationship with them. When a practitioner sets out on the journey that is clinical care with a client (whether that client is an individual, a family or a team) there is no way of knowing where that journey will take them. In this case the practitioner is a passenger, who may affect the route but cannot dictate it. As such, clinical supervision is as much about defining where the client and the practitioner are on that route, and if they are comfortable being there, as anything else. With regard to the interventions in this book, the emphasis is as much on assisting the client to drive better as it is about getting to a set destination.

This difficulty is, in turn, transferred on to the supervisor. Whereas managers have the structural support of clear policies and practice to assist them in their process, the clinical supervisor can be jumping into the unknown at every session. There are, however, structural guides that can help the supervisor to keep some boundaries with regard to the process and it is important for both parties to understand these if clinical supervision is to be supportive. As we will see, these guidelines can be extended into other meetings to provide a supportive framework around the content.

THE STRUCTURING OF CLINICAL SUPERVISION SESSIONS

Setting the process

Clinical supervision is a relationship between a practitioner defined as the supervisee and a practitioner defined as the supervisor. The supervisor will normally be someone who is recognised as having the ability, through their experience and skill base, to guide the supervisee through the reflective process. As such, however, the relationship between a supervisee and a supervisor can be seen as a reflection of the clinical relationship between a client and a practitioner. In this regard, the stages of therapeutic relationship building between a client and a practitioner as identified by Peplau (1988) can provide a very useful map to the stages of supervision also (Box 22.1)

Box 22.1 The supervision process as an adaptation of Peplau's interpersonal relationship model

Orientation: The supervisee and the supervisor meet as strangers, introduce themselves and make a decision as to whether they can work together. (Even if the two people have worked together previously it is worth remembering that undertaking supervision is very different from their previous relationship.)

Identification: The supervisee decides what they would like help with and how that help should be given and this is negotiated and agreed with the supervisor.

Exploitation: The supervisee and supervisor embark on supervision proper. The supervision is time limited in that the supervisee and supervisor agree a time for evaluation to ensure that the relationship is functioning as it should and that the agreements made in earlier stages are effective and being adhered to. If not, these should be changed or modified.

Resolution: At the ending of the supervision relationship both parties have the opportunity to evaluate, say goodbye and move on healthily.

Orientation and identification: setting the agenda

In setting the agenda for supervision it is essential that the supervisee and supervisor meet to begin the process. In this initial meeting it is useful to have the following loose blueprint as a means of understanding the supervisee's attitude to supervision and what they would like to get out of it:

◆ Introduce the model of clinical supervision:
  ● Why are you both here?
  ● What do you hope to get out of supervision?
◆ Explore supervisee's previous experience of supervision:
  ● Did the supervisee have any?
  ● Did the supervisee have useful supervision from which you can both learn?
  ● Did the supervisee have supervision that they found of little use or harmful and from which you can both learn?
◆ Clarify purpose and expectation:
  ● What can the supervisor offer?
  ● What can the supervisor not do or what do they not know?
◆ Direct supervisee to goal setting:
  ● What, if any, are the clinical needs of the supervisee?
◆ Deal with administration:
  ● Who will organise venue, frequency, note-keeping, if it is to proceed?

Setting up a supervision agreement or contract

From the orientation of both parties to working together in a collaborative manner and a clearer idea of what expectations both have, a supervision agreement or contract can be formulated. Whether this is better written down or verbally agreed is a debatable point, although most guidance now points to having some written form of agreement and monitoring it, if only to aid recall and map progress (Johns 1996, Cutcliffe 2000). In the event of a written agreement being made, the following should be included:

◆ Date of agreement and date for review
◆ Broad summary of supervisee objectives, for instance:
  ● 'For X to have space to consider assessment, intervention and evaluation of clients on caseload'
  ● 'For X to explore how to assist client A with their voice hearing'
  ● 'For X to plan and carry out a carers' group within their clinical area'
  ● 'For X to bring casework as necessary for mutual discussion and intervention planning'
◆ Administrative and conduct responsibilities of supervisee and supervisor:
  ● 'X will book the clinical room on B ward for supervision sessions'

- 'In the event of a cancellation, Y will ring X to organise a new date for supervision'
- 'X and Y will each book one hour of protected time for the supervision session'
- 'For X and Y to treat each other with respect during the supervision sessions'
◆ Administrative details:
  - Frequency of supervision (weekly, 2-weekly, monthly, etc.)
  - Duration of session (1 hour, 45 minutes, etc.)
  - Note keeping, if any, including responsibility for safekeeping.

Exploitation: the heart of the matter

The purpose of supervision is to assist the supervisee to deliver care. The content of supervision is indefinable, as care is multifaceted. As a consequence it is not possible to aptly describe the process of the supervisee exploiting the relationship to further care, and yet, for supervision to be effective, this should be the largest part of the process, in terms of both energy and time. Given the nature of the interventions outlined in this book we can make an assumption that the supervisee can exploit supervision to process clinical information in terms of assessment data, problem formulation, interventions and evaluation of these. It is also possible, however, that supervisees may want to use their time to discuss how to advocate for their client in the wider system, learn the use of a specific assessment tool, prepare clinical work for publication or just simply reflect on the experience of being with a person in distress.

It would be disingenuous, however, to present the supervisor as a passive observer of the supervisee's deliberations. Within exploitation the supervisor has the role of positively challenging the supervisee, attending to errors of thinking, reframing issues such as client resistance and generally opening up the supervisee's practice to supportive examination. For example, consider a supervisee who had completed over 15 separate assessments with one individual but who described them as non-compliant with treatment. The supervisor in this instance pointed out the anomaly in the supervisee's understanding of the client and re-examined the 'non-compliance', which turned out to be a normal reaction to misdiagnosis and overmedication. Hence the client's behaviour was reframed as a normal response rather than a pathological one. In this, the supervisor had to be mindful of how powerful a message this was for both the practitioner and the team supporting the client.

Although it is not possible to be definitive about the content of individual supervision, the reflective cycle of turning experience into learning, as outlined in Figure 22.2, gives a general guideline that highlights how supervision can be utilised by the supervisee. In this we see that the experience, whatever that

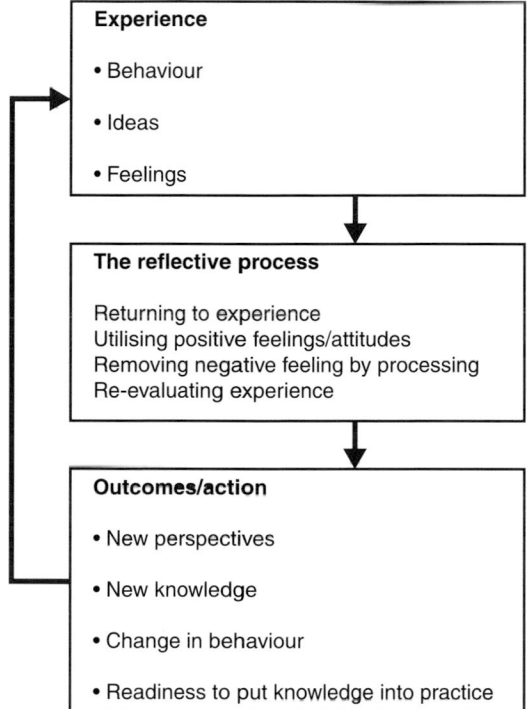

Figure 22.2 Reflection: turning experience into learning. (**Source:** adapted from Boud et al 1985.)

experience may be, is processed by examination and the supervisee can come away with new knowledge and a readiness to put this knowledge into practice.

The cyclical reflection of experience with regard to psychosocial intervention should follow the same principles that are intrinsic to the process of psychosocial interventions. In this regard we ask the supervisee to follow the same therapeutic structure as the client and/or the family. In other words, we use cognitive–behavioural principles while valuing all contributions, sharing time and space, with the expectation that all involved will be treated with respect within a non-hostile atmosphere. Thus supervision sessions, when effective, mirror individual psychosocial therapy and, to facilitate this, the agenda format set out in Table 22.2 is used and is explicitly understood by both supervisor and supervisee.

There is one final aspect of exploitation, which involves adhering to the fidelity of the model and duty of care to the client. It should be understood by both supervisor and supervisee that the supervisor has a responsibility to discuss any concerns they may have with regard to competency. Frameworks are now available to assist in this process (Sainsbury Centre 2001) and further

Table 22.2 Agenda for supervision sessions

Format	Supervisor response/framework
Personal update	How are you?
Link to last supervision session (previously supervised cases)	Before we go any further, how did you get on with… (previous objective)?
Agenda setting	What are you bringing today?
Highlight priorities	Which one of those is the main issue?
Talk about the issue until it becomes clear	Let's funnel this down, shall we? So what, where, when, who with and how often is this an issue?
Generate solutions	What can we do about this? Is this simple, measurable, achievable and realistic? How will you know it is effective? Will this have an impact on others? If so, do we need to generate solutions to these new considerations?
Assignment of new homework	So let's be clear, you are going to do what?
Summary and feedback from supervisee	Let's reflect and summarise on this session….

work is being undertaken to ensure that practitioners remain clinically competent after they have received training (Campbell 2000). Although this would appear to be a managerial function, the issue here is duty of care to the client and the supervisor's duty to inform the supervisee of their concerns in order for them to treat the client responsibly.

Resolution

All relationships end, and the nature of the ending is important. The supervision process itself should be attentive to this, ending through a continual process of evaluation of the original aims and objectives. It is important during these evaluations for the supervisee and supervisor to reaffirm their individual commitment to the process. In this way, when the time comes for the supervision to discontinue, both parties are prepared for the final evaluation and can move on.

BEYOND ONE TO ONE

So far our discussion has considered supervision as a mainly supervisee-to-supervisor structure. It is possible to also provide clinical support to practitioners in a group setting. Of the interventions discussed in this book, the area which has most employed this form of supervision is family interventions.

In group supervision for family interventions the key is to funnel down the information brought by the supervisees to a single situation that can be examined in detail. To do this there must be two parts to the supervision session. In the first part all group members are given the opportunity to feed back on any interventions that have taken place. In doing this, however, the facilitator of the group needs to understand that their role is to incorporate the whole group and not fall into the trap of holding either a briefing meeting or one-to-one supervision with an audience. Figure 22.3 illustrates the difference (Bond & Holland 1999).

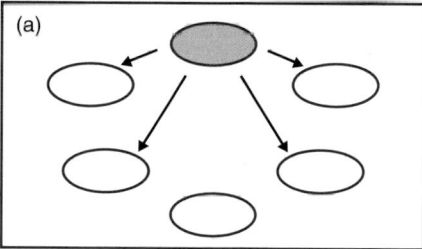

(a)

Briefing Meeting:

Facilitator finds themselves 'doing all the talking' and presenting material to the group

This is not group clinical supervision

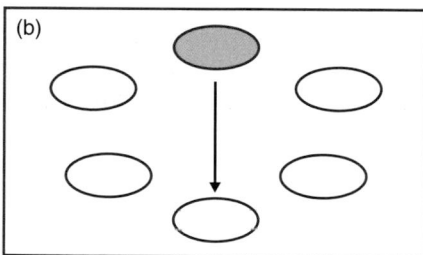

(b)

One-to-one clinical supervision with an audience:

Facilitator provides individual supervision for each member while others wait their turn

This is not group clinical supervision

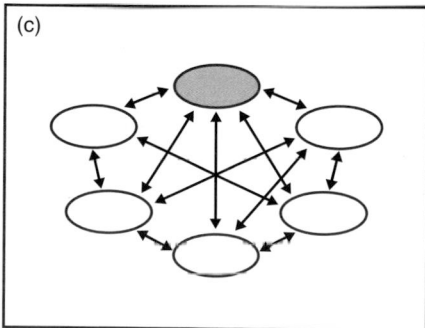

(c)

Group Clinical Supervision

The group members take turns to share an issue and reflect on it
The facilitator is not the only one with a valid opinion

In family interventions this structure can then change to allow for role play with all group members adopting roles, but it will return to this structure to process and reflect on the role play.

Figure 22.3 Facilitating group supervision: meeting format. (**Source:** redrawn from Bond & Holland 1999.)

Following this, an agreement is negotiated within the group and by the supervisor as to which particular experience generated during family sessions should be fed back and reflected upon, in the manner described in Figure 22.3. The great benefit of group supervision for family interventions is that the situation can be role-played to open out the experience for examination. Many supervisees find it valuable to role-play the families they are working with to experience receiving the interventions they are implementing. In these cases supervisees can often gain a new perspective on a family member and consider their interventions using this new information. This, however, does require the supervisor to have additional skills, such as the ability to safely coordinate role-play, selecting role players, assigning tasks for observers, setting the scene and knowing how to derole.

Even in group supervision sessions for family interventions, boundary setting and having some basic agreement as to individual responsibilities, time frames and overall objectives for the sessions is important. It is also possible to draw up a supervision agreement or contract, as described above, in order for all parties to understand the parameters of supervision and negotiate group ground rules.

PEER SUPERVISION

In the absence of a more experienced practitioner it is still possible for individual or group supervision to occur through a peer supervision process. Again there are some guiding principles that are useful when considering peer supervision (adapted from Hawkins & Shohet 1994):

- ◆ Peer groups must come to a consensus as to the objectives of the sessions
- ◆ Groups should be small and closed, with a maximum of seven members
- ◆ Ground rules and administrative duties such as sharing time, timekeeping, note-keeping and booking rooms should be negotiated at the beginning of the process
- ◆ An external person can be co-opted in to assist in evaluation
- ◆ Special care must be taken to stop the sessions becoming either a 'moaning shop' or a comfort zone with little challenging or true reflection.

In the situation where peer supervision is organised between individuals an agreement to swap supervisor and supervisee roles is an effective way of managing the process. In this case the advice above is pertinent to the management of the relationship, with the individuals having equal time in each role.

As in the more common situation of group supervision, the funnelling technique is also a useful manner in which to conduct sessions, although it is less likely that participants will feel comfortable in a role-play situation.

Despite this, there are ways in which groups can explore client work, such as one person presenting and each member offering an intervention or reflection for the presenting practitioner's consideration. In this way, equity of speaking time can be assured and each participant has the opportunity to both receive and offer support.

CONCLUSIONS

Clinical support of practitioners is essential if they are to continue to effectively practise psychosocial interventions. Additionally, there is evidence that practitioners stop delivery of the interventions if adequate clinical support is not available. Where clinical support is available it comes in the form of quality clinical supervision, as opposed to managerial supervision, which reflects the therapeutic process of psychosocial interventions, with special attention paid to ensuring that the supervisee has overall control of the process.

If the availability of psychosocial interventions is to increase it is essential that services attend to the provision of quality supervision and that psychosocial practitioners are encouraged to provide supervision as well as looking for it. If you are a practising psychosocial worker reading this chapter and think that you need supervision it is also your responsibility, therefore, to consider when you will be able to provide it.

References

Barker P 2004 Tidal model of recovery and reclamation – together we can change! Available online at www.tidal-model.co.uk/New%20developments.htm

Bond M, Holland S 1999 Skills of clinical supervision for nurses. Open University Press, Buckingham.

Boud D, Keogh R, Walker D 1985 Reflection: turning experience into learning. Kogan Page, London

Campbell A 2000 Evaluation of the West Midlands family intervention programme. Presented at Working with Families – Making it a Reality (Conference), Stratford upon Avon, 20/21 March

Cutcliffe J R 2000 To record or not to record: documentation in clinical supervision. British Journal of Nursing 6:350–355

Hawkins P, Shohet R 1994 Supervision in the helping professions: an individual, group and organizational approach. Open University Press, Buckingham

Johns C 1996 Visualising and realising caring in practice through guided reflection. Journal of Advanced Nursing 24:1135–1143

Peplau H 1988 Interpersonal relations in nursing. Macmillan, London

Sainsbury Centre 2001 The capable practitioner: a framework and list of the practitioner capabilities required to implement the National Service Framework for Mental Health. Sainsbury Centre for Mental Health, London

Wheeler M 2000 Oxleas NHS Trust clinical supervision pack. Unpublished manuscript

Index